OXFORD MEDICAL PUBLICATIONS

The New Genetics
and Clinical Practice

The New Genetics and Clinical Practice

Third Edition

D. J. Weatherall, FRS

Nuffield Professor of Clinical Medicine and
Honorary Director, MRC Molecular Haematology Unit and
Institute of Molecular Medicine, University of Oxford

Oxford   New York   Tokyo
OXFORD UNIVERSITY PRESS
1991

Oxford University Press, Walton Street, Oxford OX2 6DP

Oxford   New York   Toronto
Delhi   Bombay   Calcutta   Madras   Karachi
Petaling Jaya   Singapore   Hong Kong   Tokyo
Nairobi   Dar es Salaam   Cape Town
Melbourne   Auckland

and associated companies in
Berlin   Ibadan

Oxford is a trade mark of Oxford University Press

Published in the United States
by Oxford University Press, New York

© *D. J. Weatherall, 1991*

First edition (1982) published by the
Nuffield Provincial Hospitals Trust
Second edition 1985 Oxford University Press

British Library Cataloguing in Publication Data
Weatherall, D. J. (David John)
The new genetics and clinical practice.–3rd ed.
1. Man. Genetic disorders
616.042
ISBN 0–19–261905–5

Library of Congress Cataloging in Publication Data
Weatherall, D. J.
The new genetics and clinical practice/D. J. Weatherall.—3rd ed.
(Oxford medical publications)
Includes bibliographic references.
Includes index.
1. Medical genetics.   2. Human genetics.   3. Human chromosome
abnormalities.   I. Title.   II. Series.
[DNLM: 1. Genetics, Medical.   2. Hereditary Diseases—prevention &
control.   3. Hereditary Diseases—therapy.   QZ 50 W362n]
RB155.W33   1990
616'.042—dc20   90–7362   CIP
ISBN 0–19–261905–5 (pbk.)

Typeset by Cotswold Typesetting Ltd, Gloucester
Printed and bound in Hong Kong

Preface to the third edition

The first edition of this book originally saw the light of day because the Nuffield Provincial Hospitals Trust asked me to hazard a guess at the impact that recent developments in molecular biology might have on the care of patients with inherited diseases. Apart from a long-standing interest in thalassaemia, a common inherited disease and the one to which the new techniques of recombinant DNA technology were first applied, I had no particular qualifications for tackling this subject. However, probably because my level of ignorance of this complex field was such that at least I appreciated the plight of my fellow clinicians, the book, and its succeeding edition, seem to have been popular. For this reason, and because the field has moved so fast since the publication of the second edition in 1985, I decided to embark on a third edition. Because of the extraordinary developments in this field over the last few years this, as last time, has meant that the book has had to be almost completely rewritten.

My main objective, as in previous editions, is to interest students and clinicians, and anybody else who is involved in health care, in the field of human molecular biology and to try to give them some idea of its enormous implications for clinical practice. As the field has developed it has become apparent that there are virtually no branches of clinical medicine that will not be touched by molecular and cell biology over the next few years. It is equally clear that because of the remarkable technology that has evolved from this field, medical research has moved into the most exhilarating phase of its development. If the reader can catch just a little of this excitement my efforts will have been well worthwhile.

As in the previous editions I have used the haemoglobin disorders throughout the book as models for trying to explain how recombinant DNA technology can be applied to the study of human disease. I make no apology for this because these disorders still remain the best understood examples of how it is possible to relate the extraordinary variation of the clinical picture that we see in our patients with events at the molecular level. But I have also tried to anticipate the broader applications of this field to other areas of clinical practice and preventative medicine, and have tried to review some of the ethical and pastoral problems that will be encountered as we start to develop the technology with which to modify our genes.

I have been helped by many friends, particularly those in the Institute of Molecular Medicine, University of Oxford. I am very grateful to John Clegg, Bill Wood, Douglas Higgs, Kay Davies, John Bell, Adrian Harris, and Andrew Wilkie for reading parts of the manuscript. Andrew Wilkie also helped me to revise the gene frequencies for some of the common genetic disorders that are listed in Chapter 2; I was relieved to discover that, like me, he was unable to find the original references to many of them, the data for which appear to have been handed down from textbook to textbook over the centuries. I am also grateful to John Old, Swee Lay Thein, Veronica Buckle, and Martyn Bell for providing illustrations. Finally, I should like to thank my colleagues in the MRC Molecular Haematology Unit for continuing the thankless task of trying to keep me educated in this field, Gordon McLachlan of the Nuffield Provincial Hospitals Trust for initiating this project, the Oxford University Press for prodding me into writing a third edition, and my secretary Janet Watt for translating my late nocturnal ramblings into something approaching the English language.

Oxford   D.J.W.
June 1990

Contents

1 Introduction 1
What is the new genetics? 1

2 The frequency and clinical spectrum of genetic diseases 4
Patterns of inheritance 4
The overall spectrum of genetic diseases 10
Single gene defects 11
Chromosome abnormalities 21
Congenital malformation and common diseases: Multifactorial inheritance 25
Cytoplasmic inheritance 31
Cancer; somatic cell genetics 32
The total burden of genetic disease 32
Summary 36
Further reading 37

3 The structure, organization, and regulation of human genes 39
Structure of genes and the transmission of genetic information 39
DNA 40
The regulation of gene expression 48
How do genes make contact with the outside world? Co-ordinated gene expression 53
Many human genes are organized in families 55
The size of the human genome 69
Further reading 71

4 The techniques of gene analysis 73
Basic methods 73
Speeding up the analysis of human DNA for diagnostic purposes 91
Studying the function of isolated genes 96
Studying gene regulation 100
Further reading 101

5 Finding our way round the human genome 103
Approaches to human chromosome mapping 103

Genetic mapping   104
Some genes that have been assigned by RFLP linkage   117
Progress in genetic mapping of the human genome   118
Physical mapping techniques   120
Linking up genetic and physical maps; finding human genes   123
Reverse genetics   129
Future directions for genome mapping   133
Further reading   135

6 The molecular pathology of single gene disorders   138

Types and levels of abnormal gene expression   139
Monogenic disorders resulting from the synthesis of an abnormal
   protein   141
Molecular lesions that result in the production of reduced amounts
   of gene products   164
Phenotype/genotype relationships for mutations that alter the output of
   structural genes   185
The heterogeneity of monogenic disease   189
Summary   191
Further reading   191

7 Molecular genetics and common diseases   193

General approaches to the analysis of the molecular basis for polygenic
   disease   194
Diabetes   196
Other autoimmune diseases   198
Cardiovascular disease   200
Neuro-psychiatric disease   211
Hereditary variability in response to drugs   215
Infectious disease   217
Allergy and atopy   218
Postscript   219
Further reading   219

8 Cancer   221

Tumour viruses and oncogenes   221
Cancer suppression and 'anti-oncogenes'   235
How many mutations are required to produce a cancer cell?   242
Rare genetic disorders that predispose towards cancer   243
Viruses and human cancer   244
Tumour immunology   246
Metastatic disease   247

Molecular aspects of cancer chemotherapy   247
What is cancer? Practical applications   249
Further reading   251

 9 **Carrier detection and prenatal diagnosis of genetic
    disease**   254

The avoidance of genetic disease   254
Current methods for prenatal diagnosis   256
Sources of fetal DNA   259
How is fetal DNA analysed for single gene disorders?   261
Current progress   275
Sources of error   281
The future   282
Further reading   286

10 **Gene therapy**   288

Current methods for treatment of genetic disease   288
Gene replacement or corrective therapy   291
Other approaches to the correction of genetic diseases   305
A start at human gene therapy   307
Summary   308
Further reading   308

11 **Some broader implications of the new genetics for
    clinical practice in the future**   310

Mapping the human genome   310
Molecular pathology   312
Diagnostic uses of recombinant DNA   319
The treatment of disease   322
Other areas of research in human molecular and cell biology of future
    clinical relevance   328
Further reading   344

12 **Ethical issues and related problems arising from the
    application of the new genetics to clinical practice**   347

Specific ethical problems posed by the new genetics   347
Broader issues arising from the new genetics   360
Postscript   366
Further reading   368

Index   369

Introduction

1

● What is the new genetics?

With the increasingly successful control of environmental diseases in the developed world, disorders that are either wholly or in part genetically determined have assumed an increasingly prominent role in childhood illness and mortality. It is estimated that these conditions account for about a third of admissions to paediatric wards and are a significant cause of childhood deaths. Many of them are associated with chronic and distressing mental or physical handicap, or both. Hence genetic disease poses a considerable burden on health, social, and educational services. In addition, it causes immense stress and misery for the families of affected children. But this is not all. It is now clear that many of the major diseases of unknown cause that afflict western societies—stroke, coronary artery disease, mental illness, and diabetes, for example—have an important genetic component, and that many forms of cancer are due to inherited or acquired changes in the genetic make-up of cells. Clearly, the totality of genetic disease, or disorders in which changes in our genes play a major role, are of great importance in current clinical practice in the developed countries. The same problems will be posed for the developing world once the high mortality rates due to infection and malnutrition come under control.

Very few genetic diseases can be treated effectively. A few conditions with a genetic component, such as cleft palate, harelip, and some forms of congenital heart disease, are amenable to surgical correction. Some of the inborn errors of metabolism can be controlled by regular replacement of a missing protein or enzyme or by preventing the accumulation of toxic metabolites by appropriate manipulation of the diet. However, little can be done for the majority of inherited disorders, and pending the development of better methods of treatment, the main goal of clinical genetics has been prevention. In the past this has been approached in several different ways. As the pattern of inheritance of individual genetic diseases was clarified, it was possible to provide genetic counselling for families who already had an affected child. Screening programmes were set up for some common and easily identifiable genetic disorders, with a view to primary prevention through prospective genetic counselling. Several techniques were developed for prenatal diagnosis of genetic diseases. The first success story was the identification of various chromosome abnormalities by analysis of amniotic fluid cells. As the biochemical basis for some of the inborn errors of metabolism was determined, it became possible to carry out specific enzyme analyses on cultured amniotic fluid cells. In addition, the development of methods for fetal blood sampling allowed the prenatal diagnosis of some common inherited haematological disorders, such as the haemoglobinopathies and haemophilia.

Although these developments led to considerable progress towards the avoidance and management of genetic disease, many problems remained. When therapy was available, it was often required for life and was unpleasant or expensive, or both. While carrier detection and prenatal diagnosis of some genetic disorders was possible by these approaches, the techniques were complicated and expensive, and produced a major burden for our health services. Lack of progress in determining the cause of many common genetic disorders such as cystic fibrosis, Huntington's disease, and many others, meant that it remained often impossible to identify carriers for these conditions or to develop methods for their prevention. And despite a great deal of work, very little was learned about the way in which genetic factors contribute to the causation of common disorders such as diabetes and premature vascular disease, or how they are involved in the generation of chromosomal or congenital abnormalities. It was the advent of the 'new genetics' about ten years ago that raised the possibility that these hitherto intractable problems might be solved.

What is the 'new genetics'? As far as I know, the term was first used by David Comings, editor of the *American Journal of Human Genetics*, in commenting on a paper that outlined a novel approach to using DNA analysis for mapping the human genome, and hence had great clinical potential. He summed up his reaction to these new ideas as follows: 'since the degree of departure from our previous approaches and the potential of this procedure are so great, one will not be guilty of hyperbole in calling it the New Genetics'. Over recent years there have been remarkable advances in molecular and cell biology which have led to the development of methods for isolating and determining the fine structure of genes and for studying their function in the test tube. As these techniques have been refined and simplified it has been possible to apply them to study human genes, both in health and disease. It is now possible to start to understand many diseases in terms of their molecular pathology, a level of diagnostic precision that would have been undreamt of even ten years ago.

In the short time that has passed since some of these methods were applied to the study of human disease we have gained remarkable insights into the molecular basis for genetic disorders. Furthermore, these new developments are already having some important practical consequences for preventative medicine. In particular they have greatly broadened the scope of prenatal diagnosis, even for many genetic diseases in which the biochemical and molecular basis is still not understood. In the future, as well as leading to better approaches to prevention, they should provide definitive therapy for many genetic disorders. Finally, and perhaps most important in the long term, these new analytical techniques will broaden the scope of the genetic analysis of human disease to encompass the cell and molecular biology of a variety of the major killers of western societies, in particular vascular disease, diabetes, cancer, rheumatic disease, and the major psychiatric disorders. In effect, when we speak of the 'new genetics' ten years after the term was coined by Comings, we simply mean the study of inheritance at the molecular level.

Why should we wish to understand the genetic factors that are involved in the common disorders of middle and old age which fill our hospitals? Surely there is strong epidemiological evidence that many of them are the result of many years of bad habits, such as smoking or eating the wrong kind of diet. The fact is that we have made very little progress in understanding the underlying causes of any of these diseases. Although they are not inherited in the sense that they can be traced through generations in the same way as haemophilia or cystic fibrosis, it is quite clear that there is a tendency for all of them to run in families. Presumably this reflects the action of environmental factors set against a background of genetic susceptibility. If we were able to define the main genes involved in increasing the likelihood of having a heart attack or developing diabetes, and we could determine how their products differ from those of similar genes in non-affected individuals, we would be in a much better position to understand precisely how these conditions arise and, hopefully, how better to prevent and manage them.

When considering cancer we have to broaden the scope of what we mean by genetic disease. This is usually thought of as something that we inherit from our parents. However, throughout our lives our cells are dividing. Recently it has become apparent that many cancers result from acquired changes in the genetic make-up of cells that are passed on to their progeny and prevent them from behaving in an orderly fashion. In other words, the new genetics considers not only the molecular pathology of what we inherit from the germ cells of our parents, but also encompasses acquired changes in cells of any organ during an individual's lifespan.

When viewed in this broader context it is quite clear that human genetics, and certainly the new genetics, involves the whole of clinical practice. As well as providing us with powerful diagnostic and therapeutic tools for tackling genetic and acquired disorders it will ultimately allow us to harness many human genes for producing therapeutic agents and will yield major insights into ageing and human evolution. There is little doubt therefore that we have moved into a most exciting phase of medical research and the study of human biology.

Enough has happened in the field of human molecular biology over the last few years to suggest that the medical sciences are moving from whole-patient physiology and pathology to the study of diseases at the cellular and molecular level. In the chapters that follow I shall try to anticipate how these developments will be applied in clinical practice and discuss some of the problems that might arise from our increasing ability to dissect the human genome.

The frequency and clinical spectrum of genetic diseases

2

The main object of this book is to try to assess the impact that recent developments in molecular biology will have on the prevention and management of genetic diseases or those in which genetic factors play a part. Before doing so we need to consider the frequency and spectrum of these diseases, how they are inherited, and the load that they impose on our health services. Hopefully, this will provide a framework on which we can identify those conditions that should be amenable to analysis by these new techniques.

● Patterns of inheritance

Before looking at the spectrum of human genetic disease we must remind ourselves about what genes are and how the information that they contain is transmitted through successive generations of families. The ideas that are outlined in this book can be grasped without a formal training in genetics. However, it is helpful to have some understanding of the basic patterns of human inheritance. There are many excellent monographs on this topic, of which some are listed at the end of this chapter. The brief account that follows is for those who wish to learn something about the exciting new developments in clinical genetics, but for whom words like 'allele' and 'linkage' are no more than hazy reminders of a misspent youth.

Genes are the units of heredity. Their main function is to determine the structure of peptide chains, that is strings of amino acids that form the building blocks of enzymes and other proteins. The wide diversity of living things reflects the existence of numerous varieties of proteins. There are only 20 different naturally occurring amino acids. The tough proteins of hair and skin, and the fluid haemoglobin that fills our red cells, all consist of the same amino acids; they differ in their properties only because the amino acids are arranged in a different order in their constituent peptide chains. Amino acids have side chains that interact with each other, and hence peptide chains and the proteins that they constitute fold up into very precise shapes that are essential if they are to carry out their roles in body structure and chemistry. It follows, therefore, that the shape of a protein is dependent on the order of amino acids in its peptide chains; a gene must see to it that the amino acids of its peptide products are always in the *same* order.

Genetic information is stored in the nucleus of human cells in deoxyribonucleic acid (DNA) which is packaged up into 23 pairs of chromosomes. We shall take a closer look at the structure of DNA in the next chapter. Genes, that is regions of DNA that contain the information required to control the structure of individual peptide chains, are situated at specific sites, or loci, on chromosomes. One of a pair of chromosomes is derived from one parent. Since chromosomes exist in homologous pairs, so must their constituent genes. As the result of a mutation, an alteration of the structure of a gene, individual genes may exist in alternate forms, or alleles, only two of which can be present in one individual.

Except during the formation of gametes, that is germ cells, cells divide by a process called mitosis which is preceded by doubling of each pair of chromosomes (Fig. 1). This process ensures that the two daughter cells each acquire a set of chromosomes identical to the parental cell, i.e. a diploid pair. During gamete formation a different type of cell division occurs which is called meiosis. In this case homologous pairs of chromosomes segregate, or separate, to give progeny with half the number of chromosomes, i.e. the haploid number. Fertilization restores cells from the haploid to the diploid state. Because chromosomes segregate during gamete formation, so must genes. Since chromosome pairs segregate independently of each other, so do genes that are not on the same chromosome.

Many of the diseases that we shall be discussing later in this chapter follow a simple Mendelian form of transmission in families. In other words they obey Mendel's two laws of inheritance. First, genes are units that segregate; members of the same pair of genes, alleles, are never present in the same gamete but always separate and pass to different gametes. Second, genes assort independently; members of different pairs of genes move to gametes independently of each other. To put it in a nutshell, alleles segregate; non-alleles assort.

The consequences of these laws are beautifully simple. Take the first. If a man and a woman have identical genes at a particular locus, let us call them A, they can only produce gametes of type A, and consequently they can only have children with an AA genotype. If, on the other hand, A exists in another form, say a, and the genotype of the father is AA and that of the mother Aa, then although the father can only produce A gametes, half the mother's will be A and half will be a. The possible genotypes of the children can be worked out as follows:

		paternal gametes	
		A	a
maternal	A	AA	Aa
gametes	a	Aa	aa

It follows that half the children will have the genotype AA and half Aa. On the other hand, if both parents have the genotype Aa, then one fourth of the children will each have the genotype AA or aa, and half will have the genotype Aa, as follows:

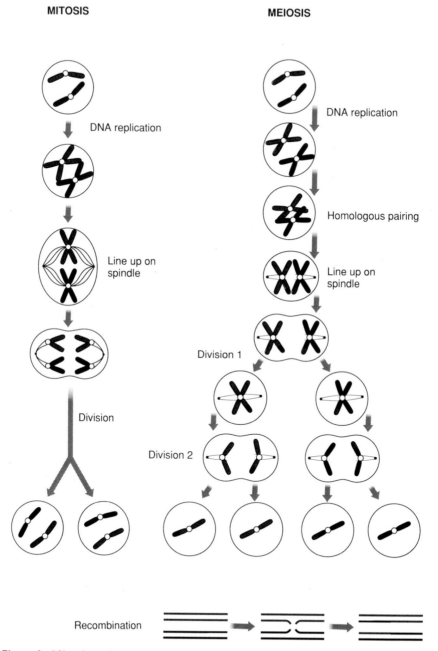

MITOSIS

DNA replication

Line up on
spindle

Division

MEIOSIS

DNA replication

Homologous pairing

Line up on
spindle

Division 1

Division 2

Recombination

Figure 1. Mitotic and meiotic cell division. The process of recombination during meiosis is illustrated schematically below.

		paternal gametes	
		A	a
maternal	A	AA	Aa
gametes	a	Aa	aa

Children with the genotypes AA and aa are called homozygotes; those with the genotype Aa, heterozygotes.

Genes are described as 'dominant' or 'recessive', terms originally invented by Mendel who defined them as follows: 'those characters that are transmitted entire, or almost unchanged by hybridization, and therefore in themselves constitute the characters of a hybrid, are termed dominant, and those that become latent in the process, recessive'. In other words, a dominant allele is one that manifests its phenotypic (recognizable) effect in heterozygotes; a recessive allele causes a phenotypic effect only when present in the homozygous state. For example, in the matings that we described above, if the a allele produced a disease in the heterozygous state it would be referred to as a dominant; if it only produced a recognizable phenotype in the homozygous (aa) state it would be defined as a recessive.

So far we have only considered single alleles. However, throughout this book we shall be interested in patterns of inheritance of more than one gene. As already mentioned, Mendel's second law tells us that the characters that are directed by different pairs of genes will appear in the next generation either together or apart, depending entirely on chance. In other words, they assort independently. There is an important exception to this rule, however. If the two genes are on the *same* chromosome, and particularly if located close together, they will tend to be inherited together; the genes are then said to be linked. However, the parental chromosomes become closely apposed at meiosis, and crossing-over of the genes between maternal and paternal chromosomes can occur, so that the two characters determined by the genes will part in some of the children (Fig. 1). Such offspring are called recombinants. The closer together a pair of genes are on the same chromosome the less will be the chance of crossing-over. Hence the number of recombinants in families is a measure of the distance between the genes. The distance separating two loci that show recombination in 1 out of 100 gametes is called a map unit, or centimorgan (named after the American geneticist T.H. Morgan).

It is often important to determine what is called the 'phase of linkage', that is whether the variant alleles at two linked loci are on the same chromosome or one on each of the homologous partners. If the two are on the same chromosome they are said to be in the coupling phase; if on opposite pairs they are said to be in repulsion. The terms *cis* and *trans* are often used to describe genes in coupling or repulsion, respectively. Thus, if we have two linked genes A and B with variant alleles a and b, the latter are in the coupled or *cis* phase when they are localized in a doubly heterozygous individual on the same chromosome, AB/ab, and in the repulsion or *trans* phase when they are localized on partner chromosomes, Ab/aB.

We shall return later to the problem of genetic linkage which plays a central role in some of the recent developments in human molecular genetics.

Of the 23 pairs of chromosomes 22 are called autosomes. The other pair are the sex chromosomes; females have two X chromosomes while males have an X and a Y chromosome. The pattern of sexual development in an embryo depends on the presence or absence of a Y chromosome. The X chromosome carries a large number of genes that control many aspects of development and function. Some of the mutant genes that we are interested in are carried on the X chromosome and hence called X-linked. Since males possess only one X chromosome, an abnormal gene that it carries cannot be paired with a normal allele; the man is said to be hemizygous for that particular mutant gene. The female in whom both members of a pair of X-linked genes are identical is said to be homozygous for that gene; if the members of a gene pair are dissimilar the woman is called a heterozygote, or carrier, for the abnormal allele.

There is another important factor to consider when we come to look at X-linked diseases. First postulated by Mary Lyon in the early 1960s was the suggestion that inactivation of one X chromosome might occur in females during early embryonic development. This would ensure that they do not have a 'double dose' of genes on the X chromosome. It is now known that this is, in fact, what happens. Since the descendants of each cell retain the same inactivated X chromosome, a proportion of cells (approximately one-half, although the proportion is variable because the inactivation mechanism is a random process that occurs during early embryonic development) have the paternal X chromosome in an active state while in the other cells the maternal X chromosome is active. Hence, a female who is heterozygous for an abnormal gene will have two types of cells, one with the normal and one with the mutant gene. In other words she is a mosaic.

Although the vast majority of diseases that we shall be considering in this book are due to abnormalities of genes carried on chromosomes, there is increasing evidence that some inherited characteristics are determined by cytoplasmic elements. Unlike sperm, eggs contain a considerable amount of cytoplasm. Mitochondria have their own DNA which is separate and distinct from nuclear DNA. We receive our mitochondrial DNA from our mothers. Quite recently evidence has accumulated suggesting that inherited abnormalities of mitochondrial DNA may account for a few human genetic diseases.

It follows from this brief outline of the patterns of inheritance that there are several types of monogenic modes of transmission of abnormal human genes: autosomal recessive, autosomal dominant, X-linked which may be recessive or dominant, and Y-linked. In addition we have to consider the possibility that a few diseases will follow a cytoplasmic mode of inheritance. How do we recognize these different patterns of inheritance in practice?

Some typical pedigrees showing different forms of inheritance are outlined in Fig. 2. Autosomal dominant disorders affect both males and females and can

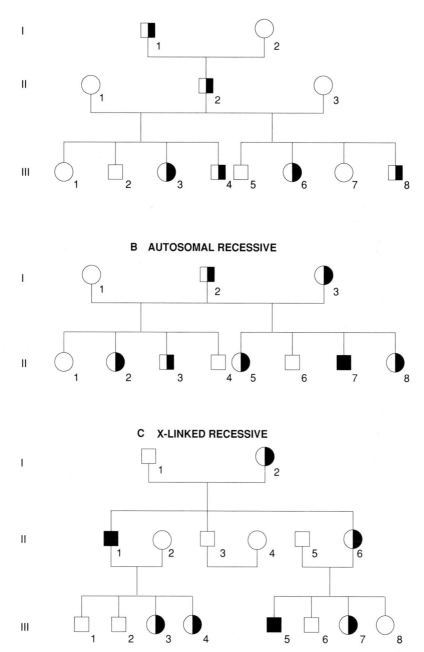

Figure 2. **Pedigrees illustrating different forms of monogenic inheritance.** □ represents male and ○ female. In the family showing autosomal dominant inheritance the open symbols represent normal individuals and half shaded symbols affected persons. In B and C open symbols are normal, half shaded are carriers (non-affected) and fully shaded are affected. Note that in the family showing X-linked inheritance, in the third generation the daughters but not the sons of the affected male, II-1, are carriers; among the children of the female carrier, II-6, half the sons are affected and half the daughters are carriers.

often be traced through many generations. Affected individuals are heterozygous for the abnormal allele which is transmitted to one-half of the offspring, regardless of whether they are male or female. The disorder is not transmitted by unaffected members of the family. Autosomal recessive disorders are found in individuals whose healthy parents both carry the same recessive gene. The risk of recurrence for future offspring of such parents is 25 per cent. Unlike autosomal dominant disorders there is usually no family history. Although the gene may be passed from generation to generation, the disorder usually occurs only in a single sibship, that is within one group of brothers or sisters. The risk of a recessive disorder occurring is increased greatly if there is parental consanguinity.

In the case of X-lined recessive disorders, only males are affected and the disorder is transmitted through healthy female carriers. Because inactivation of the X chromosome is random and occurs at an early stage during development, heterozygous females may occasionally show some features of the condition. A female carrier transmits the disorder to half her sons, and half her daughters are carriers. On the other hand, all the daughters of an affected male are obligate carriers whereas none of the sons are affected. It follows that X-linked recessive disorders cannot be transmitted by a healthy male. An X-linked dominant gene will give rise to a disorder in *both* hemizygous males and heterozygous females. The conditions are transmitted in families in a similar way to X-linked recessive genes, giving rise on average to an excess of affected females (because females have two X chromosomes). Some X-linked dominant conditions are lethal in hemizygous males and in this case there will be fewer males than expected in a family, all of whom will be healthy, and an excess of females, of whom about half will be affected.

In the case of Y-linked disorders, which are excessively rare, transmission occurs directly from father to son. In fact in most conditions in which a Y-linked inheritance has been suspected the actual mode of inheritance has turned out to be autosomal dominant, with other factors causing sex limitation.

We shall consider the evidence for the existence of cytoplasmic inheritance in a later chapter.

As we shall see later many medically important conditions appear to run in families but do not follow a pattern of inheritance that can be defined as being the result of a single gene. It is assumed in many cases that the disorders reflect the action of several genes, being influenced to a variable degree by environmental factors. These polygenic conditions have proved very difficult to analyse, despite the highly sophisticated mathematical approaches that have been developed to try and clarify their genetic transmission.

● The overall spectrum of genetic diseases

The main groups of genetic disorders are summarized in Table 1. Firstly, there are single gene defects, conditions that can be traced through families and clearly defined as following an autosomal dominant or recessive, or sex-linked pattern of

Table 1. *Genetic diseases, or conditions in which genetic factors play an important part*

Single gene disorders
Chromosomal disorders
Congenital malformations and many common diseases. Polygenic inheritance
Disorders of mitochondrial DNA. Cytoplasmic inheritance
Disorders due to somatic cell mutations

inheritance. Secondly, there are chromosome abnormalities, some of which can be related to specific clinical syndromes. The third group comprises congenital malformations and common acquired disorders, at least some of which seem to have a strong genetic component; it is clear, however, that environmental factors play an important role in the pathogenesis of many conditions that fall under this general heading. A fourth group is composed of inherited disorders of mitochondrial DNA. Finally, we must broaden our definition of 'genetic' disease to include the acquired defects of the genetic machinery of cells that appear to underlie many forms of cancer.

In the sections that follow we shall review briefly each of these groups, and then attempt to derive an approximate assessment of their overall clinical importance. The main sources for these data are summarized in the caption to Table 2 and in the report of a World Health Organization Working Party that discussed the prevention of the important inherited anaemias. It must be emphasised that the frequency figures that are outlined in these sections are, at best, gross approximations.

● Single gene defects

As we have seen, there are four well-defined monogenic modes of inheritance; autosomal dominant, autosomal recessive, and X-linked, which may also be divided into recessive and dominant. In the 1988 edition of Victor McKusick's *Mendelian inheritance in man*, the clinical geneticist's bible, 2208 proven mutant phenotypes and an additional 2136 'probables' are listed, a grand total of 4344 monogenic diseases. Of the 'definite' phenotypes 1443 are classified as autosomal dominant, 626 as autosomal recessive, and 139 as X-linked; the proportional distribution in the 'probable group' is similar.

● Autosomal dominants

A partial list of some of the more important autosomal dominant disorders is shown in Table 2. Published estimates of the total frequency of dominant disorders ranged from just less than 2, to 9, per 1000 births. This is explained, at

Table 2. *Some dominant inherited disorders (northern Europeans only)**

System	Disorder	Frequency/ 1000 births	Main clinical features
Nervous	Huntington's disease	0.20	Involuntary movement and dementia from middle life
	Neurofibromatosis	0.25	Tumours of peripheral nerves, spinal roots, and cranial nerves. Abnormal pigmentation
	Myotonic dystrophy	0.05	Several syndromes of myotonia (delayed muscle relaxation) with atrophy or other degenerative changes in various organs including eyes, heart, and gonads
	Tuberous sclerosis	0.08	Mental retardation. Epilepsy. Skin changes
Bowel	Polyposis coli	0.1	Tumours of colon which may undergo malignant change
Kidney	Polycystic disease	1.0	Progressive kidney failure
Eyes	Dominant blindness	0.1	Blindness
Ears	Dominant early childhood deafness	0.1	Deafness from infancy
	Otosclerosis	3.0	Reduced hearing from adolescence or later

Blood	Hypercholesterolaemia	2.0	Early-onset coronary artery disease
	Spherocytosis	0.2	Variable anaemia due to premature destruction of red cells
Teeth	Dentinogenesis imperfecta	0.1	Maldevelopment of teeth
	Amelogenesis imperfecta	0.02	Soft, friable enamel of teeth. Several variants
Skeleton	Diaphyseal aclasia	0.5	Multiple swellings (exostoses) at ends of bones
	Thanatophoric dwarfism	0.08	Early death with severe skeletal deformities
	Osteogenesis imperfecta	0.1	Fragile bones. Fractures. Deformity
	Marfan syndrome	0.1	Long thin extremities. Skeletal deformity. Heart disease. Eye changes
	Achondroplasia	0.04	Dwarfism. Bone deformity. Fractures
	Ehlers–Danlos syndrome	0.05	Hyperextensible joints, friable tissues
Metabolism	Acute intermittent porphyria	0.01	Acute attacks of abdominal pain and neurological disturbances
	Variegate porphyria	0.01	Light sensitivity with or without above

Sources for Tables 1–3: Carter (1977a, b, 1982), Committee on Mutagenicity of Chemicals in Food (1981), Connor and Ferguson-Smith (1988), Harper et al. (1988), Love and Davies (1989), Sykes (1989), Davies (1989).
*Published birth frequencies vary widely and figures quoted here are a gross approximation.

least in part, by the relative importance that different writers have ascribed to certain genetic disorders. For example, one of the most frequent disorders among those shown in Table 2 is monogenic hypercholesterolaemia, which does not always appear in estimates of the frequency of dominants. There are probably many forms of hypercholesterolaemia in the population, of which at least some have a polygenic basis. However, there is now good evidence for the existence of a fairly common monogenic form which is due to a genetically determined deficiency of the receptor for low density lipoproteins on cell membranes. The condition is associated with a high incidence of early death from coronary artery disease and hence is of considerable medical importance. The late Cedric Carter, whose work formed the basis for much of the data cited in these sections, emphasized the difficulty in arriving at an accurate frequency figure for disorders such as Huntington's chorea; he derived an approximate frequency of 0.5/1000, whereas most workers have given a lower estimate of approximately 0.25/1000. However, Carter believed that the higher prevalence estimates are probably justified because many cases still die undiagnosed, as is clear from the medical records of the parents of proband cases. Furthermore, some neurologists are reluctant to make the diagnosis in the absence of a history of at least one affected parent.

Some of these dominant conditions occur at a relatively high frequency, presumably because they have little effect on reproductive fitness. It is difficult to anticipate how heterogeneous they will be at the molecular level. The rarer disorders that cause severe incapacity in early life are likely to have arisen from many different mutations. On the other hand, conditions like Huntington's disease and the form of porphyria which is very common in South Africa, which seem to have a strong founder effect, may turn out to have more homogeneous molecular pathology. In this case a mutant gene is introduced into a population by one or more individuals; if their progeny remain isolated from other populations by inbreeding the particular mutation will be confined to a small subgroup which can be traced back to the founder.

● Autosomal Recessives

A list of some of the more common autosomal recessive conditions occurring in north Europeans, together with their approximate frequency at birth, is shown in Table 3. Like the dominant disorders, there is considerable variation among published frequencies. These discrepancies arise from the marked variability of incidence of particular diseases in different populations (see below) and from difficulties in arriving at a diagnosis for some of the disorders. Clearly, cystic fibrosis is by far the most common, although with widespread population movements the haemoglobin disorders are becoming increasingly important in north European populations. The high frequency of cystic fibrosis is likely to be a result of selective advantage for heterozygotes, although it is not clear why this should be the case. Given the difficulties of obtaining accurate frequency data, it

Table 3. *Some recessive disorders in the UK*

System	Disorder	Frequency/ 1000 births	Main clinical features
Metabolism	Cystic fibrosis	0.5–0.6	Viscid secretions. Chest infection
	Phenylketonuria	0.2–0.5	Mental retardation
	Tays–Sachs disease	0.004	Mental retardation. Blindness
	α_1 Antitrypsin deficiency	0.1–0.5	Liver failure in infancy. Emphysema
	Mucopolysaccharidosis (several subtypes)	0.03	Defective physical and mental development. Blindness. Large spleen
	Galactosaemia	0.02	Progressive liver failure from early infancy
	Homocystinuria	0.01	Mental retardation. Ocular and skeleton abnormalities
	Cystinuria	0.06	Renal stones
	Metachromic leucodystrophy	0.02	Paralysis. Blindness. Intellectual deterioration
Nervous	Neurogenic muscular atrophies	0.01	Progressive muscle weakness
	Friedreich ataxia	0.02	Progressive unsteadiness. Other neurological disturbances
	Spinal muscular atrophy	0.04	Progressive muscle weakness
Blood*	Sickle cell anaemia	0.1	Haemolytic anaemia
	β Thalassaemia	0.05	Severe anaemia. Bone deformity. Splenomegaly
Endocrine	Adrenal hyperplasia	0.1	Several syndromes. Include virilism in females, abnormal development of male genitalia, Addisonian crises, etc.
Ears	Congenital deafness	0.5	Deafness
Eyes	Recessive blindness	0.1	Blindness

Sources as for Table 2.
*Represents an approximate estimate based on gene frequencies in immigrant populations (Weatherall and Clegg 1981; Royal College of Physicians 1989).

is generally agreed that a figure of about 2.5/1000 is a reasonable estimate for the frequency of autosomal recessive disorders in north Europe. As we shall see later, this figure is much higher in other parts of the world.

● X-linked Disorders

The commoner X-linked disorders are summarized in Table 4. The definition of dominance or recessivity in these conditions is complicated by the inactivation of one of the X chromosomes in the cells of females during early development. It seems likely that in the few sex-linked abnormalities classified as dominant, such as oro-facio-digital syndrome, affected males die soon after conception and only genetically and phenotypically normal males survive; the diseases are transmitted from mother to daughter. The frequency of X-linked mental retardation is very difficult to define although recent work suggests that one type of this condition, the fragile X syndrome, forms a discrete group. We shall consider this later.

Table 4. *Some important X-linked disorders in northern European populations*

System	Disorder	Frequency/ 1000 males	Clinical features
Locomotor	Muscular dystrophy —Duchenne	0.3	Progressive muscular weakness leading to death, usually in third decade
Blood	Haemophilia	0.1	Bleeding after trauma
Skin	Ichthyosis	0.1	Thick skin due to excessive keratin
Brain	Fragile X syndrome	0.9	Mental retardation. Enlarged testis
Eye	Childhood blindness	0.02	Blindness

Sources as for Table 2.

In this list of the commoner X-linked conditions I have not included glucose-6-phosphate dehydrogenase (G6PD) deficiency. As will become apparent later, this is an extremely common X-linked disorder globally, although probably of quite rare occurrence in north European populations.

In severe X-linked disorders such as Duchenne muscular dystrophy, in which affected males die before reproducing, the disease would disappear if the lost genes were not replaced by new mutations. Such mutations could occur during either oogenesis or spermatogenesis. In the former case, if the ovum is fertilized by a Y-bearing sperm an affected male would be born, if fertilized by an X-bearing sperm a carrier daughter would result. Alternatively, if the mutation occurs during spermatogenesis a carrier girl will be born because sons do not normally receive their father's X chromosome.

Haldane showed that the proportion of new mutants among males with an X-linked disorder is as follows:

$$\frac{(1-f)\mu}{2\mu+v}$$

where μ = the mutation rate in female gametes per generation, v = the mutation rate in male gametes per generation, and f = the effective fertility of males. In X-linked disorders like Duchenne muscular dystrophy, in which affected males fail to reproduce, the formula becomes

$$\frac{\mu}{2\mu+v}$$

If mutations occur only in males ($\mu = 0$) no boys will be new mutants. If mutations occur only in females ($v = 0$) then half the affected boys will be new mutants and half will have inherited the abnormal gene from their mother. It follows that if mutation occurs equally in the two sexes ($\mu = v$), the proportion of new mutants among affected males will be one-third, and two-thirds of mothers will be carriers.

How do these theoretical calculations work out in practice? In one study of carrier detection for the Lesch–Nyhan syndrome, 23 mothers of 27 isolated cases were found to be carriers, while only 12–14 would have been expected if mutation rates were equal in males and females. This suggests that in this condition mutation occurs more frequently in males than females. In contrast, family studies of Duchenne muscular dystrophy show that only one-quarter of brothers are affected, suggesting that about one-half of mothers are carriers, and that mutation might be commoner in females in this condition. In X-linked disorders that are not fatal, such as haemophilia, the proportion of carrier mothers will be greater than two-thirds even if the mutation rates are equal between the sexes.

These considerations are very important when we discuss in later chapters the newer approaches to prenatal diagnosis of genetic disorders.

● Variation in frequency of single gene disorders in different populations

So far we have only discussed single gene disorders in north European races. However, the relative frequency varies considerably between populations. Some examples of the remarkable differences in the frequency of monogenic disorders between different racial groups are shown in Table 5. Well-documented examples include the high frequency of cystic fibrosis in north Europeans compared with Afro-Americans or Orientals, and the extremely high frequency of Tay–Sachs disease among Ashkenazi Jews. The reason for these discrepancies is not known. As already mentioned, there has been much speculation that the high frequency of cystic fibrosis in northern Europe may reflect heterozygote advantage for the gene in this particular environment. Whether the same applies to Tay–Sachs

Table 5. *Racial differences in frequency of genetic diseases*

Disease	Race	Frequency/ 1000 births
Porphyria	South African (White)	3.0
	Caucasians (general)	0.01
Huntington's disease	Tasmania	0.17
	Japan	0.03
Adrenogenital syndrome	Yupik Eskimos	2.0
	N. Americans	0.025
Cystic fibrosis	N. Europeans	0.4–0.5
	Afro-Americans, Orientals	0.01
Tay–Sachs disease	Ashkenazi Jews	0.17–0.4
	Sephardi Jews, Gentiles	0.001–0.003
Thalassaemia	Mediterraneans, Orientals	10–20
Sickle-cell anaemia	Africans	10–20

Source: Committee for Mutagenicity of Chemicals in Food (1981), Weatherall and Clegg (1981).

disease in Ashkenazi Jews, or whether the high frequency reflects gene drift or a founder effect, is not clear.

Of the conditions listed in Table 5, the genetic disorders of the red cell, thalassaemia and sickle-cell anaemia, reach by far the highest frequency. Indeed, information obtained over the last few years suggests that these conditions are probably the commonest single gene diseases in the world population. The World Health Organization has estimated that by the year 2000 it is likely that about 7 per cent of the world population will be carriers for one of these disorders. There is good evidence that these conditions, and the X-linked red cell enzyme disorder glucose-6-phosphate dehydrogenase deficiency, have reached their extraordinarily high frequencies because carriers are protected against *Plasmodium falciparum* malaria. This is an elegant example of balanced polymorphism. E.B. Ford has defined polymorphism as 'the occurrence together in the same habitat at the same time of two or more distinct forms of the species in such proportions that the rarest of them cannot be maintained merely by recurrent mutation'. The term 'balanced polymorphism' means that the gene frequency for the advantageous heterozygous states, for conditions such as thalassaemia and sickle-cell disease, will increase until their incidence is balanced by the loss of homozygotes from the population.

The world distribution of the thalassaemias, the most important of the haemoglobin disorders, is illustrated in Fig. 3. Data for the frequency of these conditions in different populations are summarized in Table 6. It is clear that hundreds of millions of people are carriers for the major hereditary anaemias. At least 200 000 severely affected homozygotes are born annually, approximately equally divided between sickle-cell anaemia and the thalassaemias. Based on known gene frequencies and available demographic data, it was estimated

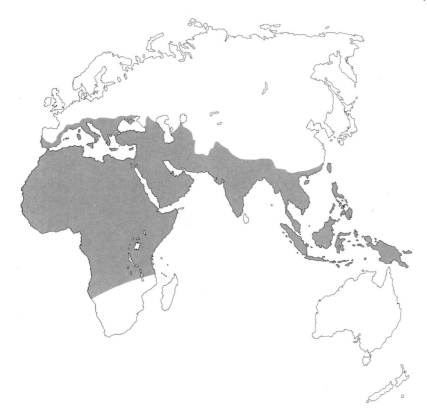

Figure 3. **The world distribution of thalassaemia.**

recently that there is an annual birth of approximately 100 000 infants with sickle-cell disease in Africa, 1500 in the USA, 700 in the Caribbean, and about 140 in the UK. Many of these children have chronic anaemia and a variety of distressing complications; the load on medical services caused by the sickle-cell disorders is very considerable.

The global data for the frequency of the thalassaemias are staggering. Consider the problem in Thailand. In a population of approximately 50 million, about 500 000 children suffer variable degrees of chronic ill-health due to the interaction of the different thalassaemia genes. Thalassaemia is a very heterogeneous disease in Thailand, as elsewhere. Homozygotes for one of the common forms (α° thalassaemia) die at birth. Homozygotes for the other common type (β thalassaemia) require regular blood transfusions to survive. The commonest haemoglobin variant is haemoglobin E, which is carried by nearly 50 per cent of the population in some parts of the country. A child who inherits β thalassaemia from one parent and haemoglobin E from the other has a condition, haemoglobin E thalassaemia, which may be almost as severe as homozygous β thalassaemia and which affects hundreds of thousands of individuals in

Table 6. *Approximate number of heterozygotes for the haemo-globinopathies throughout the world (conservative estimates) (WHO 1983)*

Haemoglobinopathy	No. of heterozygotes
β-Thalassaemia	
Asia	60.2×10^6
North Africa	2.6×10^6
Europe	4.8×10^6
Subtotal	67.6×10^6
α°-Thalassaemia	
Asia	29.4×10^6
HbE/β-Thalassaemia	
Asia	84.3×10^6
Subtotal (all thalassaemias)	181.3×10^6
Hb S-trait	
Africa	50×10^6
North Africa, South America,	
South-West Asia, Caribbean,	
India, USA	10×10^6
Subtotal	60×10^6
Total (all major hereditary anaemias)	242×10^6

Thailand. It seems likely that the disease is equally widespread in parts of southern China, Laos, Cambodia, Malaysia, and in localized areas of the Indian subcontinent.

The thalassaemias also produce a major health problem in Italy, Greece, and some of the Mediterranean island populations such as Cyprus and Sardinia. Estimates from Italy in 1979 suggested that several hundred new cases of severe thalassaemia were being added to the population each year; even with inadequate therapy affected children live for approximately 2 to 4 years and hence there were probably about 4000 severely affected homozygous thalassaemics in the country. With the availability of improved treatment the number will continue to increase. It is estimated that approximately 7 per cent of the population of the Greek mainland carry β thalassaemia and hence there are probably about 200 new cases of homozygous β thalassaemia born each year. In the island populations of Cyprus and Sardinia the carrier rate for β thalassaemia ranges from 15 to 20 per cent; approximately 1 in every 100 babies are homozygous for the condition.

It should be emphasized that these extraordinary figures for the thalassaemia problem describe the position as it was a few years ago. As we shall see in a later chapter, the development of prenatal diagnosis programmes is leading to a dramatic reduction in the numbers of new cases of severe thalassaemia in some of these countries.

Although the genetically determined haemoglobin disorders are the most important single gene disorders, glucose-6-phosphate dehydrogenase deficiency is also extremely common in some areas and has been estimated to affect probably 100 million individuals in the world population. Although the disorder is not responsible for chronic ill-health, some important clinical problems are presented including severe anaemia in response to a variety of drugs, neonatal jaundice which may lead to kernicterus with mental and physical impairment, favism (haemolysis after eating beans), and haemolytic anaemia in response to intercurrent illness.

Although the red cell disorders are particularly common in the Mediterranean, the Middle East, the Indian subcontinent, and Southeast Asia, they cannot be ignored when considering the problem of genetic disease in northern European populations and the USA. Mass movements of populations have occurred in recent years, the Vietnamese refugees for example. This, together with the large immigrant populations that are already established in Europe and the USA means that these genetic blood disorders are being seen with increasing frequency and have to be taken into account when assessing the burden of genetic disease in these countries. In the UK, sickle-cell anaemia occurs mainly in individuals of African descent, while thalassaemia occurs mainly in the Cypriot and Asian immigrant populations. It has been estimated that there are currently 300–500 β thalassaemia homozygotes in the UK and probably about 600–1000 individuals with sickle-cell anaemia. About 50 to 150 infants are born in this country each year with one or other of these conditions. We know nothing about the early childhood mortality rate for sickle-cell anaemia in the UK. It is probably not in excess of 10 per cent and therefore the chronic ill-health and complications of this condition will pose an increasing load on our medical services. Similarly, it now appears that children who are homozygous for β thalassaemia are surviving, at least until the end of the second decade. As methods for treatment improve, these children will pose an increasing load on our blood transfusion and paediatric services.

● Chromosome abnormalities

As mentioned earlier, normal individuals have 46 chromosomes, 23 pairs in which each member of the pair is of either maternal or paternal origin. Each chromosome can now be identified with certainty using special staining methods which result in a specific banding pattern; the number and relative sizes of alternating dark and light bands produced by different staining processes give each chromosome a characteristic appearance (Fig. 4).

The autosome pairs are numbered sequentially from 1 to 22, from largest to smallest. When describing chromosome morphology, cytogeneticists refer to the appearance of the chromosome during a phase of mitosis called the metaphase during which the chromosome is in a particularly compact state and hence can be examined easily under the light microscope. Each chromosome appears to be composed of two halves called sister chromatids. The word 'sister' implies that

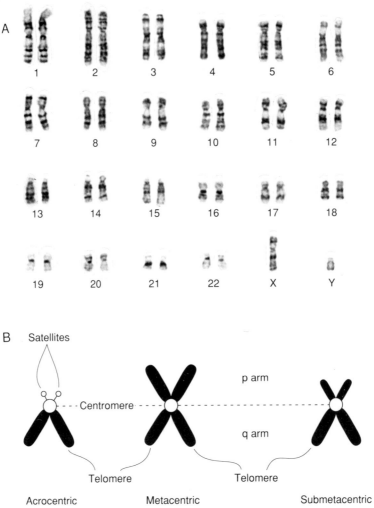

Figure 4. Human chromosomes. **A** The normal human male karyotype. The chromosomes are identified by their size, banding patterns, and position of the centromere. Trypsin–Giemsa banding. (Kindly prepared by Dr. J. Jonasson.) **B** The anatomy of human chromosomes (for details, see text).

both halves are identical and are the result of replication of an original chromosome strand. The chromatid halves are separated from each other along their lengths except at one point, called the centromere, where they are joined. The centromere divides chromosomes into two regions which are called short and long arms. The term 'metacentric' is used to describe chromosomes that have short and long arms of more or less the same length, i.e. the centromere is near the middle of the chromosome (Fig. 4). Chromosomes with centromeres very close to one end, thus making the short arm very small, are called acrocentric.

Specific sites on the arms of chromosomes are designated according to a convention which was agreed at the Paris Conference in 1971. Each of the chromosomes is divided up into band numbers; those on the short arm are designated by the lower case letter p, and those on the long arms by q. The total number of chromosomes per cell is described by an Arabic number and, if relevant, the sex chromosome constitution is indicated by one X and/or Y for each sex chromosome. Thus a normal male karyotype is written 46,XY, and a normal female 46,XX. If there is an extra chromosome its number is preceded by $+$; if one is missing by $-$. For example, trisomy 21 is written 47, $+$21. Extra material on a chromosome arm is indicated by $+$; for example, 14q$+$ means that there is extra material on the long arm of chromosome number 14. Similarly, a deletion is indicated by a $-$ sign; e.g. 11p$-$ means that there is material missing from the short arm of chromosome 11.

The situation gets even more difficult when we come to complex structural arrangements. For example, a reciprocal translocation (the exchange of chromosomal pieces) between the short arms of chromosomes 7 and 20 is denoted by t followed by parentheses containing the symbols 7p and 20p, separated by a semicolon, i.e. t(7p;20p). Finally, there is an agreed nomenclature for describing the various bands and regions of chromosomes using numbers, with the centromere as the point of reference. In designating a band, four pieces of information are needed; the chromosome number, the arm symbol, the region number, and the band number in the region. For example, 1p33 indicates chromosome 1, short arm, region 3, band 3. The terminal ends are described as ter; pter is the end of the short arm, and qter the end of the long arm.

Chromosome abnormalities are among the best defined causes of fetal loss or congenital disease. The frequency of spontaneous abortion is estimated to be between 15 and 20 per cent of all pregnancies, and of these approximately 50 per cent are associated with chromosome abnormalities. Overall, it is probable that about 6 per cent or more of all early human conceptions that lead to an identifiable pregnancy are chromosomally abnormal.

The frequency of chromosome abnormalities at birth is approximately 5.6 per 1000 (Table 7). Of these, about 2 per 1000 are due to a variation in the number of sex chromosomes, 1.7 per 1000 to variation in numbers of autosomal chromosomes, and 1.9 per 1000 are major chromosomal rearrangements. These abnormalities account for sixty or more different clinical conditions. Among the commoner and best defined are Down syndrome or mongolism (trisomy 21), Edwards syndrome (trisomy 18), Patau syndrome (trisomy 13), Klinefelter syndrome (sex chromosomes XXY) and the XO sex monosomic disorder (Turner syndrome). Trisomy 21 is the commonest of these disorders, despite the fact that as a group the sex chromosome trisomies are more frequent than the autosomal trisomies. It should be remembered that about 4 per cent of individuals with Down syndrome have received the extra chromosome 21 from a parent with a balanced translocation involving chromosome 21.

Trisomies result from fertilization of gametes carrying two copies of a particular chromosome; in the case of Down syndrome a gamete carries two

Table 7. *Some commoner chromosome disorders*

Condition	Frequency/ 1000 births
Numerical	
Sex chromosomes	
45X	0.1
47XXX	1.0
47XXY	1.3
47XYY	1.0
Autosomal	
Trisomy 21	1.4
Trisomy 18	0.1
Trisomy 13	0.1
Others	0.2
Structural	
Balanced translocation	2.0
Unbalanced translocation	0.5

Sources as for Table 2.

copies of chromosome 21. Such abnormal gametes result when homologous pairs of chromosomes fail to separate at the anaphase stage of the first or second division of meiosis, a phenomenon called nondisjunction. The only aetiological factor that has been shown to be of real importance in Down syndrome is maternal age. The maternal age curve for the disorder falls into two components, one, age-independent, which accounts for about 40 per cent of cases, the other age-dependent which accounts for the remainder. A maternal age effect has also been found with translocation forms of Down syndrome and with trisomy 13, trisomy 18, XXX and, to a lesser extent, XXY. Once a couple have had one infant with Down syndrome they carry a significantly increased risk of having another; this seems to be especially marked in the cases of younger parents.

Are there genetic or environmental factors that increase the likelihood of nondisjunction? Evidence for the existence of specific 'genes' is scanty. There is no increase in the incidence of consanguinity in the grandparents of children with Down syndrome and no increase in the frequency of the disorder has been found in inbred populations. What is the role of environmental causes? Radiation increases the risk of nondisjunction in *Drosophila*. However, there have been several studies of the effect of radiation on the incidence of Down syndrome; some show a small increase but in others the effect is insignificant. Similarly, there is no evidence to support a role for viral infection, chemicals, or the use of oral contraceptives in causing trisomy 21. There seems to be no association between aneuploidy (the presence of extra chromosomes or absence of a chromosome) and social class or race.

Chromosome rearrangements are most easily understood in terms of the breakages that give rise to them. A simple break in a chromosome with subsequent loss of the distal segment is called a terminal deletion. Two breaks involving one chromosome can produce an inversion, an interstitial deletion, or loss of the terminal segments and the formation of a ring chromosome. A break in two chromosomes and mutual exchange of the distal segments is called a reciprocal translocation. If only one of the translocation chromosomes is passed on at conception, the chromosome complement is unbalanced, with a deletion and/or partial trisomy. There is a special type of translocation, often referred to as a Robertsonian or centric fusion translocation. This is limited to acrocentric chromosomes and may follow from the loss of one of the translocation products. The long arms of the two acrocentrics become fused at a common centromere; so do their short arms but these are lost from the cell. Isochromosomes are the result of a duplication of one arm of a chromosome and loss of the other.

Chromosome breakage is usually random. However, some subjects show breakage of a non-staining chromosome region (gap) at the same site in a considerable proportion of metaphases. Sometimes these 'fragile sites' can be detected *in vitro* in a folate-deficient medium. Such sites may be inherited, for example the fragile site at the tip of the X chromosome (Xq28) which is associated with mental retardation. There is some increase in paternal and maternal ages in association with structural chromosomal abnormalities such as Robertsonian fusions and translocations. Analysis of autosomal breakpoints in humans has shown no obvious 'hot spots' with respect to breakage and exchange of chromosomes.

It is disappointing to reflect on how little we understand about the pathogenesis of these common chromosomal abnormalities. Thus, although much is known about the effects of radiation and chemicals on the genesis of chromosomal changes and malignancy, and a whole family of genetically determined conditions associated with fragile chromosomes and defective DNA repair has been defined, it is difficult to see where research related to the aetiology of the common chromosome disorders is likely to lead.

● Congenital malformation and common diseases: Multifactorial inheritance

The founders of modern genetics worked with clearly identifiable factors. Mendel's plants were either tall or short, while the fruit flies (*Drosophila*) that were used by T.H. Morgan had many traits that could be identified easily in different generations. Similarly, although there may be some variation in the expression, or penetration, from generation to generation or among affected sibships, the single gene disorders considered in the previous sections can all be traced through families in a clear-cut autosomal dominant, autosomal recessive, or X-linked fashion. However, many important diseases have a strong genetic component which cannot be classified in this way. There is increasing evidence that they result from the complex interaction of both genetic and environmental factors.

Single gene traits are described as being discontinuous, that is the mutant alleles produce clearly distinguishable phenotypes. Multifactorial traits may be discontinuous or continuous, but in either case the phenotype is determined by the interaction of several genes at different loci, each with an additive effect, together with a variable environmental component. In the case of discontinuous multifactorial traits the risk within affected families is raised above that of the general population. However, it rapidly falls towards that of the general population in more distant relatives. In the case of continuous multifactorial traits such as height and blood pressure there is a range with a continuous gradation between the two extremes. Most human characteristics are inherited in this way, and the contribution of heredity varies widely.

One of the most useful approaches for defining the genetic component of traits of this type is the study of twins. Twins occur about once in every 90 pregnancies. Of these about one-third are monozygotic, that is they arise from a single zygote which divides into two embryos, while two-thirds are dizygotic or non-identical, and result from the fertilization of two ova by two spermatozoa. It follows that dizygotic twins have on average one-half of their genes in common and have the same genetic relatedness as their brothers and sisters. Twins are said to be concordant if they both show a discontinuous trait, and discordant if only one shows the trait. In order to try to reduce the effect of environment on any particular trait it is helpful to analyse the concordance of monozygotic twins who have been reared apart from early infancy. If a condition has no genetic component the concordance rates will be similar for monozygotic and dizygotic twins. Concordance data for some continuous and discontinuous traits are summarized in Table 8. While they give some indication of 'heritability' in these common diseases the data must be viewed as only the grossest of approximations. However, one is left in little doubt of the importance of our genes in the pathogenesis of many of the common and ill-understood disorders of western society.

Another way of determining the importance of genetic factors in complex diseases is to try to assess the relative proportions of genes shared by relatives. Clearly, if a trait is determined by several genes, related individuals should show it in proportion to their genetic similarity. The similarity of different relatives in this respect is called their correlation and is measured on the scale zero to 1, where 1 is identical and zero is completely dissimilar. Table 9 shows the frequency of some discontinuous traits for differing degrees of relationship.

● Congenital malformation and mental retardation

It appears that many of the commoner congenital malformations (Table 10) follow a multifactorial or polygenic form of inheritance. For a couple who have had one child with a congenital malformation the risk of having another is

Table 8. *Twin concordance for some common diseases*

Condition	Concordance (per cent)	
	Monozygotic	Dizygotic
Cleft lip ± cleft palate	35	5
Cleft palate alone	26	6
Spina bifida	6	3
Pyloric stenosis	15	2
Congenital dislocation of the hip	41	3
Talipes equinovarus	32	3
Hypertension	30	10
Diabetes mellitus (insulin-dependent)	50	5
Diabetes mellitus (insulin-independent)	100	10
Ischaemic heart disease	19	8
Cancer	17	11
Epilepsy	37	10
Schizophrenia	60	10
Manic depression	70	15
Mental retardation	60	3
Leprosy	60	20
Tuberculosis	51	22
Atopic disease	50	4
Hyperthyroidism	47	3
Psoriasis	61	13
Gallstones	27	6
Sarcoidosis	50	8
Senile dementia	42	5
Multiple sclerosis	20	6

Modified from Connor and Ferguson-Smith (1987).

Table 9. *Frequency of discontinuous traits for differing degrees of relationship*

Condition	Frequency (per cent)			Population frequency (per cent)
	First-degree relatives	Second-degree relatives	Third-degree relatives	
Cleft lip	4	0.6	0.3	0.1
Spina bifida/anencephaly	4	1.5	0.6	0.3
Pyloric stenosis	2	1	0.4	0.3
Epilepsy	5	2.5	1.5	1
Schizophrenia	10	4	2	1
Manic depression	15	5	3.5	1

Modified from Connor and Ferguson-Smith (1987).

Table 10. *Congenital malformation*

System	Rate/10 000 births
Central nervous system	18–50
Eye	3–12
Ear	7
Heart	40–96
Respiratory system	4
Lip and palate	14
Digestive system	12–38
Genitalia	11–24
Urinary tract	9–16
Limbs	43–89
Abdominal wall	5–6

Based on Registration of Congenital Anomalies in Eurocat
Centres, 1979–83.

between 2 and 5 per cent. For example, cleft lip and palate, which are among the commonest congenital malformations, are inherited in a discontinuous multifactorial fashion. Parents are usually normal and therefore it is assumed that several genes are involved in the development of these regions. It is thought that the phenotype results from the balance between the number of defective and normally active genes that are inherited. Only when the balance towards abnormal genes exceeds a critical threshold will the malformation occur. It follows, therefore, that the further the threshold is exceeded the greater the extent of the malformation. The liability to this type of malformation, which probably reflects both genetic and environmental factors, can be represented as a Gaussian curve (Fig. 5). The threshold is indicated by the proportion of the population affected by the condition. For first degree relatives of an affected child the liability curve is shifted to the right and hence we would expect to find an increased frequency of the malformation among parents and other first degree relatives. The liability curve moves with increasing degrees of unrelatedness towards the position of the general population, with a corresponding reduction in incidence (Table 9).

It is estimated that 0.3 to 0.4 per cent of the childhood population of the UK have moderate to severe mental retardation; 2–3 per cent have a milder disability (IQ < 70). In previous sections we have mentioned some of the single gene disorders that can give rise to mental retardation. The results of three large surveys, one from England and two from Sweden, which attempted to assess the different causes of mental retardation in groups of children or teenagers are summarized in Table 11. The frequency of Down syndrome, by far the commonest single cause, was remarkably similar in the three studies. Other chromosomal disorders were much less common, although recent work indicates

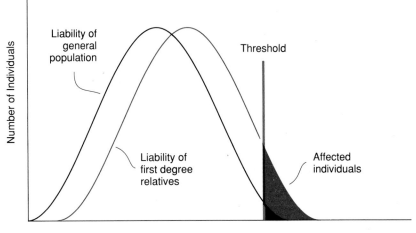

Figure 5. **The displaced liability curve in first degree relatives of a patient with a congenital disorder such as cleft lip and palate.**

Table 11. *Causes of severe mental retardation in children*

	Percentage
Known cause	
Prefertilization: Genetic	
Chromosomal: Down syndrome	32
other autosomal	2
sex-chromosomal* (average both sexes)	6
Monogenic	15
Intrauterine: environmental (maternal infection)	2
Perinatal: asphyxia/cerebral haemorrhage	7
Postnatal: meningitis/encephalitis/trauma/hypoglycaemia	2
	66
Unknown cause	
with congenital defect or dysmorphic features	14
with additional evidence of brain damage	10
without other abnormality	10
	34

Courtesy of the late Dr Cedric Carter, from Carter (1981).
*Recent data on the high incidence of the fragile-X syndrome may change this estimate.

that the fragile X syndrome, which was not included in these particular surveys, may account for up to 10 per cent of cases of mental retardation in males; some female carriers are also affected.

The monogenic causes of mental retardation include autosomal dominant or recessive and X-linked conditions. Some are associated with genetic disorders with a recognizable phenotype such as tuberous sclerosis, phenylketonuria, or macro-orchidism, while others are identified as single gene disorders simply by their patterns of inheritance. A surprisingly small number of cases are definitely related to environmental changes such as maternal infection, asphyxia during birth, or post-natal intracranial bleeding. At least a third of cases do not have any obvious aetiology, except that where there are other dysmorphic features it seems likely that there has been a serious defect early in fetal development. Since nearly 40 per cent of cases of mental retardation, in which the cause is known, are due to chromosomal abnormalities (probably more if the fragile X syndrome is included), it is likely that at least some cases for which the cause is unknown will turn out to be due to more subtle chromosomal changes that are not amendable to analysis by current cytogenetic techniques. Clearly, mental retardation, a problem of particular importance to public health, has a complex basis that includes monogenic and polygenic disorders, chromosomal abnormalities, and a number of ill-defined environmental factors.

● Common diseases of adult life

There is very good evidence for a strong genetic component to many of the common conditions that affect the populations of industrialized western societies, giving rise to much chronic ill-health and premature death. Indeed, most of the disorders that have proved so intractable to prevention or treatment and have led to the increasingly high-technology patch-up medicine that dominates our current practice, seem to be the result of environmental factors acting on genetically susceptible individuals. This is certainly true of vascular disease, diabetes, the major psychiatric illnesses, at least some of the major musculo-skeletal disorders, and the other common conditions listed in Table 8.

There are extensive data that point to the importance of genetic factors in the causation of degenerative arterial conditions, particularly premature coronary artery disease. Many studies have found within families a clustering of relatively young people with myocardial infarctions which cannot be explained adequately by environmental risk factors. In an extensive study in the United States a heritability figure of 0.56 was observed for serious coronary artery disease under the age of 55 years, even after exclusion of cases of monogenic hyperlipidaemia; having a first degree relative who has had a premature heart attack is a significant risk factor.

Genetic factors seem to be equally important in the generation of hypertension. As mentioned earlier, the distribution of blood pressure in any population is continuous and therefore hypertension is defined in rather arbitrary terms; in itself hypertension is not a disease but represents the upper 15–20 per cent of a biological variable in which there is increased risk of cerebrovascular, cardiovascular, and renal disease. Extensive family studies have demonstrated significant positive correlations between blood pressure levels among relatives, particularly in monozygotic and dizygotic twins and parent–child pairs, as well as more distantly related individuals. The results of these studies show that with increasing genetic relationship the correlations become higher, indicating that hypertension is inherited in a polygenic fashion. These studies have, in many cases, made considerable efforts to rule out the role of a common environment as the basis for familial aggregation; for example by blood pressure measurements of spouse pairs and adopted child–parent pairs. Absent or low correlations compared to positive correlations for biological relatives have usually been found. On the other hand, the lack of 100 per cent concordance for blood pressure in monozygotic twins makes it quite clear that there is an important environmental influence in setting the level of the blood pressure. High blood pressure is very unusual in primitive populations, but when they migrate to environments with the lifestyle and salt-containing diets characteristic of industrial societies hypertension becomes a common problem.

Diabetes mellitus is an extremely common condition that also has a strong genetic component. There are two forms of the condition—insulin dependent diabetes mellitus (IDDM) and non-insulin dependent diabetes (NIDDM). Elegant studies of twins have shown that the genetic component is very much stronger for NIDDM than for the insulin-dependent form of the condition. Furthermore, the latter shows a strong association with certain HLA-DR types while NIDDM shows no such correlation. These observations suggests that the basic underlying aetiology of the two forms of diabetes is different and, at least in the case of IDDM, provide us with some clues to possible direction we might take in the further analysis of the genetic component.

There is increasing evidence that genetic factors play a major role in the pathogenesis of some of the most common and important psychiatric disorders, notably schizophrenia and the bipolar affective (manic-depressive) conditions. Of course once we enter the world of psychiatry we have the added complexity of the accurate definition of phenotypes. It is likely that much of the confusion in the literature about the patterns of inheritance of psychiatric illness reflects these difficulties together with the heterogeneity of these conditions; but whatever their mode of inheritance there is overwhelming evidence for the importance of genetics in their aetiology.

● Cytoplasmic inheritance

As mentioned earlier, we receive our mitochondrial DNA from the cytoplasm of our mothers' ova. There is increasing evidence that mutations of mitochondrial DNA may underlie at least a few rare diseases. How might we recognize this unusual type of inheritance? A trait of this type always follows a pattern of maternal inheritance; but, unlike X-linked disorders, children of both sexes are affected. Subsequent generations show the trait as an autosomal dominant, but with many more affected individuals in each generation than is usual for this type of inheritance. There are many complicating factors that cause difficulties in identifying mitochondrial mutations. Because there are multiple copies in each cell, the phenotype will depend on the relative proportions of mutant and wild-type mitochondrial genomes in a particular tissue. The phenotypic effect is greatest in cells that contain only the mutant DNA, a condition called homoplasmic. In heteroplasmic cells with mixed populations of mitochondria there is scope for wide phenotypic variation. Furthermore, during cell division the proportion of mutant and wild-type mitochondrial DNA may change, a phenomenon called mitotic segregation.

We shall consider what is known about these mutations and human disease in Chapter 4.

● Cancer; somatic cell genetics

When we come to consider cancer, one of the major killers in western society, we have to broaden our definition of what we mean by genetic disease. So far we have been considering disorders that result from the abnormal function of genes that we have inherited from our parents. However, with the exception of a few rare childhood forms of the condition, cancer does not run through families in a manner that can be analysed in terms of a single gene. Cancer studies directed towards identifying a polygenic pattern of inheritance have given variable results depending on the particular type involved.

Over the last few years it has become obvious that many forms of cancer result from acquired abnormalities of the genetic machinery of cells. Throughout our lives we are constantly renewing many of our tissues and this requires the orderly division and maturation of the particular cell populations involved. It is now clear that cell division and differentiation is controlled by batteries of genes, both within the cells themselves and in related cell populations. There is increasing evidence that malignant transformation, that is the inability of a particular cell population to divide and mature in an orderly and restrained fashion, results from a breakdown of these genetic mechanisms. Thus cancer is now thought to result from a series of acquired mutations involving these fundamental cellular regulatory mechanisms. Even more interestingly, it appears that we may inherit genes that make us more likely to develop a particular cancer following a mutation of this type in a somatic cell.

● The total burden of genetic disease

A breakdown of the overall importance of genetic disease is shown in Table 12. Of course, the data give only a crude estimate and reveal very little about the

Table 12. *The total load of genetic disease. The bracketed figures indicate that they are, at best, gross approximations!*

Type of genetic disease	Frequency/ 1000 population
Single gene	
Dominant	1.8–9.5
Recessive	2.2–2.5
X-linked	0.5–2.0
Chromosome abnormalities	6.8
Common disorders with a significant genetic component*	(7–10)
Congenital malformations†	(19–22)
Total (approximate)	(37.3–52.8)

*Genetic contribution, say, one-third of such disorders as schizophrenia, diabetes mellitus, cyclothymia, and epilepsy.
†Genetic contribution, say, half of malformations like spina bifida, congenital heart disease, talipes equinovarus, cleft lip with or without cleft palate, etc.
Based on Tables 1–4 and 11, and personal communication from Professor John Edwards.

burden on the community or our health services; many of the conditions are lethal at birth or in early life while some appear only in middle life. An attempt to estimate the average disability caused, and the length of life lost by some of the more common genetic diseases is summarized in Table 13.

Another approach to assessing the importance of these disorders is to analyse the frequency of genetic disease and congenital malformation in patients in paediatric hospitals. A valuable study of this type, carried out in Montreal, analysed a sample of 12 801 admissions to a paediatric hospital between 1969 and 1970. 'Genetic' admissions accounted for 11.1 per cent, and congenital malformations 18 per cent, of the total. Overall, it was estimated that about one-third of all admissions were for diseases with a genetic component. It was also found that 70 per cent of patients with multiple admissions had genetic illnesses or congenital malformations. Based on assumptions derived from the type of gene frequency data summarized in earlier parts of this chapter, the Montreal group suggested that, with a referral population of one million for their hospital and a current birth-rate of not less than 20 000 per year, about 500 'new' patients with genetic disease or congenital malformations should have presented during the course of the survey. In fact, about eight times that number of patients were admitted in the age group of 1 day to 18 years. Only a small fraction (3.2 per cent) represented multiple admissions of the same patient. This study, and similar work carried out in other countries, leaves no doubt that genetic diseases put a serious burden on the health services.

The importance of genetic diseases in the less developed countries must not be

Table 13. *Representative estimates of overall effect of genetic disease (data supplied by the late Dr Cedric Carter)*

Condition	Birth frequency per 10 000	Average age at which impairment appears (years)	Average years of impaired life (and percentage impairment)	Years of life lost	Cause of death
Dominants					
Familial hypercholesterolaemia	20	55	10 (50)	5	Coronary thrombosis
Deafness: congenital	1	0	70 (30)	0	None
adult onset (dominant)	10	30	40 (20)	0	None
Polycystic kidney	8	30	10 (50)	30	Renal failure
Huntington's disease	5	45	15 (50)	10	Cerebral degeneration and infection
Neurofibromatosis	4	20	30 (50)	20	Cancer
Retinoblastoma (untreated) (dominant)	3	3	1 (50)	66	Cancer
Myotonic dystrophy	2	40	10 (50)	20	Dementia and infection
Blindness (dominant)	1	10	60 (50)	0	None
Tuberous sclerosis	1	5	45 (80)	20	Dementia and infection
Multiple polyposis	1	30	5 (50)	35	Cancer
Osteogenesis imperfecta	0.4	2	63 (40)	5	Infection
Marfan syndrome	0.4	30	20 (30)	20	Aortic aneurysm
Peroneal muscular dystrophy (dominant)	2	10	60 (20)	0	None
Spastic paraplegia (dominant)	0.5	20	50 (30)	0	Renal damage

Cerebellar ataxia	0.5	35	25 (50)	15	Infection
Autosomal-recessives					
Cystic fibrosis (untreated)	5	2	8 (50)	60	Lung infection
Phenylketonuria	1	0	40 (95)	30	Infection
Neurogenic muscle atrophy	1	1	4 (90)	65	Paralysis and infection
Adrenal hyperplasia	1	0	60 (30)	10	Electrolyte loss
Congenital deafness (recessive)	2	0	70 (50)	0	None
Early onset blindness (recessive)	1	5	70 (50)	0	None
Non-specific mental retardation (recessive)	5	0	50 (90)	20	Infection
X-linked recessives					
Muscular dystrophy (Duchenne type)	2	4	16 (60)	50	Debility and intercurrent infection
Haemophilia A	1	0	50 (20)	20	Haemorrhage
X-linked ichthyosis	1	0	70 (15)	0	None
X-linked forms of mental retardation	1	0	50 (80)	20	Intercurrent infection
Chromosomal anomalies					
Down syndrome	12	0	35 (95)	35	Associated malformation or infection
Edwards syndrome	1	0	1 (100)	69	''
Autosomal structural aneuploidy	5	5	20 (95)	50	''
XXX	5	5	65 (30)	0	None
XXY	5	5	65 (30)	0	None
XYY	5	5	65 (20)	0	None

underestimated. Because of the high infant mortality rates due to infection and malnutrition the incidence of genetic disease is difficult to assess. However, as social circumstances and medical services improve, these conditions assume a greater importance, particularly in populations in which there is a high gene frequency; thalassaemia in the Mediterranean region for example. The burden that a very common genetic disease can pose for a community is graphically illustrated by some cost analyses which were made for the problem of thalassaemia in Cyprus where, as medical services have improved, many severely affected children now survive. It was estimated that if all children with severe transfusion-dependent β thalassaemia were kept alive and treated by regular blood transfusion and iron chelating drugs to remove excess iron derived from the transfused blood, in 20 years time half the entire health budget of the island would be directed towards treating this one disease. There is no doubt that in many parts of the Indian subcontinent and Southeast Asia the inherited blood diseases will assume a very serious public health problem once the current high infant and early childhood mortality rates due to environmental factors are reduced.

Since we understand so little about the genetic factors involved in the common diseases of western society, it is impossible to provide any useful information about their relative role in creating the total load of common and intractable diseases in these communities. In a later chapter we shall develop the theme that it is only through an understanding of the genetic component of these conditions that we can hope to prevent and manage them more logically and hence reduce the enormous financial burden that is being placed on the health services of western society. It is our continued inability to understand the basic cause of these conditions that has led to the current expansion of high technology medicine and the major crises in health care that have affected nearly all the developed countries in recent years.

● Summary

Genetic disease and congenital malformations occur in approximately 2 to 5 per cent of all live births, account for up to 30 per cent of paediatric admissions to hospital, and are an important cause of death under the age of 15 years. In countries in which single gene disorders reach an unusually high frequency due to the action of natural selection, an even greater health burden will be caused by genetic disease once the high neonatal and childhood mortality rates due to malnutrition and infection are reduced. There is an important genetic component to most of the common diseases of western societies and increasing evidence that many forms of cancer result from acquired defects of the genome of particular cell populations.

Inherited diseases produce a major burden on our health services. It is not possible to measure the human misery caused by these disorders; the strain on a family with one or more children with a chronic, untreatable disability is incalculable. Although many families manage to cope with a situation of this kind, the stresses are too much for others. There is a high incidence of broken marriages among the parents of children with genetic disability; attention is focused on the disabled child, often to the exclusion of its siblings. The main load of coping with these children often falls on one parent. Despite the best explanations that can be given by physicians, parents often feel a considerable amount of guilt about having a child with a genetic disorder and, again, this engenders stress between husband and wife.

The pastoral component is mentioned in closing only to emphasize the uniqueness of these disorders among the diseases of childhood. They are common and particularly distressing. In terms of the total importance of genetic factors in disease they represent only the tip of the iceberg of human genetic diversity, which can be identified due to a major effect on the phenotype. There remains the enormous range of genetic heterogeneity which may be of great importance in determining individual susceptibility to most of the common diseases that affect human populations.

● Further reading

Bodmer, W.F. and Cavalli-Sforza, L.L. (1976). *Genetics, evolution and man.* W.H. Freeman and Company, San Francisco, CA.

Bundey, S. (1984). X-linked disorders. In *Antenatal and neonatal screening*, (ed. N.J. Wald), pp. 106–27. Oxford University Press.

Carter, C.O. (1977a). The relative contribution of mutant genes and chromosome abnormalities to genetic ill-health in Man. In *Progress in genetic toxicity*, (ed. D. Scott, B.A. Bridges, and F.H. Sobels), pp. 1–14. Elsevier/North Holland Biomedical Press, Amsterdam.

Carter, C.O. (1977b). Monogenic disorders., *J. Med. Genet.*, **14**, 316–20.

Carter, C.O. (1982). Contribution of gene mutations to genetic disease in humans. In *Progress in mutation research* **3**, (ed. K.C. Bora *et al.*), pp. 1–8. Elsevier Biomedical Press, Amsterdam.

Clinical Genetics Society Working Party on Prenatal Diagnosis in Relation to Genetic Counselling (1978). Provision of services for the prenatal diagnosis of fetal abnormality in the United Kingdom. *Bull. Eugen. Soc.* Suppl. 3, 1–31.

Clinical Genetics Society Working Party on Prenatal Diagnosis in Relation to Genetic Counselling (1982). The provision of regional genetic services in the United Kingdom. *Bull. Eugen. Soc.* Suppl. 4, 1–21.

Committee of Mutagenicity of Chemicals in Food, Consumer Products and the Environment (1981). *Guidelines for the testing of chemicals for mutagenicity.* Her Majesty's Stationery Office, London.

Connor, J.M. and Ferguson-Smith, M.A. (1988). *Essential medical genetics*, 2nd edn. Blackwell Scientific, Oxford.

Davies, K.E. (ed.) (1989). *The fragile X syndrome.* Oxford University Press.

Edwards, J.H. (1988). The importance of genetic disease and the need for prevention. *Phil. Trans. R. Soc. Lond. B*, **319**, 211–227.

Emery, A.E.H. and Mueller, R.F. (1987). *Elements of medical genetics*, 7th edn. Churchill Livingstone, London.

Gardner, R.J.M. and Sutherland, G.R. (1989). *Chromosome abnormalities and genetic counselling*. Oxford University Press.

Hames, B.D. and Glover, D.M. (1988). *Molecular immunology*. IRL Press, Oxford.

Harper, P.S., Quarrell, W.J., and Youngman, S. (1988). Huntington's disease: prediction and prevention. *Phil. Trans. R. Soc. Lond. B*, **319**, 285–98.

Levitan, M. (1989). *Textbook of human genetics*, 3rd edn. Oxford University Press.

Lewin, B. (1990). *Genes*, IV. Oxford University Press.

Love, D.R. and Davies, K.E. (1989). Duchenne muscular dystrophy: the gene and the protein. *Mol. Biol. Med.*, **6**, 7–18.

McKusick, V.A. (1988). *Mendelian inheritance in man*, 8th edn. Johns Hopkins University Press, Baltimore, MD.

Nevin, N.C. (1988). Prevention and avoidance of congenital malformations *Phil. Trans. R. Soc. Lond. B*, **319**, 309–14.

Rothwell, N.V. (1989). *Understanding genetics*. Oxford University Press.

Royal College of Physicians, London (1989). *Prenatal diagnosis and genetic screening. A report*.

Scriver, C.R., Beaudet, A.L., Sly, W.S., and Valle, D. (eds) (1988). *The metabolic basis of inherited disease*, 6th edn. McGraw-Hill, New York.

Scriver, C.R., Neal, J.L., Saginur, R., and Clow, A. (1973). The frequency of genetic disease and congenital malformation among patients in a pediatric hospital. *Can. Med. Assoc. J.*, **108**, 1111–15.

Stamatoyannopoulos, G., Nienhuis, A.W., Leder, P., and Majerus, P.W. (eds) (1987). *The molecular basis of blood diseases*. Wiley, New York.

Sykes, B. (1989). Inherited collagen disorders. *Mol. Biol. Med.*, **6**, 19–28.

Vogel, F. and Motulsky, A.G. (1987). *Human genetics*, 2nd edn. Springer-Verlag, Berlin.

Weatherall, D.J. and Clegg, J.B. (1981). *The thalassaemia syndromes*, 3rd edn. Blackwell Scientific, Oxford.

World Health Organization (1983). Report on the community control of hereditary anaemias. Memorandum from a WHO Meeting. *Bull. World Health Org.*, **61**, 63–80.

The structure, organization, and regulation of human genes

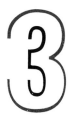

Over the last few years the genes of a wide range of species have been characterized at the molecular level. In this chapter we shall focus on the function and structure of human genes and what is known about their regulation and organization. Those who wish to augment this brief introduction to molecular genetics should consult the monographs and reviews cited in the short bibliography at the end of this chapter.

● Structure of genes and the transmission of genetic information

Enzymes and other biologically important proteins consist of one or more peptide chains folded into a three-dimensional structure, the exact shape of which is critical for their normal function. The shape and stability of enzymes depend on the interactions of the different amino acids from which they are constructed. The genetic information that determines the order of amino acids in a peptide chain, and hence the structure of the protein of which it forms a part, is encoded in the DNA constituting the gene for that chain. This information is transported from the nuclei of cells to their cytoplasm by means of a type of ribonucleic acid (RNA) called messenger RNA (mRNA) which has a structure exactly complementary to that of the DNA from which it is copied, or transcribed. The process whereby a protein chain is synthesized on an mRNA template is called translation. Thus, the flow of genetic information in cells can be written.

$$\text{DNA} \xrightarrow[\text{transcription}]{} \text{RNA} \xrightarrow[\text{translation}]{} \text{PROTEIN}$$

● General organization of the genetic control of protein synthesis and structure

The amino acid sequence of any particular peptide chain is determined by the order of bases of the DNA forming its structural gene; one gene equals one peptide chain. As we shall see later, there are occasional exceptions to this rule. DNA carries its information in the form of a three letter code; different arrangements of three bases code for particular amino acids. Such coding triplets are called codons. Messenger RNA is transcribed from DNA strands by the action of an enzyme called RNA polymerase II. Because of the rules of base pairing it is a mirror image of the DNA from which it is copied. After various processing steps, mRNA moves from the nucleus to the cytoplasm of the cell where it acts as a template for protein synthesis. This takes place on polysomes, groups of ribosomes that have become attached to mRNA and carry the growing peptide chains. Amino acids do not bind directly to mRNA, but first become attached to another type of RNA called transfer RNA(tRNA). Each tRNA molecule is specific for a particular amino acid and for an appropriate mRNA codon. A transfer RNA molecule binds to its particular codon on mRNA through its anticodon, a group of three nucleotides carried by the tRNA and which has a sequence complementary to the particular mRNA codon. Successive tRNAs carry their amino acids to the mRNA template and hence a peptide chain is gradually built up, with each of its constitutional amino acids in the correct position. The regulation of the rates of peptide chain synthesis can be modified by either the rate of transcription of their messenger RNAs or by the speed at which these messenger RNAs are translated in the cell cytoplasm.

To understand the transmission of genetic information we have to consider the structure of the different components of this system, and how each of the steps involved in the movement of genetic information from DNA to the cell cytoplasm, and the subsequent assembly of proteins, is regulated.

● DNA

DNA molecules consist of two chains of nucleotides bases wrapped around each other (Fig. 6). There are four bases, adenine (A), guanine (G), cytosine (C), and thymine (T). The building blocks of each chain are deoxyribonucleotides, which consist of a base, deoxyribose, and phosphate, covalently joined. The backbone of DNA, which is constant throughout the whole molecule, consists of deoxyribose molecules linked by phosphates (Fig. 6). The variable part of a DNA chain is the sequence of bases which can be in any order along the sugar phosphate backbone. Because of their particular shapes, A always pairs with T, and C with G; the bases (and hence the chains or strands) are linked by hydrogen bonds. Genetic information is encoded by the order of the bases; it is a triplet non-overlapping code in which three bases determine a particular amino acid.

To understand the function of DNA, it is helpful to note a few key points relating to its structure, as shown in Fig. 6. First, the phosphate can be attached to either of the two hydroxyl groups on deoxyribose which are numbered by convention 3' and 5'. Second, the two chains are coiled up in a helical fashion around a common axis. They have opposite polarity, that is they run in opposite directions, one chain 5'→3' and the other 3'→5'. The bases are on the inside of the helix whereas the sugar phosphate backbone is on the outside. Finally, the sequence of bases along one of the DNA chains determines the sequence of bases along the other, i.e. the two strands are complementary to each other.

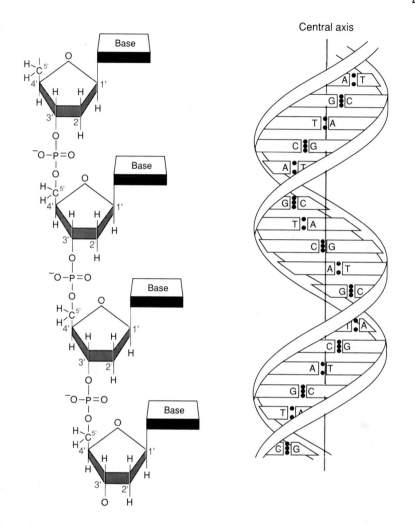

Figure 6. **The structure of DNA.** The diagram in the right is a model of the Watson–Crick DNA double helix. The two bands represent the sugar phosphate backbones of the two strands, which run in opposite directions. The vertical line represents the central axis round which the strands wind. The position of the four nucleotide bases, C, A, T, and G, is shown, together with the hydrogen bonds (●) which link them together. The diagram on the left represents the structure of part of a DNA chain. It shows the chain-linked deoxyribose and phosphate residues which form the sugar-phosphate backbone.

DNA replication is an extremely complex process whereby the strands are separated and each one is copied to produce a new daughter strand. Since one of each parent strand remains intact after replication the process is said to be 'semi-conservative'. Through the action of enzymes called DNA polymerase each new strand is synthesized in a 5′→3′ direction by the stepwise addition of the four deoxyribonucleoside triphosphates; these bases are added to complementary bases on the parental template strand so that the replication process produces two identical copies of the original molecule.

● Gene structure

It used to be thought that a gene consists simply of a length of DNA that contains sufficient nucleotide triplets to code for the appropriate number of amino acids in the peptide chains of that gene. It is now apparent that this is not the case. In fact, almost all mammalian genes that have been analysed so far have their coding sequences interrupted by sequences of unknown function called intervening sequences (IVS), or introns, at varying positions along their length (Fig. 7). Their number and size, often considerably longer than the coding sequences or exons, varies from gene to gene. For example, in the case of the human globin genes there are two introns, whereas in the gene for α collagen there are more than 50! In all mammalian genes the dinucleotides GT and AG are found at the 5′ and 3′ ends of

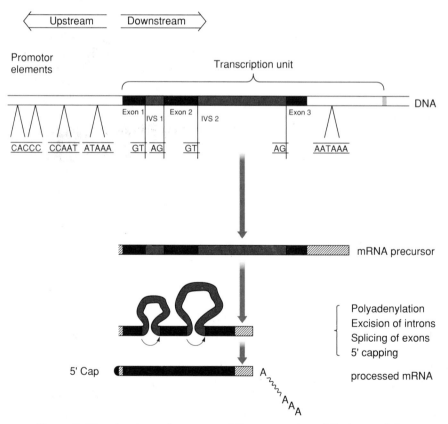

Figure 7. The structure of a gene and the processing of its transcript.

the introns, and sequences close to these dinucleotides have also been highly conserved during evolution. We shall return to the functional significance of these sequences when we discuss the processing of messenger RNA.

Why do we carry all these stretches of apparently useless DNA in our genes? The answer to this intriguing question is not yet known although there is no shortage of hypotheses! One of the more attractive relates to the way in which proteins may have been put together during evolution. It has been observed that introns tend to separate regions of genes that code for different functional domains of proteins. In this context a domain is defined as a discrete, continuous part of a peptide sequence that can be equated with a particular function. Many proteins look like patchwork quilts, consisting of various 'pieces' of sequence that have homology with a diverse variety of other proteins. For this reason it has been suggested that introns may have provided a means for speeding up evolution. The chopping out of intervening sequences might, the idea goes, facilitate the juxtaposition and hence joint expression of DNA sequences which may previously have been widely separated throughout the genome and then brought together by genetic recombination. In other words, introns may have increased the speed at which selection for functionally important proteins has occurred.

At the 5' and 3' ends of genes there are specific triplets which determine the initiation (ATG) and termination (TAA, TAG, or TGA) of protein synthesis on mRNAs. There are also sequences of varying lengths at both ends which determine the structure of non-translated regions of mRNA. As we shall see later the highly conserved AATAAA sequence in the 3' non-coding region of all mammalian genes is critical for normal processing of mRNA.

Most mammalian genes have blocks of sequences in their 5' flanking regions which are similar to those found in *Drosophila* and many other species. The first of these, ATA, located about 26–30 nucleotides upstream (to the left in a DNA strand reading left to right) from the RNA initiation or CAP site (see below), is a sequence that was originally found in the histone gene cluster of *Drosophila* and called the Goldberg-Hogness box; the second, CCAAT, is found about 72–77 nucleotides upstream from the beginning of the gene. These regions, and another with the structure CACCC, which is about 87–95 nucleotides upstream from the beginning of a gene, are involved in the regulation of transcription of mRNA. For this reason they are called promotors, or upstream promotor elements, regions of DNA to which RNA polymerases bind and initiate gene transcription.

● Transcription and processing of messenger RNA

Messenger RNA is synthesized on its DNA template in a 5'→3' direction by the action of enzymes called RNA polymerases. When the latter bind to double-stranded DNA they cause a localized separation of the two DNA strands, but only one of these is copied into RNA. Chemically, RNA is similar to DNA except for two differences: the sugar of DNA is deoxyribose while in RNA it is ribose, and instead of thymine RNA contains the closely related pyrimidine, uracil. The synthesis of RNA on DNA templates is very similar to the process of DNA replication and involves the formation of complementary base pairs. As in the case of DNA duplication, G pairs with C, but when mRNA is being made on a DNA template A pairs with U instead of T.

The primary transcript is a large mRNA precursor which contains the entire gene complex including exons and introns (Fig. 7). This molecule undergoes a series of processing steps before it is ready for delivery to the cell cytoplasm. The introns are cut out and the exons spliced together. This is a remarkable achievement, particularly when we remember that in the case of the α2 collagen gene 51 exon transcripts must be linked together with complete precision; a mistake involving even one base may make the mRNA untranslatable. As mentioned earlier the 5' exon/intron junction always has the bases G and T whereas the 3' junction has A and G. There appear to be conserved or concensus sequences near the 5' and 3' splice junctions which are called the 'donor' and 'acceptor' sites respectively. The precise details of the complex mechanism whereby the introns are cut out and the exons are joined are still being worked out. The process appears to occur in two stages. First, the mRNA precursor is cut at the 5' splice site to generate two intermediates, a linear first exon and a branched lariat-shaped molecule containing the intron and second exon. Second, the 3' splice site is cleaved, the lariat intron released, and two exons joined. This process involves the interaction of a number of enzymes and other nuclear proteins.

As well as cutting and splicing, mRNA undergoes further processing while still in the nucleus. It is chemically modified at its 5' end by the addition of a CAP structure, so-called because the formation of a 5'-5' pyrophosphate linkage in effect seals off the 5' end of the mRNA. It is also modified at its 3' end by the attachment of a string of adenylic acid residues (polyA) which may serve to stabilize it during its passage into the cytoplasm. The site of polyA addition is related to the highly conserved AATAAA sequence shown in Fig. 7. It seems quite likely that during its time in the nucleus and for much of its time in the cytoplasm the mRNA precursor and its processed product are associated with various protein molecules which may serve to stabilize and protect them from nuclease attack.

● Protein synthesis

Once in the cell cytoplasm mRNA acts as a template for protein synthesis (Fig. 8). Amino acids cannot interact directly with nucleic acids and, as mentioned earlier, are brought to mRNAs attached to another type of molecule called transfer RNA(tRNA). There is a family of different tRNAs, each specific for a different amino acid and with three bases (anticodons) which are complementary to the appropriate mRNA codons for their particular amino acids. Protein synthesis occurs on ribosomes, each of which consists of two different-sized

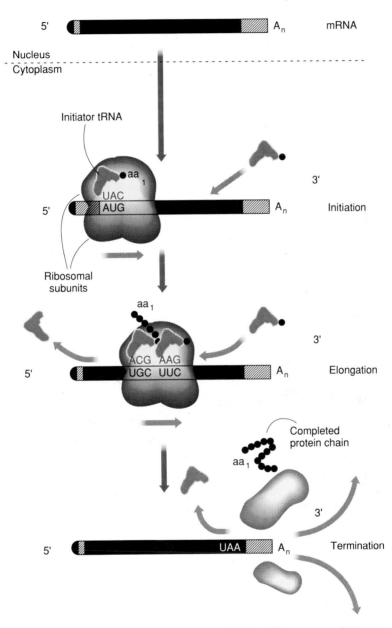

5' ━━━━━░░░ A_n mRNA

Nucleus
Cytoplasm

Initiator tRNA

aa$_1$

UAC
5' ░AUG━━━━━░░░ A_n Initiation

Ribosomal
subunits

aa$_1$

3'

ACG AAG
5' ━━━UGC UUC━━━░░░ A_n Elongation

Completed
protein chain

aa$_1$

3'

5' ━━━━━UAA░░ A_n Termination

Figure 8. The different steps in the translation of messenger RNA.

ribonuclear protein subunits. The initiation of protein synthesis is achieved when a ribosome is bound to the region of the initiation codon, AUG, and when an initiator tRNA base pairs with this codon. AUG is the codeword for methionine. There are two types of methionine transfer RNAs, one that can initiate protein synthesis, while the other inserts methionine in the appropriate place in the growing chain.

Initiation involves the formation of a complex consisting of several initiation factors, ribosomal subunits, and initiator tRNA. A second tRNA then binds to the next codon along and a peptide bond is formed between the two amino acids carried by these tRNAs. The first tRNA is then released. This cyclical process, which involves the shifting of the growing chain between specific donor and acceptor sites on the ribosomes, is then repeated in a $5' \rightarrow 3'$ direction from codon to codon until a specific termination codon (UAA, UAG, or UGA) is reached. The completed peptide chain is then released from the last tRNA molecule and the ribosomal subunits fall off the mRNA. Most mRNAs can carry several ribosomes at any one time; the mRNAs with ribosomes attached along their length (polysomes) appear like strings of beads in the cell cytoplasm.

It seems likely that proteins start to fold and form their complex tertiary structures as they are synthesized on the ribosome/mRNA complex. Some peptide chains constitute subunits that must combine with other subunits to form definitive proteins. And some proteins have to undergo a considerable amount of post-translational modification before they are functional. Insulin, for example, is first synthesized as a molecule called preproinsulin which is 110 amino acids long. The first 24 amino acids constitute a signal peptide which facilitates entry of the molecule into the endoplasmic reticulum; many secreted proteins have signal or leader peptides of this type. The signal peptide is cleaved to produce a shorter molecule called proinsulin. A sequence of 35 amino acids called the connecting peptide, or C-peptide, in the middle of the proinsulin chain is then removed to yield an A chain of 21 amino acids and a B chain of 30 amino acids. The A and B chains are then joined to each other by disulphide bonds formed during the initial stages of protein synthesis.

● The genetic code

The term 'genetic code' is used to describe the relationship between the sequence of bases in DNA or its RNA transcript and the sequence of amino acids in proteins. As mentioned earlier, amino acids are encoded by groups of three bases called codons. Of the 64 possible coding triplets (Fig. 9), 61 specify particular amino acids whereas the other three codons, UAA, UAG, and UGA are signals for chain termination. Thus, since only 20 different amino acids occur naturally in proteins, most of them must have more than one codeword; in other words, the genetic code is degenerate. It is also universal; with the exception of mitochondrial DNA, the same codons are used to code for the same amino acids in all living organisms.

First position (5' end)	Second position				Third position (3' end)
	U	C	A	G	
U	Phe	Ser	Tyr	Cys	U
	Phe	Ser	Tyr	Cys	C
	Leu	Ser	Stop	Stop	A
	Leu	Ser	Stop	Trp	G
C	Leu	Pro	His	Arg	U
	Leu	Pro	His	Arg	C
	Leu	Pro	Gln	Arg	A
	Leu	Pro	Gln	Arg	G
A	Ile	Thr	Asn	Ser	U
	Ile	Thr	Asn	Ser	C
	Ile	Thr	Lys	Arg	A
	Met	Thr	Lys	Arg	G
G	Val	Ala	Asp	Gly	U
	Val	Ala	Asp	Gly	C
	Val	Ala	Glu	Gly	A
	Val	Ala	Glu	Gly	G

Figure 9. The genetic code. The codons are given as they appear in mRNA. The abbreviations for the different amino acids are the first three letters of each amino acid except in the case of Asn, asparagine; Gln, glutamine; Ile, isoleucine; and Trp, tryptophane.

● Exceptions to the one gene–one peptide chain rule

As knowledge about the organization of the genetic control of human proteins has evolved it has become clear that, although one gene–one peptide chain holds for many genes, the rule has been modified in some very subtle ways to meet a variety of different needs. As we shall see in the next section, many proteins are made up of different subunits. Each subunit is quite commonly encoded by genes on different chromosomes, which of course does not break our rule. Nor does the fact that different forms of the enzyme amylase may be produced by the use of different promotors, or that some peptide chains may have multiple enzymic activities. But there is an increasing number of examples of cases in which mRNA processing may actually change the original message encoded by a gene.

One well-characterized way of making more than one use of mRNA is by differential splicing, so that different proteins are synthesized in particular tissues, a particularly popular activity among neuropeptides and muscle proteins. Another mechanism for changing the template is called mRNA editing. In this case, by an unknown mechanism, U's are inserted or removed. So far, this has only been observed in the mitochondria of trypanosomes, parasites that cause sleeping sickness. Another remarkable example of post-transcriptional modification of mRNA is a C→U conversion that occurs in the pre-mRNA for human apolipoprotein B. This change, the mechanism of which is not yet understood, creates a stop codon resulting in a shortened but functional protein. Apparently this is how it is possible to synthesize two different apolipoproteins, B-100 and B-48, using one gene. We shall consider the functions of these proteins in Chapter 7.

Very recently an even more surprising example of human mRNA modification has emerged. One of the subunits of glucose-6-phosphate dehydrogenase (G6PD) appears to be chimeric. The C-terminal 479 amino acid residues are encoded by the X chromosome; the N-terminal 55 residues are encoded by a gene on chromosome 6. Remarkably, it has not been possible to find a 'fusion' mRNA for this protein. How is it made? Do ribosomes hop from one message to another, or are the two peptide products joined together after they have been synthesized? Both mechanisms raise formidable problems for the cell, and for human geneticists if this work is confirmed!

Another apparent exception to the Mendelian patterns of inheritance that, by and large, are reflected in the events at the molecular level considered in this chapter is the observation that the expression of certain genes is determined by whether they are inherited from the male or female parent. This fascinating phenomenon is called *parental imprinting*. At the present time very little is known about the molecular basis for imprinting, though recent studies suggest that it may reflect the degree of methylation of different genes, or regions of chromosomes. We shall look further at the role of methylation in gene regulation in the sections that follow.

These few examples of the subtleties of what can happen before and after a gene is transcribed emphasize how much remains to be learnt about gene action; nothing can be taken for granted.

● The regulation of gene expression

Every cell in our body contains the complete complement of genes necessary to make an entire human being. Since most of our organs are made up of cells with very specialized functions it follows that only a small proportion of their genes must be active. Furthermore, many genes are required to function only at specific phases of development and they must be activated and switched off at the appropriate times. Also individual genes must be so regulated that they produce just the right quantity of product for the physiological requirements of their cells. The accuracy required for the regulation of particular genes varies widely according to the function of their products. For example, it appears that some genes are switched on in most tissues at all stages of development. It may well be that these so-called housekeeping genes do not require very precise regulation. On the other hand genes that control highly specialized proteins like haemoglobin, which change their structure at specific developmental stages and must be synthesized in very precise quantities, require very much tighter regulation. Although considerable progress has been made in working out the regulation of genes in prokaryotes, much less is known about these highly complex functions in higher organisms. Before we consider this problem we must try to understand how our genes are packaged together in the nuclei of our cells.

● Chromatin

So far in this chapter we have talked about genes as if they are simple linear strands of DNA. As we shall see later, there is about two metres of DNA in every cell in the body. It follows, therefore, that our DNA must be remarkably compressed in the nucleus of our cells. In fact DNA does not exist in the form of naked strands but complexed with histones and other proteins to form chromatin. Histones are highly basic proteins which have very similar amino acids in higher organisms, and are classified according to their amino acid composition. Octomers containing two each of histones called H2A, H2B, H3, and H4 form a core around which helical DNA is wrapped, apparently twice, to form beaded bodies called nucleosomes. A further order of packaging of chromatin occurs in which a helical assembly of nucleosomes forms a structure called an elementary fibre, a compact arrangement of six nucleosomes. The organization of these structures into chromatin fibres, which can be seen under the electron microscope, is shown in Fig. 10.

● The anatomy of gene activation and repression

One of the results of this remarkable degree of packaging is that the transcriptional activity of the genome of individual cells is quite limited. For example in the erythroid cells of the marrow, the progenitors of red blood cells, only a few per cent of the total DNA sequences capable of being expressed are active. This variability in activity of different regions of DNA is reflected by major alterations in chromatin structure which can be demonstrated experimentally as an increased sensitivity to digestion by various nucleases, notably DNase 1. There is an increased sensitivity to this enzyme in long regions of DNA surrounding active genes and there are specific regions of even greater sensitivity which correlate with active transcription. Although these observations tell us that regions of DNA are potentially active, for example at different stages of development, they beg the question of what it is that brings about these alterations in chromatin structure.

Another indicator of the state of activity of our genes is their degree of methylation. As a general rule actively transcribed genes are hypomethylated, and vice versa. Methylation occurs mainly at the C residue of CG dinucleotide sequences. While hypomethylation of 5′ flanking DNA appears to be a necessary prerequisite for the normal expression of many genes it is not the primary signal; there are many examples of genes that are hypomethylated but not expressed.

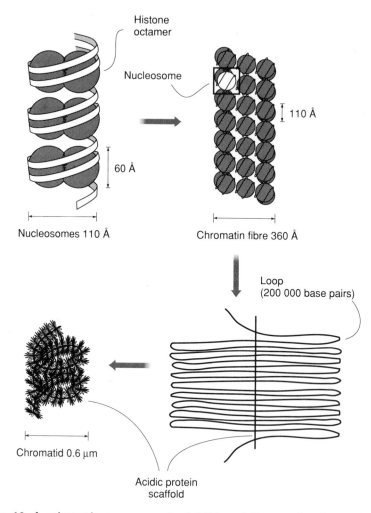

Figure 10. **A schematic arrangement of DNA and its associated protein in the nucleosome, chromatin fibre and chromatid.** Modified from Connor and Fergusson-Smith (1987).

Perhaps the methylation state should be looked on as a permissive control of gene expression rather than a positive expression signal.

Virtually nothing is known about how these alterations in chromatin configuration and DNA packaging lead to the conformational changes that result in genes being available for transcription. Recent studies suggest that chromatin in higher organisms is organized into a series of loops, anchored to a protein matrix. It appears that each loop represents a unit of replication and, incidentally, a unit of function in that the loop as a whole may be in a potentially active or repressed transcriptional state. Furthermore, it is becoming apparent that there is a relationship between the timing of DNA replication and the transcription of genes in different cells. For example, as mentioned earlier one of the X chromosomes in females is inactivated. It turns out that the DNA in these cells is replicated late in the cell cycle. On the other hand, the housekeeping genes, which were also alluded to earlier, are generally found in early replicating DNA. It appears that the timing of replication is related to the transcriptional competence of sets of genes. Thus at the chromatin level it is likely that a number of control elements are involved in transcription, one involving the timing of replication and another that controls chromatin conformation.

● Regulatory sequences and DNA binding proteins

When we get down to the level of DNA itself our knowledge of regulation is equally hazy. As mentioned earlier, the highly conserved boxes of DNA sequence in the 5′ region of mammalian genes are necessary for normal gene expression because they provide binding sites for the regulatory signals for RNA polymerase II. In addition to these well-defined promotor sequences another class of sequences has been found which appears to be involved with the regulation of gene activity and tissue specificity of gene expression. These so-called enhancer sequences may lie within the transcription unit of structural genes or at a considerable distance from them. Although there is evidence that they may become apposed to the promoter sequences by alterations in DNA configuration, the mechanism whereby they increase the output of structural genes or determine tissue specificity remains to be worked out.

Over the last few years there has been an enormous amount of activity directed towards defining elements of DNA that may subserve regulatory functions. The work is based largely on systematic mutational analyses of structural genes and has shown quite unequivocally that, as well as the promotor and enhancer elements that we have already discussed, each gene in an animal cells has a remarkable array of positive and negative *cis* elements. Many of these sequences are found within several hundred base pairs of the initiation site of the structural gene but others can exert control over great distances, up to 30 kb. It is also clear that the importance of an individual *cis* element can vary in different cell types and in response to different physiological signals, presumably because the DNA binding factor or factors that recognize these sites vary in abundance in different tissues. Overlapping or superimposed binding sites for multiple factors can result in different positive and negative factors competing for sites. Some of the *cis* elements seem to act as silencer regions that can block the activity of *cis*-linked enhancers. The property that all these *cis* regions of DNA have in common is that their action is mediated through their interaction with a family of DNA-binding regulatory proteins.

In the last few years techniques have been developed for the purification from nuclear extracts of a variety of DNA binding proteins. The binding properties have also been utilized as a way of screening expression libraries for complementary DNA clones that encode them. The determination of the general properties of DNA binding proteins is an area of research that has generated some of the more colourful terminology of molecular biology. Several different structural motifs have been proposed for the DNA binding domains of these proteins; helix-turn-helix, zinc fingers and leucine zippers, for example. The helix-turn-helix structure is, as intimated by its name, two α helices separated by a β turn. Amino acid residues in one of the α helices make direct contact with a group in the target DNA. These proteins are best characterized in their role in the early development of *Drosophila*. There are several types of zinc fingers. For example, one family of these proteins is composed of nine repeated units of about 30 amino acid residues. Each unit always contains two pairs of cysteines and histidines which serve as a tetrahedral co-ordination site for a single zinc ion; the amino acids between these sites jut out like a finger. Zinc fingers are found in a wide variety of DNA binding proteins in species ranging from yeast to man. Leucine zippers consist of four to five leucine residues spaced exactly seven residues apart, every two turns of an α helix. They have been found in a number of DNA binding proteins including the products of oncogenes (see Chapter 8).

It is now apparent that the DNA binding proteins are the product of a large gene family and that during evolution they have evolved into a remarkably diverse series of molecules with individual patterns of regulated post-translational modifications, binding affinities, binding sites, and interactions with other regulatory proteins. Several individual classes of these proteins have been defined and at least some of their physiological roles are being worked out. Although very little is known about their regulation and interaction some recent progress has been made, particularly in the field of developmental genetics. The pattern that is emerging is of a complex regulatory network between genes that code for the proteins controlling the transcription of structural genes and external signals that activate or repress these genes. Since we now have the capacity to isolate the genes for the regulatory proteins it should be possible to start to understand how these complex networks actually work.

So far we have restricted the discussion of our ideas about gene regulation to factors that might alter the rates of transcription of individual genes. It should be remembered, however, that regulation could also be mediated at the level of nuclear RNA processing, by differential rates of mRNA turnover, by variation in the rates of translation of individual mRNAs and, indeed, by the rates of processing the final protein products. However, from the very limited information that is available about the control of human genes it looks as though the bulk of regulation occurs at the transcriptional level.

It appears, therefore, that the control of gene regulation is a multi-step process requiring fundamental alterations in the configuration of chromatin, the action of a complex series of regulatory proteins that bind to and activate or repress individual genes, the co-ordinated activity of these DNA binding proteins and their genes with internal and external regulatory signals, and, perhaps, some fine tuning at the levels of mRNA processing and translation. Clearly a lot of work will have to be done to convert this complicated jigsaw into anything like a complete picture of how we regulate our genes. Even when we understand how individual genes are controlled there will remain the problem of how it is possible to co-ordinate in a synchronized fashion the output of genes for the various subunits of proteins. As already intimated, genes do not function *in vacuo*; their activity has to be synchronized in a highly co-ordinated fashion throughout different tissues. To achieve this end there must be mechanisms whereby genes in individual cells can respond to regulatory signals from without.

● How do genes make contact with the outside world? Co-ordinated gene expression

To co-ordinate the complex mechanisms of growth, differentiation, and metabolism of the millions of cells in the tissues and organs of a human being a highly sophisticated communication network has evolved. In many cases this involves the activation or repression of the activity of genes by external signals. It is useful to consider these extracellular regulatory pathways in terms of the distance over which a particular signal must act.

In *endocrine signalling*, the highly specialized cells of the endocrine organs synthesize hormones, substances that act on a distant set of target cells. In *paracrine signalling* the target cell lies close to the signalling cell and the signalling molecule affects only cells that are adjacent to it. A good example is the conduction of an electric impulse from one cell to another through the action of chemical neurotransmitters. Finally, *autocrine signalling* is a term used to describe the response of cells to substances that they themselves release. This type of regulation is particularly important with respect to the growth factors required for normal cellular growth and maturation, and which are becoming of particular interest in the cancer field.

The ways in which the external regulatory molecules used for cell to cell signalling act vary widely but can be categorized into two main mechanisms. First, lipid soluble hormones, for example steroids or thyroxine, diffuse across plasma membranes and interact directly with proteins in the cytosol or nucleus. Second, small peptide hormones, growth factors, and other external regulatory molecules bind specifically to cell surface receptors, a process that then initiates a complex series of intracellular events.

Once steroid hormones are released from their carrier proteins, they diffuse across the plasma membranes of their target cells and bind reversibly to specific hormone receptor proteins in the cytosol. In the bound configuration receptor proteins acquire an affinity for DNA that leads to their accumulation in the nucleus. Here the complex binds to chromatin and regulates the transcription of a number of different genes; information is accumulating about the specific DNA sequences involved.

On the other hand, hormones or growth factors that bind to specific receptors on the cell surface rely for their activity on a series of intracellular messenger molecules, a process called signal transduction. For example, adrenalin or glucagon, by binding to their surface receptors trigger the activation of adenylate cyclase with the subsequent elevation of the intracellular concentration of 3-, 5-cyclic AMP. The interaction between the receptors and the cyclase is mediated by a specific transducing protein called protein G which binds guanosine triphosphate (GTP) in response to the hormone binding to its receptor. The G-GTP complex in turn dissociates into subunits and hence activates adenylate cyclase. Cyclic AMP action is mediated by a cyclic AMP-dependent protein kinase which is capable of activating a variety of enzymes. The activity of insulin and many growth factors is also mediated through receptor binding and activation of intracellular protein kinases, in this case with tyrosine specificity. These second messenger systems are all ultimately dependent on the action of protein kinases which are able to transfer the terminal phosphate group of ATP to serine, threonine, and tyrosine residues of particular proteins; the phosphorylated form of many enzymes is much more active than the unphosphorylated state. These processes are all reversible when the level of the particular hormone or other signalling agent is reduced and the level of cyclic AMP falls.

In fact there is a variety of intracellular second messages including calcium and specific phospholipids. For example, stimulation by nerve impulses causes the release of calcium and an increase in its intracellular concentration. The latter triggers contraction and also the breakdown of glycogen which leads to prolonged contraction. It is now clear that many hormones bind to receptors and cause an increase in intracellular calcium, largely by triggering the release of calcium from the endoplasmic reticulin. It appears that phosphatidyl-inositol 4,5-biphosphate is an intracellular transducer, or second messenger, which couples receptor–hormone binding to calcium release. Furthermore one of the products of its hydrolysis, 1,2-diacylglycerol, is able to diffuse in the membrane and activate a protein kinase, protein kinase C which has, as its substrate, several proteins essential for the control of cell growth.

Some of these complex interactions which involve the transfer of information from cell surface receptors to intracellular messages are summarized in Table 14. It will be apparent, even from this very brief description, that specificity of cellular regulation is mediated by the interaction between receptors and mediators. Thus cellular differentiation reflects the appearance of particular receptors on the cell surfaces at different stages of development and during different states of function. Although cellular regulation must involve many hundreds of genes for mediators and receptors, the fact that different receptors utilize similar intracellular messenger systems provides an extremely efficient mechanism for the control and co-ordination of gene expression in complex multicellular organisms.

It is apparent, therefore, that studies of the regulation of cellular activity, whether by the direct interaction of intracellular hormones and their receptors with DNA, or mediated via complex transduction systems following the interaction of regulatory molecules with surface receptors, provide some important insights into how genes or their products are involved in the regulation of cellular functions (Table 14). It is becoming apparent that mutations involving the critical regulatory molecules, be they growth factors, receptors, intracellular

Table 14. *Examples of signal transmission via receptors (modified from Mitchell 1988)*

Receptors with intrinsic ion channels	*Receptors that inhibit adenylate cyclase*
Acetyl choline (nicotinic receptors with Na^+ channel)	Adrenergic (α_2)
	Acetyl choline
GABA* and glycine (with Cl^- channels)	*Receptors that activate phosphatidyl-inositol 4,5-biphosphate hydrolysis*
Receptors with intrinsic protein kinase activity	Adrenergic (α_1)
	Gonadotrophin releasing hormone
Platelet derived growth factor	Angiotensin
Epidermal growth factor	Thyrotrophin releasing hormone
Insulin and insulin-like growth factors	
Receptors that activate adenylate cyclase	
Adrenergic $(\beta_1$ and $\beta_2)$	
Thyroid stimulating hormone	
Parathyroid hormone	
Glucagon	

*GABA $= \gamma$ aminobutyric acid

messengers, or DNA binding proteins, may have profound effects on the regulation of cell growth and maturation. We shall return to this question in a later chapter when we consider recent concepts about the molecular basis of cancer.

● Many human genes are organized in families

Many human genes are organized in families. A group of homologous genes with similar functions is called a multigene family. The more grandiose title of supergene family has been used to describe sets of multigene families and single-copy genes of common ancestry which are not all necessarily involved in identical function. Since even molecular biologists have questioned whether there is such an entity as a 'supergene' it is now the fashion to describe such systems as gene superfamilies. These gene families include many of particular interest in clinical practice, for example those that control the haemoglobins, the immune system, cytochromes involved in the detoxification of drugs and environmental carcinogens, and the blood clotting factors.

Since the globin multigene family and the superfamily of immunoglobulin-related proteins are so well understood, and are of such major importance in the later chapters of this book, I shall describe them briefly here. They provide elegant examples of the way in which large numbers of specialized genes have evolved from what was probably a single primordial ancestor.

● The genetic control of human haemoglobin

The multigene family that controls the human haemoglobins is shown in Fig. 11. The structure of haemoglobin changes during development, an adaptive process designed to meet differing oxygen transport requirements at various stages of fetal maturation.

All the human haemoglobins have a tetrameric structure. Adult and fetal haemoglobins have α chains combined with β chains (Hb A; $\alpha_2\beta_2$), δ chains (Hb A$_2$; $\alpha_2\delta_2$, the minor adult haemoglobin), or γ chains (Hb F, or fetal haemoglobin; $\alpha_2\gamma_2$). In embryonic life the α chain counterparts, ζ chains, combine with ε or γ chains to form Hbs Gower 1 ($\zeta_2\varepsilon_2$) or Portland ($\zeta_2\gamma_2$) and α and ε chains combine to form Hb Gower 2 ($\alpha_2\varepsilon_2$). This complexity reflects the fact that in late embryonic and early fetal life the ζ, ε, α, and γ genes are active at the same time. Haemoglobin F is a mixture of two different molecular species. There are two varieties of γ chains which differ in their amino acid composition at position 136, where they have either glycine or alanine; γ chains with glycine at position 136 are called $^G\gamma$ chains and those with alanine at this position are called $^A\gamma$ chains. The $^G\gamma$ and $^A\gamma$ chains are products of separate gene loci. During human development the ζ and ε genes are activated first, followed by the α and γ genes in the fetus, and then just before birth by the δ and β genes.

The α-like globin genes lie in a linked cluster on chromosome 16 and the β-like genes on chromosome 11. Long before the advent of recombinant DNA technology the order of these genes had been guessed from studies of families with mutant haemoglobins. These early predictions are now known to be correct. The globin genes have been isolated from libraries and their fine structure and linkage relationships defined (Fig. 10). The α and ζ globin genes form a cluster, in the following order 5′-ζ-$\psi\zeta$-$\psi\alpha$-$\alpha2$-$\alpha1$-θ-3′. The β gene family is arranged in the following order: 5′-ε-$^G\gamma$-$^A\gamma$-$\psi\beta$-δ-β-3′. The loci designated $\psi\alpha$, $\psi\beta$, and $\psi\zeta$ are called pseudogenes, i.e. they have sequence homology with the α, β, and ζ genes but have mutations that prevent their expression. It seems likely that they are evolutionary remnants of once active globin genes. It is interesting to note that haemoglobin genes comprising these families occur in the order in which they are expressed during development.

By comparing the structure of the different globin chains, and more recently their neucleotide sequences, it has been possible to build up a picture of the evolutionary history of the globin gene family. It is believed that the α and β genes arose from a single ancestral gene approximately 450 million years ago. In human beings as well as in birds and mammals the α and β gene clusters subsequently became established on different chromosomes. The ζ/α split was probably the most ancient of the subsequent duplications and was followed by the β/γ duplication about 200 million years ago, and the γ/ε duplication about 100 million years ago.

The evolutionary history of the gene cluster reflects the adaptive changes required by human haemoglobin as an oxygen carrier at different stages of

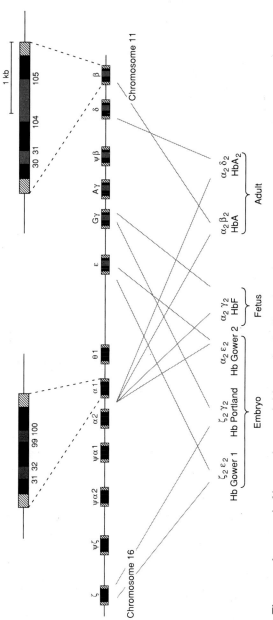

Figure 11. The genetic control of human haemoglobin synthesis. The α1 and β genes are expanded to show the arrangements of flanking regions (hatched), exons (black), and introns (unshaded).

development. Haemoglobin is an allosteric protein, that is it undergoes alterations in configuration which are essential for normal function. The oxygen binding properties are reflected in the well-known sigmoid oxygen-dissociation curve, which means that haemoglobin can bind oxygen tightly in the lungs and release it rapidly when a lower partial pressure of oxygen is encountered in the tissues. Furthermore, the oxygen affinity of haemoglobin can be modified according to physiological needs, the curve shifting to the left or right in response to pH, temperature, and carbon dioxide levels. Some of these adaptive changes are the result of binding small molecules, notably 2,3-diphosphoglycerate. They require the interaction of two unlike pairs of globin chains, α and β in the adult for example; a haemoglobin molecule made up of identical chains has a hyperbolic oxygen dissociation curve and is incapable of delivering oxygen at physiological tensions or in partaking of any of these complex adaptive processes. Fetal haemoglobin has a higher oxygen affinity than adult haemoglobin, an adaptive response to the oxygen requirements in fetal life. Thus we can see how, by a series of gene duplications followed by mutations which modify the function of particular forms of haemoglobin, it has been possible for us to arrive at our present state of evolution in which we have different haemoglobins adapted specifically to varying physiological needs at particular stages of development.

Of course the development of this beautifully regulated series of changes in our haemoglobin constitution poses further problems in trying to understand how our genes work. We have to explain how the genes for different pairs of globin subunits, α and β for example, which are coded on different chromosomes are so regulated that neither pair is produced in excess. We also need to understand how the various loci are switched on and off at different stages of human development. At the present time we have very little idea about the mechanisms that underlie these regulatory functions.

● The immune system: the immunoglobulin gene superfamily

The immune system, together with the scavenger cells of the marrow and tissue macrophage system, is our major defence against infection. It is made up of large numbers of lymphocytes, cells that have a unique cell-surface receptor allowing them to bind a foreign protein or antigen. There are two main types of lymphocytes: B cells which make circulating antibodies, and T cells which constitute the cellular component of the immune system involved in local reactions to invading organisms and in modifying the responses of other lymphocytes. The binding of a foreign antigen to a lymphocyte initiates a response designed to eliminate that antigen. As part of this process, some of the lymphocytes differentiate into memory cells so ensuring an enhanced future response to the same antigen.

The major conceptual difficulty that faced immunologists for many years is how the body can produce the extraordinarily large number of antibodies in response to the diverse series of antigens that might be encountered during a lifetime. In addition they had to explain how the immune system is able to recognize self from non-self antigens so that, except in certain diseases, an immune attack is not mounted on itself.

Of the many models that have attempted to explain the generation of antibody diversity, it is the remarkably intuitive clonal selection theory, initiated by Niels Jerne and worked out in detail by MacFarlane Burnet, which has stood the test of time and is undoubtedly correct. The idea is that the body continually elaborates B lymphocytes that have immunoglobulin molecules on their surface, that all these molecules on any one cell have the same binding specificity, and that for any particular antigenic determinant there is only a small subset of the entire pool of B cells that has the appropriate binding specificity. Thus when a foreign antigen enters the circulation it will combine with *pre-existing* immunoglobulins, but only on those B cells that have the appropriate specificity. The interaction of antigen and antibody on the B cell surface then triggers these cells into multiplication, synthesis, and ultimately, secretion of their specific antibodies. In other words the particular antigen will *select* from an enormous pre-existing pool of B lymphocytes only those with the appropriate specificity, and then cause their proliferation into a large population of cells. Such is the basis for the clonal selection theory which, of course, implies the existence of a very large repertoire of pre-existing immunoglobulin molecules on individual B cells. The requirement for the generation of such enormous antibody diversity, and for providing a similar degree of flexibility of T cell function, has led to the evolution of the immunoglobulin multigene family.

In recent years much has been learnt about the organization of the immunoglobulin gene family and about the genetic mechanisms for the production of antibody diversity. Much less is known about the basis of tolerance to self antigens; we shall address this complex topic when we discuss autoimmune disease in a later chapter.

● B cells and antibody production

Each clone of B cells makes antibody molecules with unique antigen binding sites. A proportion of these molecules are inserted into the lymphocyte membrane, where they act as surface receptors for antigen. When the latter binds to these sites, B cells are 'switched on', proliferate, and synthesize large amounts of soluble antibody with the same antigen binding site as the cell of origin. Antibodies are Y-shaped molecules composed of two identical heavy (H) chains and two light (L) chains (Fig. 12). They are divided into five different classes, IgA, IgD, IgE, IgG, and IgM, each with a distinctive H chain (α, δ, ϵ, γ, and μ, respectively). There are two main types of L chain (κ or λ), which can associate with any class of H chain.

When an antigen is encountered for the first time the antibody class that is made is IgM. One of the major functions of IgM is activation of the complement system, a complex family of proteins able to kill cells to which antibody is bound.

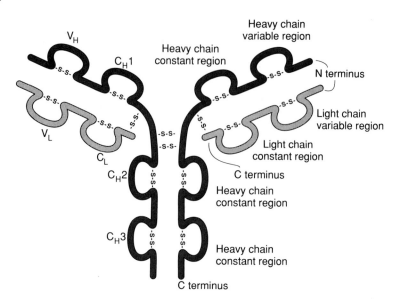

Figure 12. **Schematic representation of an immunoglobulin molecule.**

IgG is the main serum antibody; like IgM it stimulates both complement and macrophages. IgE is found mainly in tissues where, complexed with antigen, it activates the release of histamine from specialized cells called mast cells. This is the basis of many allergic reactions, although its physiological role is not absolutely clear. IgA binds to a receptor on many epithelial surfaces and is transported across epithelial cells. For example, it is secreted in large amounts into the intestinal lumen. IgA probably represents the body's first line of defence against infection by organisms at body surfaces. IgD occurs on the surface of many cells but its function is not yet clear.

The structure of an antibody molecule is illustrated in Fig. 12. Both L and H chains have variable (V) amino acid sequences at their N-terminal ends and a constant (C) sequence at their C-terminal ends. The V_H and V_L regions are involved in antigen binding, whereas the C_H and C_L regions subserve effector functions such as complement fixation. L chains have a constant region of about 110 amino acids and a variable region of about the same size. The N-terminal variable region of the H chain is also about 110 amino acids long but the constant region comprises about 330–440 amino acids depending on the class. The variable regions of the L and H chains each contain three hypervariable regions which together form the antigen binding sites. In effect these regions form a binding pocket into which individual antigens can fit. Each chain is composed of repeating folded domains; an L chain has one variable region (V_L) and one constant region (C_L) domain, while an H chain has one variable region (V_H) and three or four constant region (C_H) domains.

A great deal is known about the genetic control of antibody molecules and about the remarkable rearrangements that their genes undergo to provide the structural diversity required of the immune system. Immunoglobulin genes are the product of three separate gene families encoding the κ, λ, and H chains respectively. Like the globin gene clusters described earlier, they are on different chromosomes. The κ gene family is on chromosome 2, the λ family on chromosome 22, and the H chain family on chromosome 14. The arrangement of these gene clusters is shown in Fig. 13.

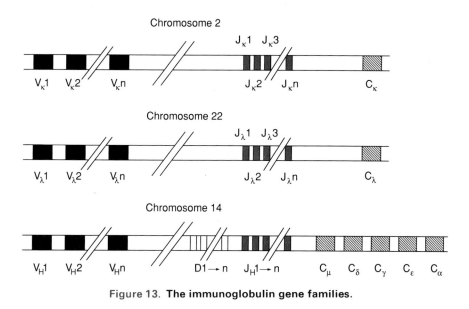

Figure 13. **The immunoglobulin gene families.**

The immunoglobulin gene clusters consist of one or more constant (C) gene segments and sets of variable (V) and joining (J) gene segments. For the light chains there are V_κ, $V_\lambda J_\kappa$, and J_λ gene segments. At all stages of development the J segment lies next to the C segment from which it is separated by an intron. During B cell development the V segment of the gene, which in embryonic cells lies many kilobases upstream from the J and C segments, is translocated so that it comes to lie next to the J segment, thus generating a V-J-intron-C sequence. This DNA is then transcribed into a large RNA precursor from which the introns are later removed. The exons are then spliced together to produce mRNA molecules in which the V, J, and C sequences are joined together. These molecules are then translated into light chain polypeptides. The genetic control of κ light chains is illustrated in Fig. 14.

The precise organization of the light chain genes varies between the κ and λ families and there is also considerable interspecies variability. For example, in all species studied so far λ proteins have not one but multiple constant regions, each with its own J_λ region. Humans have many C_λ regions and presumably many V_λ. On the other hand there appears to be less diversity among λ light chains than κ

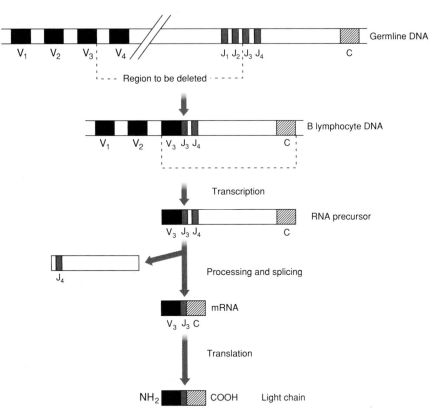

Figure 14. **A schematic representation of the rearrangements which occur during B cell maturation and which lead to V-J-C joining.**

light chains. However, the general principles of the complex rearrangements that involve the light chain loci and their products are similar for both classes.

Things get even more complicated when we come to the genetic organization and rearrangements of the genes for the heavy chains. A J gene segment is involved, but in addition some of the amino acids in the third hypervariable region of the V_H region are coded for by another region called a D (diversity) gene segment. In other words heavy chain diversity is determined by three gene families, V, J, and D, unlike light chains which have only V and J determinants. By a series of site-specific recombination events a D segment can be joined to any V_H and any J_H gene segment to create a functional V_H gene. There may be hundreds of V_H segments, up to twenty D segments, and four J segments. Furthermore, when D joins to J_H or V_H to D, a few nucleotides not present in either sequence are slipped in, the so-called N region.

The various joining reactions that we have described involve highly conserved recognition sequences of two types. One is a heptamer followed by an 11- or 12-

base spacer with a random sequence and an AT-rich nonomer; the other has a similar heptamer followed by a 21- to 23-base spacer.

We can now start to envisage the extraordinary potential for ontogenetic generation of antibody diversity. First, there are multiple germ-line genes; perhaps 100 to 300 V_H and V_κ gene segments, 10 or more D gene segments and multiple J_H and J_κ segments. A great number of combinations can serve to amplify V gene diversity. For example, any V_κ can join with any J_κ, and any V_H to D, and any D to J_H, and so on. Furthermore, at least two types of somatic alteration of these sequences can occur. The first is known as junctional diversity: the process of V gene formation appears to be relatively imprecise and the joining of gene segments can occur at a number of positions at their boundaries. Although the penalty for such imprecision is the generation of frameshift and termination codons (see Chapter 6), the overall effect is to increase the diversity at the V_L-J_L, V_H-D, and D-J_H junctions. Furthermore, somatic mutations occur throughout the V_H and V_L segments as well as in their flanking sequences.

What are the genetic mechanisms that determine the types of antibodies that are produced? For example, we have already seen that all classes of antibody can be made in a membrane-bound form or in a soluble form ready for secretion. In the case of IgM, the only difference between the two types is in the C-terminal end of the μ chain; the membrane-bound μ chains have a hydrophobic carboxyl-terminus which holds them in the lipid bilayer of the plasma membrane, while the μ chains of secreted molecules have a hydrophilic tail which allows them to leave the cell. It turns out that this simple structural transformation is achieved by differential splicing of the C_μ mRNA. Furthermore, although B cells begin their antibody synthesizing activities by making IgM, they can eventually switch to making other classes of antibodies such as IgG or IgA. Again, this seems to involve differential splicing with the production of two species of mRNA molecules, each with the same V_H sequence: one has a C_μ sequence and the other a C_δ sequence. In addition, the cell can rearrange its DNA so that any C_H gene can be placed 3′ to a V_H gene. This type of DNA rearrangement is called class switching.

● T cells and the MHC system

There appear to be at least two, and probably more, functionally distinct subclasses of T cells which make up the cellular immune system. Firstly, there are cytotoxic T cells which directly kill foreign or virus infected cells. Secondly, there are helper T cells which aid B cells in making antibody responses, help other T cells to make cell-mediated immune responses, and release lymphokines which mediate effects such as macrophage activation. Finally, there are the less well-defined suppressor T cells which may inhibit the responses of B cells and other T cells. Helper and suppressor T cells interact with their target lymphocytes by recognizing foreign antigen or receptor idiotypes (determinants on variable regions of L and H chains which are associated with the antigen-binding sites of antibodies) on the target cell-surfaces.

While B cells bind foreign antigen directly, T cells can only bind antigen presented to them on the surface of another cell where it is recognized along with molecules of the major histocompability complex (MHC). In man the MHC is better known as the HLA complex, of particular medical interest in that it is involved in tissue typing for organ transplantation. The nature of the receptor on the T cell surface and the problem of its dual recognition of foreign antigen and molecules of the MHC system has been one of the most intractable puzzles of modern immunology and has only very recently been solved. To examine it in outline it is necessary to describe what is known about the structure of the T cell receptor and of the MHC molecules with which it interacts.

Receptors on most T cells consist of two polypeptide chains, α and β, linked to each other and associated on the plasma membrane with a collection of invariant proteins called CD3 (Fig. 15). The latter are thought to play an important role in transmitting the information that the T cell receptor is occupied. The gene families that are responsible for regulating the structures of the α and β chains of the T cell receptor are on chromosomes 14 and 7 respectively. The T cell receptor α and β chains are encoded by genes that are the products of rearrangements of

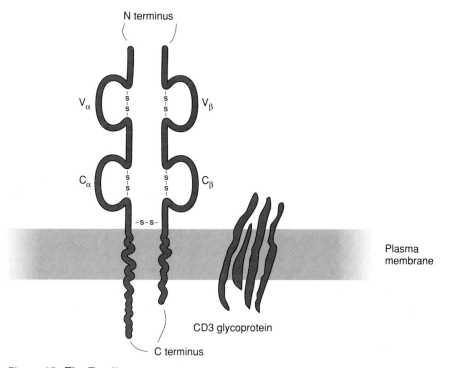

Figure 15. The T-cell receptor. Both α and β chains consist of a constant and variable domain. The heterodimer former by these two chains is part of a multichain complex that also includes the three or four invariant polypeptides recognized by CD3 monoclonal antibodies.

several germ-line genes of the same general pattern described earlier for the immunoglobulin genes. The α chain genes probably include at least 50 different V region genes and a similar number of J region genes. Their random association is responsible for the production of at least 2500 different mature α chains and there is the possibility for even more diversity because, as in the case of the immunoglobulin genes, nucleotides not encoded in the germ-line can be introduced, or germ-line encoded nucleotides can be deleted, at the point of V-J joining. We have already described the occurrence of such N regions in the heavy chain immunoglobulin genes. The β genes are constructed from the joining of about 80 V regions to one or two D regions and one of 13 J regions. Because of the flexibility of the N regions it has been estimated that at least 4000 different β sequences are possible. Overall, therefore, the T cell receptors have more than 10^7 different sequences, a number not far off that estimated for the immunoglobulin molecules. Thus even though the genes for the α and β chains of T cell receptors do not seem to undergo somatic mutation they have an enormous propensity for identifying different antigenic structures.

The human MHC or HLA gene complex lies on the short arm of chromosome 6 (Fig. 16). There are two major classes of human MHC antigens (the proteins of the complement system which are encoded for in the same complex are called class III). First, there are the HLA class I antigens (A, B, and C) which are the counterpart of the H2-K-DL antigen system in mice, and second there are the class II or DR antigens. It turns out that cytotoxic T cells recognize antigens in association with class I products, A, B, and C, while helper T cells identify antigens in association with the class II proteins.

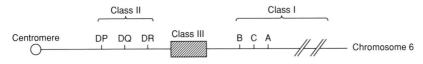

Figure 16. **The HLA–DR complex on chromosome 6.**

The genes of the HLA–DR complex on the short arm of chromosome 6 encode single peptide chains (Fig. 17). Those of the class I molecules are inserted into plasma membranes with a short hydrophilic (water repellant) C-terminal segment inside the cell, a short segment that transverses the cell membrane, and a large N-terminal segment that is exposed to the exterior. The latter is divided into three separate domains, α1, α2, and α3, which show some homologies with the immunoglobulin domains. α1 and α2 are the more variable and express the main polymorphic differences. These proteins are found on the surface of almost all nucleated somatic cells where they are non-covalently associated with a small

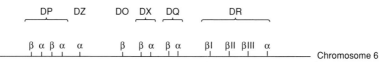

Figure 17. **A map of the class II genes of the human HLA–DR region.**

protein called β2 microglobulin which is encoded by a gene on a different chromosome and shows structural similarity to immunoglobulin molecules. Recently the crystallographic structure of the class I molecules has been solved. As expected the β2 microglobulin and α3 portion of the heavy chain are next to the membrane while the α1 and α2 domains sit on top of them. They are orientated into a groove with sides formed by α helices and a floor that is composed of several pleated sheets.

The MHC class II molecules are also membrane glycoproteins, but in this case are expressed on the surface of macrophages and B lymphocytes. They consist of an α chain and a β chain each of which have two extracellular domains (Fig. 18a). The domains that lie next to the membrane (α2 and β2) are thought to fold to form immunoglobulin-like structures while the structures of the α1 and β1 domains are not yet known. It seems likely that they will turn out to be similar to those of the class I molecules, in that they fold up together to form a peptide binding site. The genes that control the class II molecules are in the HLA–D region, which spans about 1100 kilobases. It contains three subregions, DP, DQ, and DR, each of which has at least one expressed α and β chain gene (Fig. 17). These molecules are extremely polymorphic and each gene has many alleles.

Given this information about the structure of the T cell receptor and the class I and II molecules of the HLA–DR system, it is possible to start to understand how T cells interact with macrophages during antigen presentation. There is increasing evidence that antigens are not presented intact to T cells but that they are first broken down into peptide fragments containing 10–20 amino acids. It seems very likely that these small peptides fit into the antigen binding grooves of the class I and, presumably, class II molecules (Fig. 18b). If the bound antigen is in the appropriate steric configuration the α and β chains of the T cell receptor will fit this complex, and subsequent conformational changes in the receptor lead to T cell activation. How T cells learn not to respond to self antigen, and the mechanism whereby they are primed to this critical function in the thymus remains to be determined.

During the search for the genes encoding the α and β chains of the T cell receptor a third class of rearranging T cell-specific genes were discovered which were called γ. This has led to the identification of a third family or lineage of lymphocytes, distinguished by the presence of a novel receptor using anti-γ peptide antibodies. It has been found that the γ chain is associated with a second variable chain called δ. In most tissues, cells that bear the γ/δ receptors are present in very small numbers. However, it turns out that lymphocytes that are found within most surface epithelia express γ/δ receptors and it appears that this newly recognized class of T cells is involved in the surveillance of these important regions.

● A gene superfamily

The immunoglobulin gene superfamily is summarized in Fig. 19. It is believed

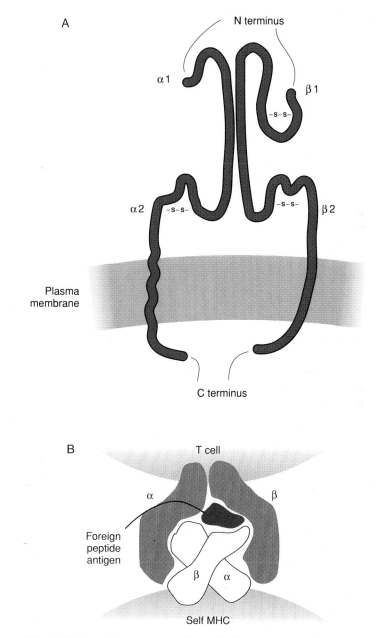

Figure 18. A Schematic representation of the structure of a human class II molecule. B A representation of the binding of a T-cell receptor to antigen plus a class I or II MHC molecule.

68

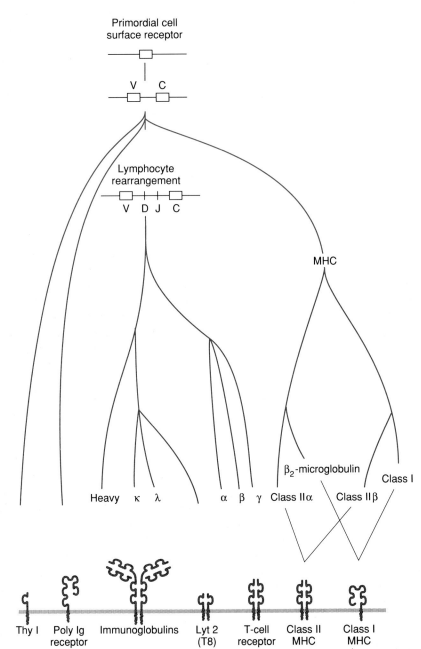

Figure 19. **The super-family of immunoglobulins and related gene products of the immune system.** Modified from Hood *et al.* 1985.

that a primordial cell surface receptor diversified into variable and constant regions and that this molecule then diverged in a number of directions which ultimately led to the immunoglobulin genes, the gene families for the T cell receptor, and the different classes of genes that make up the MHC or HLA–DR system in man. Ultimately this remarkable gene family provided a compartmentalized immunological defence system with the properties of specificity and diversity required for a combined humoral and cell-mediated immune system (Table 15).

● The size of the human genome

If we are going to search for genes that are involved in human disease we ought to have some idea of the size of the human genome and hence of the magnitude of the task.

In each human cell, double-stranded DNA, distributed among the 23 pairs of chromosomes, consists of about $3–3.5 \times 10^9$ base pairs, which corresponds to a total length of about two metres. For those who are statistically minded it is interesting to reflect that there are approximately 3×10^{12} cells in the body; since there are about two metres of DNA in each cell this means that a human being has about 6×10^{12} metres of DNA. Joined end to end it would reach to the moon and back nearly 8000 times! Thus, when we wish to analyse a single human gene of, say, 1000–2000 bases, we are embarking on a search among an amount of DNA sufficient to contain up to three million of them. This problem has been likened to looking for something the height of an ant compared with that of Mount Everest.

At first sight these numbers suggest that gene hunting will be impossible and that the human genome is far too large ever to be mapped. However, a closer consideration of the different types of DNA in mammalian cells suggests that things may not be quite as bad as they seem. First, highly repetitive DNA sequences with no obvious function may account for as much as 50 per cent of the total of 3×10^9 nucleotide pairs in the human haploid genome. Furthermore, we have already seen that the proportion of base pairs contributing to the part of a gene that actually directs protein structure is only a relatively small fraction of the total length of the gene, that is if we include its introns and flanking regions. If we assume that about 50 per cent of the total DNA is in functional clusters, that the average gene product has a size of about 300 amino acids corresponding to approximately 1000 base pairs, that an average gene cluster size is about 15 genes, and that the coding ratio (the proportion of base pairs in a gene cluster which direct the structure of their protein products) is about 1:30, then the total number of clusters is $1.5 \times 10^9/30 \times 15 \times 1000$ or about 3300. This may be an underestimate, but it seems likely that the total number of clusters will be in the range of 3000 to a maximum of, say, 15 000, and hence the total number of different protein products may be in the order of 50 000 to 200 000. Furthermore, the overall complexity of the genome will be less than this if account is taken of the organization of gene clusters into related families. As we have seen earlier in this

Table 15. *Summary of immune defence system (modified from Janeway 1988)*

Location of pathogen	Type of immunity	Receptor	Recognition	Ligand	Accessory systems	Function	Location
Extracellular	Humoral immunity B lymphocytes	Surface immunoglobulin	IgM	Bacterial surface	Complement	Lysis	Intravascular
			IgG	Bacterial surface bacteria, virus virus, toxin	Complement phagocytes	Lysis engulfment neutralization	Tissue fluids
						Vascular changes killing	
			IgE	Antigens, allergens parasitic worms	Mast cells eosinophils		
			IgA	Virus, toxin bacterial adhesins, virus	—	Neutralization block adherence	Sub-epithelial Epithelial surfaces
Intracellular	Cell-mediated immunity T lymphocytes	CD3α/β	CD4$^+$T	Extracellular protein fragment, class II MHC	B lymphocyte	B cell activation	Somatic
			CD4$^+$T	Fragment of intracellular bacteria, class II MHC	Macrophage	Macrophage activation	Somatic
			CD8$^+$T	Fragment of cellular or viral protein, class I MHC	—	Target cell killing	Somatic
Intracellular	Cell-mediated immunity T lymphocytes	CD3γ/δ	V$_\gamma$5/V$_\delta$ CD4$^-$CD8$^-$	?	?	?Killing	Epidermis
			V$_\gamma$6V$_\delta$ CD8$^+$	?	?	?Killing	Intestinal epithelium
			V$_\gamma$/V$_\delta$ CD4$^-$ CD8$^-$	Ig, MHC, ?	?	?Killing	Somatic

chapter some of these, like the globin genes, are small but others, such as the immunoglobulin supergene system, will be much larger.

As mentioned in the previous chapter, McKusick's catalogue of Mendelian inheritance lists over 4000 entries. If the basic number of genetic functions in terms of gene clusters is in the order of 5–10 000 then the proportion of these that have already been identified as mutants causing disease may be quite high.

Having convinced ourselves that we possess a manageable number of genes, and that learning something about the majority of them may not be out of the question, we still have the daunting task of finding a particular gene among enough DNA to contain several million. In the next chapter we shall see how recent advances in molecular biology have made this possible.

● Further reading

Alberts, B., Bray, D., Leven, J., Raff, M., Roberts, K., and Watson, J.D. (1989). *Molecular biology of the cell*, 2nd edn. Garland Publishing Inc., New York.

Alt, F.W., Blackwell, K., and Yancopoulos, G.D. (1987). Development of the primary antibody repertoire. *Science*, **238**, 1079–87.

Bodmer, W.F. (1986). Human genetics: the molecular challenge. *Cold Spring Harbor Symp. Quant. Biol.*, **51**, 1–14.

Borst, P., Benne, R., and Tabak, H.F. (1989). A fused chimeric protein made in human cells. *Cell*, **58**, 421–2.

Brennan, S.O. (1989). Propeptide cleavage: evidence from human proalbumins. *Mol. Biol. Med.*, **6**, 87–92.

Brown, T. A. (1989). *Genetics: A molecular approach*. Van Nostrand Reinhold, Amsterdam.

Bunn, H.F. and Forget, B.G. (1986). *Hemoglobin; Molecular, genetic and clinical aspects*. W.H. Saunders, Philadelphia, PA.

Cedar, H. (1988). DNA methylation and gene activity. *Cell*, **53**, 3–4.

Dilworth, S. M. and Dingwell, C. (1988). Chromatin assembly *in vivo* and *in vitro*. *BioEssays*, **9**, 44–9.

Durell, J., Lodish, H., and Baltimore, D. (1986). *Molecular cell biology*. Scientific American Books Inc.

Emery, A.E.H. (1984). *An introduction to recombinant DNA*. Wiley, Chichester.

Ferguson-Smith, M.A. (1988). Progress in the molecular cytogenetics of man. *Phil. Trans. R. Soc. Lond. B.*, **319**, 239–48.

Gasser, S.M. and Laemmli, U.K. (1987). A glimpse at chromosomal order. *Trends Genet.*, **3**, 16–22.

Goldman, M.A. (1988). The chromatin domain as a unit of gene regulation. *BioEssays*, **9**, 50–3.

Hames, B.D. and Glover, D.M. (1988). *Molecular immunology*. IRL Press, Oxford.

Hood, L., Kronenberg, M., and Hunkapiller, T. (1985). T cell antigen receptors and the immunoglobulin supergene family. *Cell*, **40**, 225–9.

Janeway, C.A. (1988). Frontiers of the immune system. *Nature*, **333**, 804–6.

Lewin, B. (1990). *Genes*, edn IV. Oxford University Press.

Marrack, P. and Kappler, J. (1987). The T cell receptor. *Science*, **238**, 1073–9.

Mitchell, P.J. and Tjain, R. (1989). Transcriptional regulation in mammalian cells by sequence-specific DNA binding proteins. *Science*, **245**, 371–8.

Mitchell, R.H. (1988). How do receptors on the cell surface send signals to the cell interior? *Basic molecular and cell biology*, pp. 90–100. British Medical Journal, Latimer and Trend Co. Ltd., Plymouth.

Ptashne, M. (1986). Gene regulation by proteins acting nearby and at a distance. *Nature*, **322**, 697–701.

Stryer, L. (1989). *Molecular design of life*. W.H. Freeman, New York.

Swain, J.L., Stewart, T.A., and Leder, P. (1987). Parental legacy determines methylation and expression of an autosomal transgene: a molecular mechanism for parental imprinting. *Cell*, **50**, 719–27.

Waldmann, T.A. (1987). Immunoglobulin and T-cell receptor genes and lymphocyte differentiation. In *The molecular basis of blood diseases* (ed. G. Stamatoyannopoulos, A.W. Nienhuis, P. Leder, and P.W. Majerus), pp. 245–70. W.B. Saunders Company, Philadelphia, PA.

Warren, G. (1988). Sorting signals and cellular membranes. In *Basic molecular and cell biology*, pp. 83–9. British Medical Journal, Latimer and Trend Co. Ltd., Plymouth.

Watson, J.D., Hopkins, N.H., Roberts, J.W., Ateitz, J.A., and Weiner, A.M. (1987). *Molecular biology of the gene*, 4th edn. Benjamin Cummings Pub. Inc., California.

Weatherall, D.J., Clegg, J.B., Higgs, D.R., and Wood, W.G. (1988). The hemoglobinopathies. In *The metabolic basis of inherited disease*, 6th edn., (ed. C.R. Scriver, A.L. Beaudet, W.S. Sly, and D. Valle), pp. 2281–366. McGraw-Hill, New York.

Wickens, M.P. and Dahlberg, J.E. (1987). RNA-protein interactions. *Cell*, **51**, 339–42.

The techniques of gene analysis

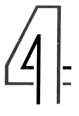

In this and the following chapter we shall consider some of the methods of recombinant DNA technology that have particular application to medical practice. The reader who wishes to augment these brief outlines with more detailed accounts is referred to several recent reviews and monographs aimed at the non-specialist which are cited at the end of this chapter.

Although modern molecular biology is a highly sophisticated pastime encompassing a wide breadth of ingenious new analytical methods, it is not necessary to have a detailed knowledge of its technical niceties to appreciate its value for medical application. However, readers who come to the field with no previous knowledge of molecular genetics will find it helpful to understand the principles underlying the methods that are central to the problems of searching for human genes and mapping the human genome. In particular they need to appreciate how it is possible to find individual genes using gene probes, how genes can be cloned and produced in quantities sufficient to determine their sequence and function, and how it is possible to transfer genes into foreign cells so that both normal and abnormal gene action can be studied in the test tube.

● Basic methods

● Molecular hybridization and gene probes

The two strands of DNA can be dissociated and reassociated *in vitro*, for example by heating and cooling. It is also possible to form hybrids of double-stranded DNA/RNA molecules in this way. The reannealing reactions are highly specific, and under suitable conditions of salt concentration and temperature occur only between DNA or RNA strands that have identical or almost identical base sequences. Thus, if we wish to look for a particular gene buried away in a large amount of DNA, we must first construct a length of DNA with an identical sequence so that it will anneal to the gene but not to the rest of the DNA. This is the principle behind using gene probes to find genes that we are interested in.

In 1970 an enzyme, RNA-dependent-DNA-polymerase or reverse transcriptase, was isolated from certain RNA tumour viruses. Reverse transcriptase can be used to synthesize a DNA copy (complementary DNA, or cDNA) from any messenger RNA (mRNA) that can be isolated from mammalian cells. Furthermore, if radioactive bases are added to the reaction the synthesized cDNA can be labelled and hence used as a hybridization probe to 'look for' complementary sequences in either genomic DNA or in cellular RNA by DNA/DNA or DNA/RNA hybridization. When these techniques were first developed they were used to study hybridization in solution. Later, it became possible to apply this method to DNA immobilized on nitrocellulose filters.

At first, cDNA probes were prepared from partially purified RNA which might consist of several different mRNA molecules. However, it soon became possible to clone cDNA sequences in bacterial plasmids. This is done by synthesizing a second DNA strand on a newly synthesized cDNA using a bacterial DNA polymerase. In this way small cDNA duplexes are made which can be incorporated into plasmids and hence grown in bacterial cells. One of the main disadvantages of cDNA probes is that, because they are made from mRNA, they will only identify exon sequences. As we shall see later, it is now possible to clone fragments of genomic DNA into plasmids or bacteriophage and to amplify individual genes in *Escherichia coli*, and hence to make genomic probes.

In order to radioactively label DNA to make a hybridization probe a technique called nick translation is used; the principle of this reaction is shown in Fig. 20. DNA can serve as a template primer for the enzyme DNA polymerase I if it contains a single-stranded break (nick) with a 3′-OH terminus. Appropriate nicks can be introduced into duplex DNA with various nucleases. The DNA is

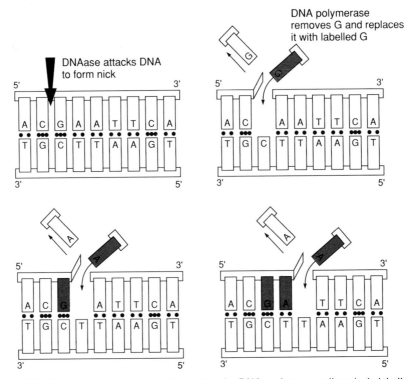

Figure 20. Nick translation. A technique whereby DNA probes are radioactively labelled.

labelled by incorporating ^{32}P-labelled deoxyribonuclease 5-triphosphatases (dNTPs) at the 3'-OH terminus of the nick by the action of DNA polymerase I. In this way it is possible to prepare highly radioactive probes. More recently it has become possible to use oligonucleotide-primed labelling for this purpose.

● Oligonucleotide probes

The gene probes that we have been describing are relatively large molecules that identify individual genes or parts of them. For this reason they hybridize with long stretches of complementary sequences but are not capable of recognizing single base changes or similar small structural alterations. As we shall see later, the ability to identify base changes in mutant genes is essential for determining the molecular pathology of human disease. To solve this problem a slightly different approach was devised which makes use of short, synthetic DNA fragments called oligonucleotides which are constructed specifically to detect single base changes in DNA.

It turns out that a single nucleotide mis-match between an oligonucleotide and a cloned gene is detectable by molecular hybridization under very carefully controlled conditions; the mis-match sufficiently destabilizes the DNA hybrid as compared with the perfect match. Probes of about 19 nucleotides (19-mers) corresponding to a particular region of a gene are prepared. Two probes are made; one has the normal sequence, while the other is identical except for a single altered base corresponding to the particular mutation. By carefully regulating the hybridization conditions, it is possible to arrange things so that the 'normal' probe hybridizes to the normal but not to the mutant DNA, while the 'abnormal' probe hybridizes to the mutant but not to the normal DNA (Fig. 21).

Of course, oligonucleotide probes have many uses other than as diagnostic agents. We shall describe their value in screening libraries for particular genes later in the chapter.

● DNA fractionation: restriction endonucleases

Fractionation of DNA became possible after the discovery of a family of bacterial enzymes called restriction endonucleases (Table 16). They are named after the particular bacterium from which they are isolated. These enzymes do not cleave DNA at random but do so only where a particular sequence of bases occurs in the molecule. The restriction enzymes used most commonly in genetic engineering recognize signals consisting of four, five, or six bases, sometimes palindromes, as shown in Fig. 22. Some enzymes cleave both strands at the same point leaving blunt ends, while others make cuts which are offset, producing cohesive or 'sticky' ends. The latter name derives from the fact that DNA spliced in this way tends to reassociate by base pairing (see Fig. 22). The number of times a particular enzyme cuts DNA is inversely related to the number of bases in the recognition

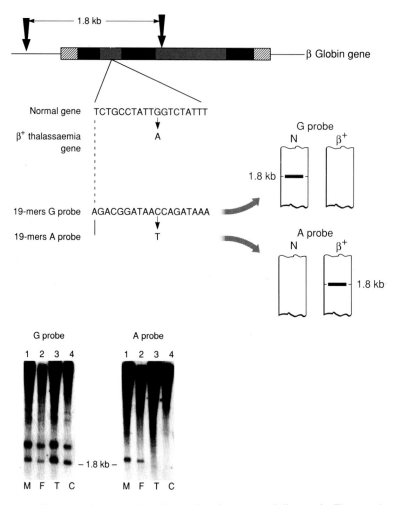

Figure 21. The use of oligonucleotide probes for prenatal diagnosis. The mutation that is being analysed is the G→A change at position 110 in the first intervening sequence of the β globin gene which causes the common variety of β⁺ thalassaemia in Mediterranean populations. Two probes, each 19 nucleotides long, are made. One has the normal sequence (G probe); the other has the same sequence except for the G→A change (A probe). The region of DNA to be studied is part of a 1.8 kb restriction enzyme fragment, as indicated. The patient's DNA and normal DNA are digested with the appropriate enzyme and the mixture is separated and hybridized with both G and A probes. Under appropriate conditions the G probe hybridizes to the abnormal but not to the normal (β⁺) DNA; the A probe hybridizes to the abnormal but not to the normal DNA. The gel shows an analysis of this kind. Lanes 1 and 2 are from heterozygous parents (M and F), lane 3 from a fetus at risk for homozygous β⁺ thalassaemia (T), and lane 4 from a normal control DNA (C). The fetus was normal.

Table 16. *Some restriction endonucleases and their recognition sequences and cleavage sites (*). Py = pyrimidine, Pu = purine, N = any base*

Enzyme	Organism	Cleavage site (*) 5′					3′
Tetranucleotides							
*Alu*I	*Arthrobacter luteus*	A	G	*	C	T	
*Hae*III	*Haemophilus aegyptius*	G	G	*	C	C	
*Hpa*II	*Haemophilus parainfluenzae*	C	*	C	G	G	
*Mbo*I	*Moraxella bovis*	*	G	A	T	C	
*Taq*I	*Thermus aquaticus*	T	*	C	G	A	
*Msp*I	*Moraxella species*	C	*	C	G	G	
Pentanucleotides							
*Ava*II	*Anabaena variabilis*	G	*	G	$\frac{A}{T}$	C	C
*Dde*I	*Desulfovibrio desulfuricans*	C	*	T	N	A	G
*Eco*RII	*Escherichia coli R.245*	*	C	C	$\frac{A}{T}$	G	G
*Hinf*I	*Haemophilus influenzae* Rf	G	*	A	N	T	C
Hexanucleotides							
*Ava*I	*Anabaena variabilis*	C	*	Py	C	G	Pu	G
*Bal*I	*Brevibacterium albidum*	T	G	G	*	C	C	A
*Bam*HI	*Bacillus amyloliquefaciens* H	G	*	G	A	T	C	C
*Bgl*II	*Bacillus globigii*	A	†	G	A	T	C	T
*Eco*RI	*Escherichia coli* RY13	G	*	A	A	T	T	C
*Hae*II	*Haemophilus aegyptius*	Pu	G	C	G	C	*	Py
*Hinc*II	*Haemophilus influenzae* Rc	G	T	Py	*	Pu	A	C
*Hind*III	*Haemophilus influenzae* Rd	A	*	A	G	C	T	T
*Hpa*I	*Haemophilus parainfluenzae*	G	T	T	*	A	A	C
*Hsu*I	*Haemophilus suis*	A	*	A	G	C	T	T
*Pst*I	*Providencia stuartii*	C	T	G	C	A	*	G
*Sac*I	*Streptomyces achromogenes*	G	A	G	C	T	*	C
*Sal*I	*Streptomyces albus*	G	*	T	C	G	A	C
*Sma*I	*Serratia marcescens*	C	C	C	*	G	G	G
*Xma*I	*Xanthomonas malvacearum*	C	*	C	C	G	G	G
*Sph*I	*Streptomyces phaeochromogenes*	G	C	A	T	G	*	C
Heptanucleotides							
*Mst*II	*Microcoleus species*	C	C	*	T	N	A	G	G

Modified from Emery (1984).

site. It also depends on the base composition and sequence of a particular length of DNA. For example, the enzyme *Msp*I recognizes only four bases 5′-CpCpGpGp-3′. It cuts relatively infrequently in human DNA because the dinucleotide CpG is under-represented.

Apart from fractionating DNA, the discovery of restriction endonucleases

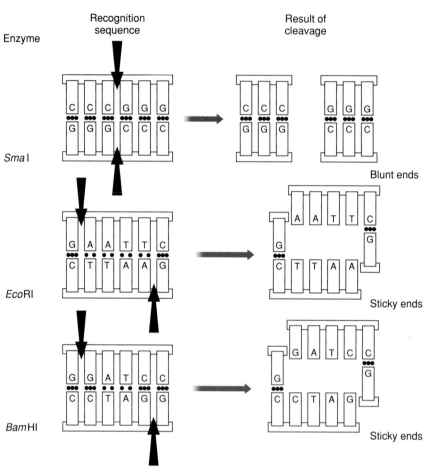

Figure 22. **Some restriction enzymes which are commonly used for analysing human DNA.**

provides us with an extremely valuable approach to analysing genetic diversity. As we shall see in the next chapter, scattered throughout the human genome there are harmless base changes which may either produce new restriction endonuclease sites, or remove pre-existing ones. This variability is inherited in a simple Mendelian fashion. The inherited difference in the size of DNA fragments generated in this way, called restriction fragment length polymorphisms (RFLPs), provides a large number of linkage markers for following mutant genes through families. In addition to these single point polymorphisms there are regions of the genome in which the length of DNA between specific restriction enzyme sites varies considerably between different persons; again the variability is inherited. These so-called hypervariable regions also offer a rich source of genetic markers. Throughout this book we shall encounter many examples of the importance of these polymorphisms, particularly when we come to consider the application of recombinant DNA technology to prenatal diagnosis or to the analysis of complex gene families.

● Gene mapping

Restriction endonuclease mapping, or gene-mapping, has become a major tool for analysing genetic diseases. It is impossible to over emphasize its importance in the development of human molecular genetics. DNA is obtained from any available tissue, often from peripheral-blood white cells, and after purification is digested with a particular restriction enzyme. The mixture of different sized fragments is then subjected to electrophoresis on agarose gel. After separation of the fragments according to their size, the DNA in the gel is denatured by alkali treatment and the separated fragments are then transferred to a nitrocellulose filter by a process called Southern blotting (Fig. 23), named after its inventor, Edward Southern. The filter is then exposed to a radioactively labelled gene probe. The position of the fragments containing the gene to be analysed is then determined by autoradiography. By using a series of different enzymes which cleave DNA either within or outside the gene or genes that we are studying, and by orientating the fragments with respect to each other, it is possible to build up what are called restriction enzyme maps of the areas of the genome (Fig. 23). We shall examine how this sophisticated form of jigsaw puzzling is applied to the study of genetic disease in later chapters.

The power of this technique for the study of human disease is quite extraordinary; the white blood cells from as little as 5 ml of blood provide sufficient DNA to analyse any normal or mutant gene for which we happen to have a probe.

● Gene cloning

If we are to study the fine structure of normal and abnormal genes it is necessary to isolate them. This is achieved by gene cloning. The idea is to insert foreign DNA, that is the DNA containing our gene, into an appropriate vector, a DNA molecule capable of replicating in a bacterial cell. Replication of the inserted fragment along with the vector in the bacterium makes it possible to amplify and isolate the foreign DNA.

Four main classes of vectors are used for gene cloning in the bacterium *E. coli*: plasmids, single-stranded bacteriophage, bacteriophage λ, and cosmids. Each type of vector has its own particular advantages. Cloning in plasmids was the first approach to isolating human genes and, because of its relative simplicity, is a particularly useful model for understanding the principles involved.

80

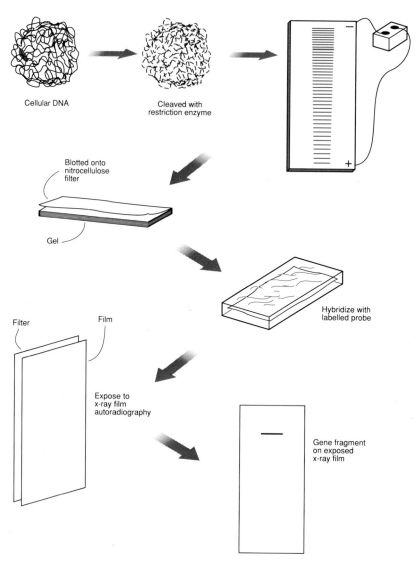

Figure 23. **Restriction enzyme mapping (Southern blotting).**

Plasmid vectors

Plasmids are extremely simple organisms that live and replicate in the cytoplasm of bacteria. They are best known to the clinical world as the vehicles for transferring antibiotic resistance between bacteria, and consist of a closed circle of DNA. A plasmid that is often used for cloning is illustrated in Fig. 24. It has an origin of replication, which ensures that it can be replicated in a bacterium by exploiting the bacterial DNA-synthesizing machinery. It usually contains one or

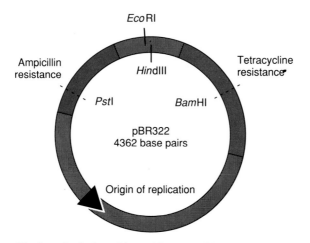

Figure 24. **A typical plasmid used in recombinant DNA technology.**

two genes for antibiotic resistance, and sites for restriction enzymes, with which cleavage opens up the DNA circle and produces a linear molecule with offset ends. The DNA to be inserted into the plasmid is fragmented by the same endonuclease, and plasmid and DNA fragments are mixed and associate with each other randomly by virtue of the 'sticky ends' of the DNA; a permanent union is achieved by adding an enzyme called DNA ligase (Fig. 25). Of course, some plasmids rejoin to form the original circular DNA but others, recombinants, incorporate the foreign DNA. Suitable bacteria are then transformed by the reformed plasmids, that is the plasmids and bacteria are mixed and a small number of the former enter the bacterial cytoplasm. Only a proportion of the bacteria are transformed by plasmids and some may contain several copies of the same plasmid. Those containing recombinants can be selected by various microbiological tricks such as allowing the plasmid to confer antibiotic resistance to the bacteria, hence favouring their growth on selective media. Bacterial colonies can be screened by hybridization with appropriate gene probes for the presence of the foreign DNA inserts; such a clone, when identified, can be isolated and grown to yield large quantities of the particular piece of DNA that is required.

Bacteriophage vectors

Although plasmid vectors have been used widely for cloning human genes they suffer from the major disadvantage that they can only accommodate fragments of foreign DNA of approximately 10 kb or less. In order to accommodate larger fragments, or to generate cloned material that is in a suitable state for sequencing, it has been necessary to use bacteriophage (phage for short), viruses that infect bacteria. Bacteriophage are some of the most intensively studied micro-organisms in the field of molecular genetics. Each phage particle consists of a

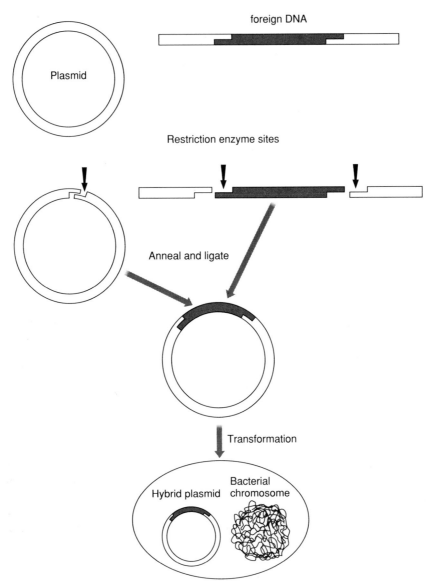

Figure 25. **The construction of a bacterial plasmid containing a foreign DNA insert for propagation in a bacterial cell.**

head and a tail and has a protein coat surrounding a central core of DNA. It attaches itself to a bacterium by means of its tail and injects its DNA into the host, after which the phage DNA circularizes by the joining together of its two ends, which are referred to as COS sites (cohesive end sites). Some types of phage can now undergo two alternate pathways, or phases, of replication. Either their genomes become integrated into the bacterial chromosome and then replicate along with it, the lysogenic phase. Or, alternatively, the circular DNA of the phage may undergo replication independently of the host DNA and generate large numbers of particles which then burst from the host cell and invade other bacteria, a process called the lytic phase. Phage spread from one bacterial cell to another, and in so doing give rise to clear areas, or plaques, in a confluent layer of cultured bacteria, each plaque indicating that bacteria are infected with phage particles. These remarkable properties of bacteriophage have been utilized to produce many different cloning vectors.

One of the most widely studied phage, bacteriophage λ, has some 60 genes all of which have been mapped in detail, and the complete sequence of its 48 000 base pairs is known. The family of genes that are involved in the lysogenic phase of its life cycle lie in the middle of the genome and, since the phage must replicate in the lytic phase in order to be used as a cloning vehicle, can be deleted and substituted. Using this general approach over 100 vectors have been derived from phage λ, including the families of λgt (generalized transducing) and Charon phage, the latter named after a rather depressing figure in Greek mythology. These vectors all have restriction sites in sequences that are not essential for replication and lysis and that can be replaced by the genes we wish to clone.

Another particularly useful variety of phage cloning vectors are made up of single-stranded DNA, notably the M13 family. They have the particular virtue that, being single stranded, cloned DNA can be generated directly for sequencing by the Sanger method described later in this chapter. And they have other major advantages, notably for the study of site-directed mutagenesis.

Cloning larger DNA fragments

As it became necessary to introduce larger fragments of DNA for cloning even more sophisticated vectors were developed. One particularly useful group are called cosmids. A cosmid is an artificial vector produced by genetic engineering and consists of plasmid DNA packaged into a phage particle. Essentially, it is made up of a circular duplex of DNA containing various antibiotic resistance genes, a number of restriction sites, and the COS sites of phage λ. The great advantage of cosmid cloning is that it is possible to introduce fragments of DNA of up to 50 kb or more.

As human molecular genetics has evolved over the last few years thoughts have turned to the possibility of cloning even larger pieces of DNA than those that can be accommodated in cosmids. This problem has particular relevance to mapping the human genome, a topic that is considered in more detail in the next chapter. Quite recently a particularly promising approach to solving this problem has been developed which makes use of yeast rather than *E. coli* for cloning.

Of the many achievements of yeast genetics in recent years the ability to take apart and put together entire chromosomes is one of the most remarkable. It has been possible to exploit this technology in a novel way to develop cloning vectors called yeast artificial chromosomes (YACs). It turns out that these ingenious pieces of genetic engineering can accommodate human DNA fragments of hundreds of kilobases in length. Essentially, YACs consist of bacterial plasmids, just like those described earlier, but which in this case carry two yeast telomeres (chromosome tips), a yeast centromere and autonomously replicating sequences (ARS), selectable markers, and a cloning site. The ARS sequences, found in most eukaryotes, provide the necessary origins for replication. These bits and pieces are used to generate two arms as shown in Fig. 26. One arm contains a telomere and a selectable marker, the other another marker and both a centromere and a telomere. The insertion of large fragments of DNA into these arms, followed by transformation into yeast and selection, gives rise to synthetic chromosomes. Despite their large size the cloned fragments appear to yield a faithful representation of the original genomic DNA from which they were isolated.

We shall consider the application of yeast cloning to the problems of human genome mapping in the next chapter.

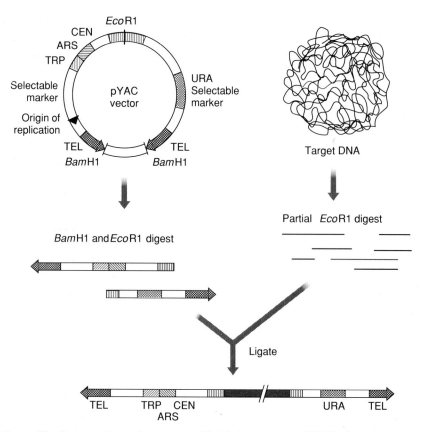

Figure 26. **Construction of a yeast artificial chromosome (YAC) cloning system.** A plasmid containing inverted repeats of telomeric (TEL) sequences together with a centromere sequence (CEN) and various selectable markers provide the two vector arms. These constructs are introduced into yeast where they function as artificial chromosomes.

● Gene libraries

Using these general approaches it is possible to prepare what are called gene libraries. There are two main types: genomic and cDNA. The former is a collection of fragments of DNA contained within self-replicating vectors which represent the entire genome of the individual from which the DNA was made. On the other hand a cDNA library, though also a collection of small pieces of DNA, represents only that DNA that is transcribed into mRNA in the particular cells from which the latter was isolated.

Genomic libraries are constructed by first digesting DNA with a restriction endonuclease that cuts frequently. For example the enzyme *Sau*3AI identifies the sequence 5′ . . . GATC . . . 3′. The digestion reaction can be controlled so that the average size of the DNA products is approximately 20 000 bp, that is the DNA is only partially digested. A particular advantage of the construction of partial-digest libraries is that they contain a series of overlapping clones covering the genome. The DNA is then fractionated by size, and fragments in the range of 18–20 kb are selected. Using this approach a relatively random collection of large uniformly sized DNA fragments from the genome can be generated. The mixture is then cloned in bacteriophage λ, and using appropriate concentrations of vector, insert fragments, and so on, it is possible to produce enough independently packaged recombinant phage to ensure that nearly all the sequences in the genome will be present. For example, for a typical mammalian genome of 3×10^9 bp, approximately 7×10^5 recombinants of an average size of 20 kb are required to ensure a 99 per cent probability that any given DNA sequence will be present in the library. This large collection of bacteriophages can then be amplified and stored to form a permanent genomic library.

Libraries can also be prepared in cosmid vectors provided that the initial partial digestion of genomic DNA is adjusted so that the average size of the pieces is approximately 40–45 kb (Fig. 27). In this case cosmid vectors are prepared (see previous section) and ligated to appropriate-sized pieces of DNA. These constructs are then packaged into λ particles. Cosmid libraries have the advantage of larger insert size, although rearrangements may occur.

Quite recently several YAC libraries have been constructed which promise to be of particular value for studies directed at mapping large regions of human DNA.

● Screening libraries and other approaches to finding particular genes

Gene libraries prepared from plasmids or bacteriophages may contain hundreds of thousands of different recombinants, each representing roughly one gene attached to a plasmid or bacteriophage DNA. In order to select a particular colony or plaque containing a desired gene from a bacterial plate a technique called colony hybridization is used (Fig. 28). A nitrocellulose filter is placed over the bacterial colonies or phage plaques. This absorbs a small amount of DNA

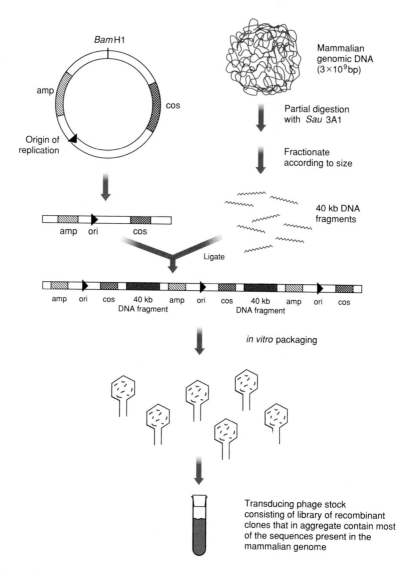

Figure 27. The construction of a genomic library in a cosmid vector. The various steps involved are described in the text.

from the colonies. The DNA is denatured and the filter is then incubated, together with a radioactive DNA probe of identical sequence to that of the gene that is being looked for, under hybridization conditions. After the excess probe has been washed away the filter is exposed to an x-ray plate; the position of the colony is indicated by a mark on the plate.

Much of the early work in applying recombinant DNA technology to human

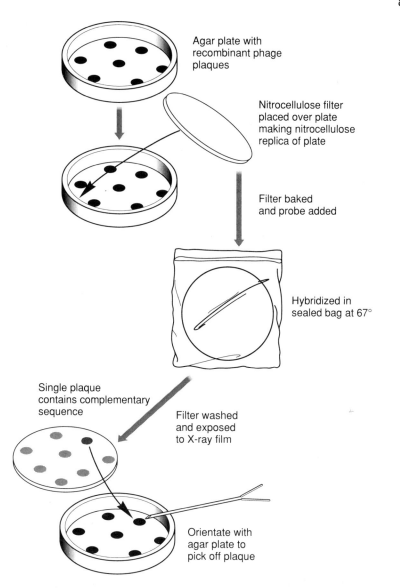

Agar plate with
recombinant phage
plaques

Nitrocellulose filter
placed over plate
making nitrocellulose
replica of plate

Filter baked
and probe added

Hybridized in
sealed bag at 67°

Single plaque
contains complementary
sequence

Filter washed
and exposed
to X-ray film

Orientate with
agar plate to
pick off plaque

Figure 28. Identification of phage plaques containing a particular gene by plaque hybridization.

genetics made use of the haemoglobin system. The reason is fairly self-evident. The genetics of normal human haemoglobin and its pathological variants was well-defined long before recombinant DNA technology came of age! The RNA in human reticulocytes is almost entirely globin mRNA. Hence, using a few simple tricks it was relatively easy to make purified mRNA for single globin chains and thus to make ^{32}P-labelled cDNA probes for the genes that direct the synthesis of the different haemoglobin subunits. It was then possible to isolate the globin genes from libraries of human DNA and to characterize their arrangement and fine structure.

While these approaches were highly successful for analysing the human haemoglobin disorders, they were not applicable to the isolation of many other genes, particularly those whose mRNAs constitued only a very small percentage of the total RNA of the cells in which they are expressed. In such cases it was necessary to devise a remarkably ingenious variety of techniques in order to isolate particular genes of interest. One of the most popular but which is possible only if at least a little is known about the amino acid sequence of the particular gene product, is to synthesize oligonucleotide probes with sequences deduced from the structure of the particular protein. The amount of potential mismatch can be reduced by choosing sequences rich in amino acids such as phenylalanine, tyrosine, and cysteine, which are encoded by only two different triplets. Oligonucleotide probes can be used for this purpose in two ways; for direct screening, the probe is incubated with radioactive ATP and polynucleotide kinase which attaches the radioactive phosphate to the 5′ end of the oligonucleotide, thus rendering it highly radioactive. The other approach involves the use of the oligonucleotide as a primer after incubation with the total mRNA preparation together with reverse transcriptase. In theory, at least, the cDNA synthesized from such a primer is complementary only to the mRNA against which it was directed.

Often nothing is known about the amino acid sequence of the product of a particular gene that is being sought. One way round this difficulty is by immunological purification of the appropriate mRNAs. Newly formed proteins start to form their three-dimensional structures as they are being assembled on ribosomes. If a suspension of polyribosomes is incubated together with antibodies against the particular protein product of a gene that we wish to find, antigen/antibody complexes form only with those polyribosomes that are producing the particular protein. By using a form of affinity chromatography that includes staphylococcal protein A, it is possible to harvest the polysomes that are bound to the antibody, and then to isolate the mRNA from the polyribosomes.

Other ingenious approaches for screening make use of *in vitro* translation. They include the so-called 'hybrid arrest' and 'hybrid selected translation' techniques, and are based on the principle that mRNA will not direct synthesis of a peptide in a cell-free translation system if it is hybridized to DNA. DNA is prepared from appropriate clones and hybridized to total mRNA, after which the mixture is incubated in a cell-free system, i.e. a mixture that contains all the ingredients required for protein synthesis, and the products are analysed by electrophoresis or immunologically. They are then compared with the translation products of non-hybridized mRNA. The translation of the protein of interest will identify which particular clones contain the DNA that is being looked for.

Another way of isolating human genes is to transfer human genomic DNA into mouse fibroblasts by techniques to be described in a later section. Those genes coding for proteins that are expressed on the cell surface, such as T cell-specific antigens, can be identified on the transformed mouse fibroblast membrane by fluorescent-antibody screening of the cell population. By using preparative fluorescent activated sorting techniques it is possible to obtain a population of cells enriched for those clones. The principle of using the expression of surface-related proteins to isolate particular genes has been developed along a number of ingenious lines. For example, it has been possible to make DNA libraries in particular expression vectors (see page 98) and to obtain transient expression in a variety of cell lines, particularly COS cells. A variety of functional approaches have been designed to 'capture' either surface or soluble ligands and hence to select for appropriate cells and obtain pure cDNA for genes of interest.

Finally, it may be possible to isolate mRNA sequences of particularly low abundance by enrichment of polyA mRNA by subtractive hybridization before differential screening of cDNA libraries. This novel approach was used to isolate the T cell receptor gene. The idea is that a particular gene may be expressed in some cell populations but not in others, T cells and B cells in the context of this particular gene. Single-stranded cDNAs prepared from mRNAs from one cell type are subtracted by hybridization to messenger RNA from another. Non-hybridizing, cell-specific cDNA is separated from hybridizing cDNA on hydroxyapatite columns and then used to screen vector libraries.

● Gene sequencing

Once genes could be isolated by cloning, the development of methods for DNA sequencing made it possible to determine the molecular basis for many single gene diseases. The two main approaches were developed independently by Maxam and Gilbert in the USA and Sanger in England. While both require the initial fractionation of DNA, from then on they are fundamentally different. Maxam and Gilbert use a degradative technique, while Sanger uses a synthetic method based on randomly stopping synthesis of a chain at every point along a strand, rather than breaking it.

For the Maxam–Gilbert method (Fig. 29) the DNA is cut with a restriction enzyme into fragments which are then sorted by size. Batches of identical fragments, which have been radioactively labelled at one end, are then divided into four lots and subjected to cleavage with specific reagents which attack DNA at one (or two) of the four bases. Under the conditions used to cleave the DNA each molecule is likely to be cut at only a small number of sites, but in the total mixture every position should be attacked. The result is a series of labelled fragments, the length of which reflects the position of the base that was cleaved relative to the radioactively labelled end. The digestion products are separated by electrophoresis in parallel tracks on the same gel under conditions in which mobility depends primarily on fragment length; the result is a series of bands generated by each specific reagent. The DNA sequence is read directly from a

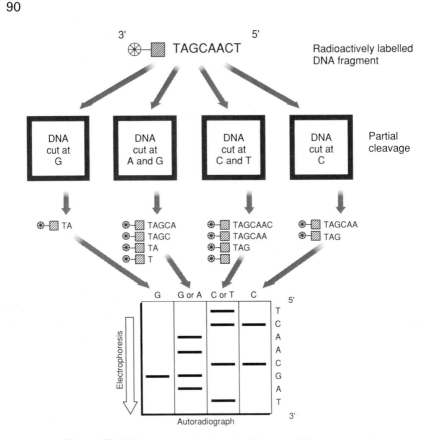

Figure 29. DNA sequencing by the Maxam–Gilbert method.

radioautograph of the gel. For example, in the case of the G-specific reaction the presence of a fragment in any particular size position indicates the presence of a G residue at that position in the sequence. An example is shown in Fig. 29. The procedure is repeated with fragments generated by other restriction enzymes, and by identifying overlapping regions the sequences of the different fragments can be ordered correctly.

The Sanger method depends on the *in vitro* synthesis of a DNA fragment copied from a piece of cloned DNA on to a radioactively labelled primer. In this case, instead of using a base-specific chemical cleavage, the growing chain is blocked at various points by adding specific nucleotide analogues. Again four batches are prepared and incorporation of analogues for each of the four different bases results in the generation of a series of radioactive fragments, each terminating at a position in the growing chain where a particular nucleotide residue would normally be added. Like the Maxam–Gilbert method, the fragments are separated according to size in parallel tracks on the same gel.

Using either of these methods it is now possible to sequence genes in a few weeks. Not surprisingly, considering that thoughts are now turning to large-scale projects such as sequencing the human genome, there is currently much interest in automated technology for DNA sequencing. One recently developed system is based on the Sanger method but with modifications that use various fluorescent dyes instead of radioactive chemicals to label the primers. Because the primers for the sequencing reaction in each of the four batches are labelled with different dyes, the products of all the enzymatic reactions can be run together in a single lane on the polyacrylamide gel. A laser beam activates the dyes, and fluorescence detectors read the DNA sequence at the bottom of the gel as each fragment appears. The sequence is then determined directly by a computer.

A variety of commercially developed variations on this theme have already appeared. Currently, most of them are based on manual enzymatic sequencing reactions and it is only the electrophoresis and gel reading that are automated. However, several systems are being developed that promise to automate the entire process. Not satisfied with all this activity several companies are attempting to introduce robotics into the field of DNA sequencing. For example, a robot has been developed to purify and isolate synthetic oligonucleotides for use as probes in cloning DNA. Undoubtedly, sequencing vast lengths of DNA becomes exquisitely boring after a while and the introduction of robots into the field will assume increasing importance, particularly if projects like sequencing the entire human genome are to be contemplated. At the time of writing, automated DNA sequencing is becoming a major industry; while none of the current methods is entirely satisfactory it seems unlikely that this will be the case for long.

● Speeding up the analysis of human DNA for diagnostic purposes

Most of the classical methods (i.e. those that are more than five years old) of gene mapping and sequencing that we have been examining are fairly time-consuming. For example, simple gene mapping can take a week or more, and cloning and sequencing a single human gene, depending on its size, takes considerably longer. As recombinant DNA technology has been applied to the diagnosis of human disease it has become apparent that more rapid methods of DNA analysis are required. Over the last few years there have been a number of major advances in the development of rapid analytical methods for studying DNA sequences which are already finding their way into medical research and clinical practice.

● DNA amplification

Quite recently a technique called the polymerase chain reaction (PCR) has been developed which allows the amplification of any short DNA sequence over a period of a few hours. Such is its power that it is possible to amplify sufficient DNA from one or two cells to obtain a genetic diagnosis within 24 hours!

The principle behind PCR is illustrated in Fig. 30. The idea is to attach short DNA primers flanking the region of interest, one on each and opposite ends of the two pairs of homologous strands. These primers are used to direct the enzyme DNA polymerase to copy each of the strands in opposite directions. Repeated cycles of enzymatic amplification increase the quantity of the targetted DNA region more than 2000-fold. By the development of a heat-stable DNA polymerase it has been possible to carry out repeated rounds of DNA synthesis at an elevated temperature. This greatly improves the amplification of targetted DNA over background DNA which may also be amplified as a result of cross-hybridization of other DNA regions with a synthetic primer at lower temperatures.

This technique permits the direct visualization of stained DNA fragments on gels and thus radioactive probes are not needed to define specific gene fragments. And it is possible to amplify DNA from blood or tissue samples without previous

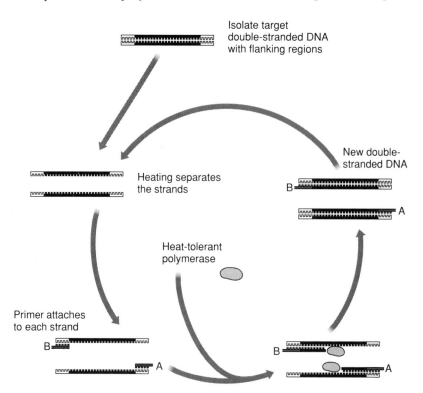

Figure 30. **The polymerase chain rection.** Specific DNA sequences are amplified in the following way. The double-stranded DNA is heated and the separated chains are allowed to bind the primers. The latter then initiate the sequences of two new chains complementary to the originals. This series of events is repeated 20–30 times, with each cycle giving a doubling of the DNA.

purification. By combining PCR amplification with the use of specific oligonucleotide probes, as described earlier, it is possible to identify single base mutations very rapidly. We will return to the practical applications of this remarkable new technology when we discuss the uses of recombinant DNA for carrier detection and prenatal diagnosis in a later chapter.

● Rapid gene sequencing and detection of point mutations

The development of the polymerase chain reaction (PCR) has led to a variety of new approaches for sequencing human genes, all of which bypass the need to clone the particular genes of interest. For example, starting with genomic DNA it is possible to amplify a particular gene or part of a gene that is to be sequenced. Having isolated the fragment, with the use of appropriate primers it is possible to obtain an abundance of double-stranded template which can then be used directly for dideoxy sequencing by the method of Sanger as described earlier (Fig. 31). A variety of variations on this theme have been developed, all of which allow the rapid sequencing of DNA starting out with as little as a nanogram of genomic DNA.

The power of this new technology for the detection of mutations in human DNA is enormous. It is possible to screen even relatively large genes, for example the gene for coagulation protein factor IX, by preparing PCR primers for nucleotide sequences in each exon together with adjacent intron sequences and for some internal sequences, and directly sequencing the amplified DNA thereby screening a large part of the coding region of the gene. Another rapid approach for the identification of mutations using PCR is called the amplification refractory mutation system (ARMS). This is based on the observation that, in many cases, oligonucleotides with a 3'-mismatched residue will, under appropriate conditions, not function as primers in the PCR. In essence, this method makes use of two primers. The 'normal' one is refractory to PCR on 'mutant' template DNA; the mutant sequence is refractory to PCR on 'normal' DNA. The difference between normal DNA and that with a particular mutation is identified by size differences of the amplified fragments.

While these new techniques have largely replaced the need for other rapid screening methods for point mutations, several have been developed over the last few years which may be of value under certain circumstances. One approach is designed specifically for identifying single base changes in messenger RNA. It is based on the principle that single point mismatches in hybridizing RNA molecules can be identified by the enzyme RNase (Fig. 32). Similar approaches have been developed for the detection of single base changes in DNA. At least some base mismatches in duplexes formed between normal DNA and DNA containing a single base change will favour denaturation of the duplex which can be detected by a reduction in its mobility in a gel run under appropriate denaturing conditions. The mismatch duplex denatures more rapidly than a perfect match and thus becomes immobile earlier in the denaturation gradient.

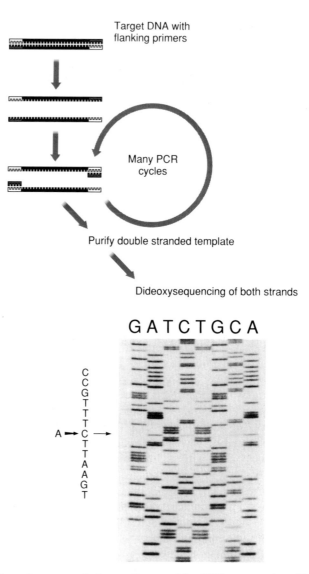

Figure 31. The polymerase chain reaction used for DNA sequencing. About 30 cycles of PCR provide a source of double stranded nucleic acid for dideoxy sequencing using the Sanger method.

● Non-radioactively labelled gene probes

Hitherto the gene probes that have been used for isolating and studying human genes or fragments thereof have been radioactively labelled, as described earlier in this chapter. But this has several disadvantages. First, it is expensive and,

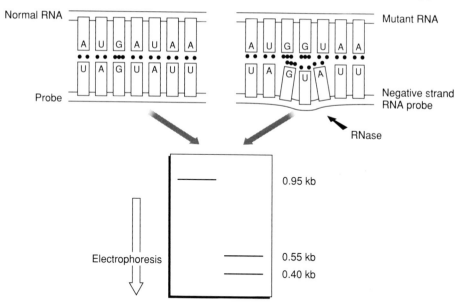

Figure 32. Screening for a mutation using a normal negative-strand RNA probe. The different sized RNase cleaved fragments are detected by gel electrophoresis and radioautography.

particularly in the case of oligonucleotide probes, requires very high specific-activity radioactive isotopes. In addition the radioactive signal has to be identified and this usually means the use of an x-ray plate and a varying amount of time for development depending on the strength of the signal. All these problems could be overcome by the use of non-radioactive sources of probe labelling, provided that the appropriate signal could be developed rapidly.

One approach that is being pursued is the use of biotinylated nucleotides as non-radioactive probes (Fig. 33). Biotin-labelled analogues of TTP and UTP can be enzymatically incorporated into DNA or RNA. The biotin incorporated into the probe can be coupled to avidin, and antibodies that identify the biotin/avidin complexes can be raised and labelled by immunofluorescence, immuno-peroxidase, or immunocolloidal gold. However, this method seems to have a limited capacity for detecting single copy sequences compared to the use of radioactive isotopes. However, the use of polymers containing bovine alkaline phosphatase and biotin promises to be more reliable. Currently these avidin-activated probes give a good though short-lived colorimetic signal.

Although these methods are still at an early stage of development, it seems very likely that they will ultimately be successful and gradually replace the use of radioactively labelled probes, at least for day-to-day diagnostic purposes in clinical laboratories.

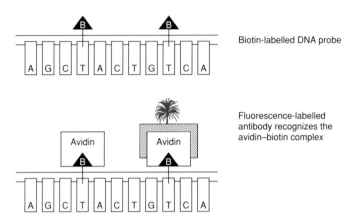

Biotin-labelled DNA probe

Fluorescence-labelled
antibody recognizes the
avidin–biotin complex

Figure 33. Non-radioactive labelling of DNA probes. The first step is to biotin-label the DNA probe. This can be identified by attaching avidin to the biotin and then fluorescently labelling the avidin with appropriate antibodies that will identify the avidin–biotin complex.

● 'Dot–blot' technology

Because it is now possible to amplify DNA so rapidly, and to define single point mutations in amplified DNA with oligonucleotide probes, it has been possible to analyse point mutations without the necessity of running DNA on gels; the DNA is simply spotted on to a nylon filter and probed with appropriate oligonucleotides. Such 'dot–blot' technology, if combined with non-radioactively labelled probes, provides a very rapid and simple laboratory approach to the diagnosis of genetic disease (Fig. 34). This procedure can be automated; undoubtedly this is the way that diagnostic genetics will move in the next few years.

● Studying the function of isolated genes

Once it was possible to isolate and sequence normal and mutant genes by cloning techniques it became important to analyse their function by introducing them into 'foreign' cells. Several approaches have been used. First, using what are called transient expression systems it is possible to insert genes into cells and to study both the quantity and structure of their transcripts. Second, genes can be introduced into established cultures of cells of the appropriate lineage. For example, human haemoglobin genes can be inserted into mouse erythroleukaemia cell lines where they are integrated into the genome to produce stably transfected lines. Another approach is to insert chromosomes containing the gene of interest into a 'foreign' cell. Finally, genes can be introduced by microinjection into fertilized eggs so that their patterns of integration and expression can be studied over several generations.

One of the earliest methods for transferring cloned genes is based on the

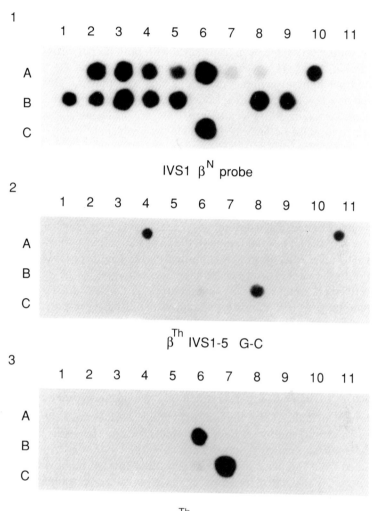

1

	1	2	3	4	5	6	7	8	9	10	11

A

B

C

IVS1 β^N probe

2

	1	2	3	4	5	6	7	8	9	10	11

A

B

C

β^{Th} IVS1-5 G-C

3

	1	2	3	4	5	6	7	8	9	10	11

A

B

C

β^{Th} IVS1-1 G-T

Figure 34. 'Dot–blot' screening for mutations of the β globin gene in β thalassaemia. The two β thalassaemia mutations that are being searched for are IVS 1, position 1 G→T, and IVS 1, position 5 G→C. An oligonucleotide probe against the normal sequence is used as a control. 1, 2, and 3 are duplicate dot blots of PCR amplified genomic DNA. There is no DNA in A1, A9, B7, B10, B11, and C1-5, C9-11. The controls for β^{Th} IVS 1-5 G→C and β^{Th} IVS 1-1 G→T probes are C8, and B6 and C7, respectively. A4 is heterozygous and A11 homozygous for the β IVS 1-5 G→C mutation.

principle of the cellular uptake of calcium microprecipitates of DNA. Although very selective, it is relatively inefficient; the rate of transfection is probably only about one cell out of 10^5. For this reason it is necessary to favour selectively the growth of cells that have taken up the foreign DNA. Various ingenious tricks have been used. For example, mouse cells that lack the thymidine kinase gene (Tk$^-$ cells) can be transfected to a Tk$^+$ phenotype and in this way are readily identified in selective media in which Tk⁻ cells are unable to grow. Furthermore, it is possible to simultaneously transfect cells using more than one gene. For example, mouse cells have been transfected with both herpes virus Tk genes and rabbit globin genes. It appears that variable numbers of the Tk genes are integrated per haploid genome at various sites and that the globin genes are expressed at a low level in cells selected by this type of approach. However, all these methods of inserting genes into cells are inefficient, and it has been necessary to look for better ways to tackle the problem.

Several types of vectors have been used to study the expression of human genes in mammalian cells in culture. At least some of them seem to satisfy the important criteria for experiments of this type, i.e. that the genes being studied are accurately transcribed from their own promotors and that the RNA transcripts are correctly spliced. Two main groups of vectors have been used, recombinant viruses and plasmids. Recombinant viruses have been constructed by the substitution of the inessential region of the viral genome with the human gene of interest. However, this approach is limited by the length of DNA that can be inserted into the virus. Better results have been achieved by the use of so-called SV40-derived plasmid vectors. SV40 is a particularly well-characterized monkey DNA tumour virus (SV stands for simian virus). It has been possible, by some ingenious genetic engineering, to construct vectors that consist of part plasmid and part SV40 sequences. One such vector consists of a derivative of the plasmid pBR322, which we have already met, into which is inserted the SV40 replication origin and a 72 base repeat which functions as an enhancer sequence. The presence of at least one copy of these tandemly repeated sequences has been found to be essential for the efficient function of some of the SV40 genes and of foreign genes introduced into these constructions. This vector is very effective for studying the transcription of human globin genes in Hela cells or Cos cells, standard cell lines than can be easily grown in the laboratory. Another vector, constructed from the plasmid pBR322 and fragments of the bovine papilloma virus genome, is also useful for studying the expression of certain human genes.

A number of physical methods for introducing genes into cells have been developed. One approach of this kind, called electroporation, involves subjecting cells to a strong electric field; it appears that pores in the cell membrane are opened up which allow the introduction of DNA fragments. This method is also relatively inefficient although there have been recent technical improvements which suggest that it may be a useful addition to the armamentarium for studying gene action.

Another way of analysing human genes in a 'foreign' environment is by direct chromosome transfer by cell fusion. For example, there is an established mouse erythroleukaemia (MEL) cell line that can be induced to synthesize haemoglobin with a variety of agents. Cells can be persuaded to fuse together by the action of certain viruses. If MEL cells are fused with human erythroid or non-erythroid cells the hybrid cells tend to lose human chromosomes. If the genes that we wish to study are on a chromosome that carries a selective marker it is possible, using specific media for growing the cells, to select fused cells that contain only mouse chromosomes and the one human chromosome in which we are interested. After induction with an appropriate agent, the human genes become active and are expressed in these fused cells. These models are particularly useful for studying putative regulatory molecules that may be involved in the activation or repression of human gene loci. They may be developed as stable cell lines or the expression of the human genes can be studied immediately after fusion in transient heterokaryons, cells that contain intact nuclei from both cell types. The latter approach is used for the study of cytoplasmic regulatory molecules.

Finally, it is possible to study human genes in *in vivo* systems. The idea is to inject genes into fertilized eggs and allow them to be expressed in the animal as it develops, and since such introduced genes may find their way into the germ cells of the animal, to follow its fate in subsequent generations (Fig. 35). This so-called transgenic approach to studying gene function has received an enormous amount of attention in recent years. The most commonly used animal is the mouse although a variety of other species have been utilized in this way.

Early attempts at transgenic gene transfer were disappointing. Introduced genes seemed to be inserted in a random way and often were not expressed. However, as knowledge has accumulated about the precise size and sequence of the DNA fragments that must be injected, many successful experiments have been carried out and a great deal has been learnt about the important regulatory sequences involved in gene expression.

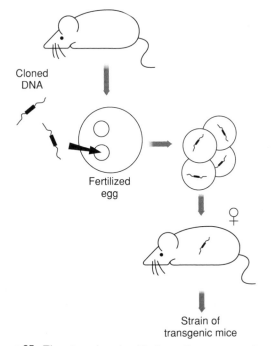

Cloned
DNA

Fertilized
egg

Strain of
transgenic mice

Figure 35. The steps involved in breeding transgenic mice.

There are now numerous examples of how the transgenic mouse model can be used to study gene expression. For example, the gene for growth hormone has been introduced in a construction in which it was linked to the promotor region of a metallothionine gene. Metallothionines are metal binding proteins the synthesis of which can be stimulated by feeding a diet rich in metals. In this particular experiment mice that received such a diet became giants; growth hormone had been produced because its gene had been 'driven' by the metallothionine promotor which had responded to the metals in the diet. In another important experiment it was found that the human globin genes could be expressed in a tissue-specific way and at physiological levels provided that the genes that were introduced contained a sequence located many kilobases upstream from the structural gene. This intriguing result suggested that there is a tissue-specific enhancer sequence that is necessary for the normal expression of the human globin genes. Even more interestingly from the medical point of view, it has been possible to 'cure' certain mouse anaemias that are due to defective globin chain synthesis by introducing normal globin genes by the transgenic approach. The transgenic model has also been used to find genes that are critical for development and has allowed the definition of genes that increase susceptibility to a variety of tumours. Quite recently genes for different haemo-poietic growth factors were introduced in this way so that their physiological properties can be analysed.

A number of variations on the transgenic model have been developed. One which is proving extremely valuable for studying the developmental regulation of genes makes use of embryonic stem (ES) cells. These murine cells can be grown easily in culture and it is possible to manipulate their genomes in a variety of ways. For example, by site-directed recombination, which we will describe in more detail in Chapter 10, it is feasible to induce mutations in particular genes. By attaching a selectable marker to the DNA which is used to induce the mutation, adequate numbers of ES cells with their genomes altered in this way can be obtained. It is then possible to inject these cells into blastocysts which can then be placed into foster mothers. In this way it is possible to breed chimeric offspring with cells derived both from the injected embryo and the ES cells. These animals can be bred again and the action of the mutated gene analysed in subsequent generations. This technique is being used widely for the study of genes that may be of importance in early development and is also providing useful information about the action of oncogenes.

Enormous progress has been made in developing the transgenic animal models for studying the regulation and expression of mammalian genes. We shall come across some of the information gained in this way in later chapters.

● Studying gene regulation

A real understanding of abnormal human gene action will depend, ultimately, on a detailed account of how genes are regulated. As pointed out in Chapter 3, it is now clear that this in an extremely complicated process, mediated at several levels: changes in chromatin structure, the interaction of regulatory proteins with DNA, the co-ordinated activity of these proteins, and a complex network of regulatory pathways which allow the genes of individual cells to respond to endogenous and exogenous signals.

In recent years methods have become available which are making it possible to dissect some of these control mechanisms. We have already seen how genes or chromosomes can be transfered into other cells to study their function. By some ingenious genetic engineering it is possible to remove particular sequences or to change their position or orientation, and hence to define their function. This is how various promotor and enhancer sequences, as defined in Chapter 3, were characterized.

It has also been possible to initiate studies of regulation at the chromatin and regulatory protein/DNA level. In Chapter 3 we saw how the recognition of specific regulatory sequences by DNA requires accessibility, and that nuclease hypersensitive sites may reflect 'open windows' that allow enhanced access of proteins to these sequences. Several methods have been developed to define these regions. The simplest involves the digestion of nuclei with DNase I followed by direct end-labelling of the resulting purified double-stranded DNA. A variety of techniques have been developed towards fine mapping of the structure of these sites, under the general title of genome footprinting. For example, end-labelled or uniformly labelled single-stranded probe can be connected to the sequences of interest, the complexes treated with single-strand-specific nucleases, and the mixture resolved on appropriate gels. It is clear that hypersensitive sites contain multiple sites of variable sensitivity to nuclease cutting, and that such substructure is related to the presence of *trans*-acting proteins.

A start has been made in purifying some of these regulatory proteins from nuclear extracts and in defining regions of DNA to which they bind by so-called gel retardation assays. By attaching these regulatory sequences to appropriate 'reporter genes' it has been possible to analyse their function, as promotors for example, in appropriate cell lines, and to make a start in defining the action of mutations of these regions. Clearly, the next step will be to isolate the genes for the *trans*-acting regulatory proteins, a *tour de force* that has already been achieved for one of the regulatory proteins for the human globin genes. Now that this is possible it should allow us to make a start in understanding how genes are regulated, and hence how batteries of genes are controlled during cellular growth and differentiation.

● Further reading

Andreason, G.L. and Evans, G.A.G. (1988). Introduction and expression of DNA molecules in eukaryotic cells by electroporation. *Biotechniques*, **6**, 650–61.

Benz, E.J. (1989). Introduction to molecular genetics and recombinant DNA technology. In *Methods in hematology; Molecular genetics*, pp. 1–20. Churchill Livingstone, Edinburgh.

Brown, T.A. (1989). *Genetic cloning*. Van Nostrand Rheinhold, Amsterdam.

Burke, D.T., Carle, G.F., and Olson, M.V. (1987). Cloning of large segments of exogenous DNA into yeast by means of artificial chromosome vectors. *Science*, **236**, 806–12.

Casky, C.T. (1987). Disease diagnosis by recombinant DNA methods. *Science*, **236**, 1223–9.

Caskey, C.T., Gibbs, R.A., Witkowski, J.A., and Hejtmancik, J.F. (1988). Diagnosis of human heritable defects by recombinant DNA methods. *Phil. Trans. R. Soc. Lond. B.*, **319**, 353–60.

Cooke, H. (1987). Cloning in yeast: an appropriate scale for mammalian genomes. *Trends Genet.*, **3**, 173–4.

Craig, R.K. (1988). Methods in molecular medicine. In *Basic molecular and cell biology*, pp. 7–16. British Medical Journal, Latimer and Trend Co. Ltd., Plymouth.

Davies, K.E. (ed.)(1988). *Genome analysis, a practical approach*. IRL Press, Oxford.

Davies, K.E. and Read, A.P. (1988). *Molecular basis of inherited disease*. IRL Press, Oxford.

DePamphilis, M.L., Hermon, S.A., Martinez-Salas, E. *et al.* (1988). Microinjecting DNA into mouse ova to study DNA replication and gene expression and to produce transgenic animals. *Biotechniques*, **6**, 662–81.

Eisenstein, B.I. (1990). The polymerase chain reaction: a new method of using molecular genetics for medical diagnosis. *New Engl. J. Med.*, **322**, 178–82.

Emery, A.E.H. (1984). *An introduction to recombinant DNA*. Wiley, Chichester.

Fritsch, E.F. and Maniatis, T. (1987). Methods of molecular genetics. In *The molecular basis of blood diseases*, (ed. G. Stamatoyannopoulos, A.W. Nienhuis, P. Leder, and P.W. Majerus), pp. 1–27. W.B. Saunders Company, Philadelphia, PA.

Glover, D.M. (1984). *The mechanics of DNA manipulation*. Chapman and Hall, London.

Jordan, B.R. (1988). Megabase methods: a quantum jump in recombinant DNA techniques. *BioEssays*, **8**, 140–5.

Kingsman, S.M. and Kingsman, A.J. (1988). *Genetic engineering*. Blackwell Scientific Publications, Oxford.

Landegren, V., Kaiser, R., Caskey, C.T., and Hood, L. (1988). DNA diagnosis—molecular techniques and automation. *Science*, **242**, 229–37.

Old, R.W. and Primrose, S.B. (1985). *Principles of gene manipulation*, 3rd edn. Blackwell Scientific, Oxford.

Newton, C.R., Graham, A., Heptinstall, L.E. *et al.* (1989). Analysis of any point mutation in DNA. The amplification refractory mutation system (ARMS). *Nucl. Acids Res.*, **17**

Palmiter, R.D. and Brinster, R.L. (1985). Transgenic mice. *Cell*, **41**, 343–5.

Saiki, R.K., Gelfand, D.H., Stoffel, S., Scharf, S.J., Higuchi, R., Horn, G.T., Mullis, K.B., and Erlich, H.A. (1988). Primer-directed enzymatic amplification of DNA with a thermostable DNA polymerase. *Science*, **239**, 487–91.

Saiki, R.K., Scharf, S., Faloona, F., Mullis, K.B., Horn, G.T., Erlich, H.A., and Arnheim, N. (1985). Enzymatic amplification of β-globin genomic sequences and restriction site analysis for diagnosis of sickle cell anaemia. *Science*, **230**, 1350–4.

White, T.J., Arnheim, N., and Erlich, H.A. (1989). The polymerase chain reaction. *Trends Genet.*, **5**, 185–9.

Finding our way round the human genome

Human geneticists have long dreamt of the day when they will have a complete map of the human genome with the precise position of all our genes arranged along their respective chromosomes. In the last few years recombinant DNA technology has so facilitated the process of human gene mapping that it now seems certain that this dream will be a reality within the forseeable future. Because this particular application of recombinant DNA technology has been so central to many of the success stories of human molecular genetics that are described in subsequent chapters, it is important to understand the principles behind these new approaches to gene hunting.

● Approaches to human chromosome mapping

As early as 1927 J.B.S. Haldane reasoned that if it were possible to map 50 or more inherited characters they could be used as markers for predicting whether children would carry genes for important disorders such as Huntington's disease. Similarly, in 1956 John Edwards pointed out that given sufficient genetic markers it should be possible to carry out prenatal detection of genetic diseases and hence reduce the transmission rate of disorders determined by autosomal dominant genes.

Why do we need genetic markers of this type? In fact, the idea is beautifully simple. Supposing we want to follow the progress of a particular genetic trait through a family but we have no way of identifying it. The thing to do would be to find a gene that we could easily identify and which was linked to the gene for the trait that we are looking for. If the two are so closely linked that they will always pass together through successive generations we now have a 'handle' on the gene that we can't identify; if the marker gene is inherited so must our gene that is closely linked to it. And, of course, if we know the chromosomal location of our marker gene then it follows that the gene that we cannot identify must be close to it on the same region of the particular chromosome.

The first gene to be assigned to a human chromosome was that for colour blindness, deduced to be on the X chromosome by Wilson and his colleagues at Columbia University in 1911. Several other X-linked traits were identified over subsequent years, but another 57 years passed before the first gene was assigned to an autosome, the Duffy blood group to chromosome 1 by a group at Johns Hopkins University in 1968. This *tour de force* was achieved by establishing linkage between the Duffy locus and a normal variation in chromosome 1 that segregated in a simple Mendelian manner in the family studied by the Johns Hopkins team. With the development of chromosome banding techniques, somatic cell genetics, and high resolution cytogenetics, progress in assigning genes to chromosomes moved more quickly in the early 1970s, and by 1976 at least one gene had been assigned to each of the 24 autosomes. More recently the field has expanded dramatically, and by the end of 1987 at least 1215 expressed genes had been assigned to specific chromosomes, 365 of which are known to be the site of mutations that cause disease. Much of this success has stemmed from the use of the physical mapping methods of somatic cell genetics in combination with new techniques of genetic mapping derived from the recombinant DNA field.

It has been apparent for a long time, therefore, that the acquisition of a map of the human genome is one of the central objectives of human genetics. Given sufficient linkage markers it should be possible to carry out carrier detection and prenatal identification of most important genetic diseases. Furthermore, once we have a detailed map it should be possible, using linkage analysis, to discover the chromosomal location of genes for disorders of which we know nothing about the cause. Indeed, we might even determine the cause of these diseases; establish a linkage, find the gene, discover what its product does, and hence work backwards to determine the underlying molecular defect. Genetics in reverse, as it were. As recently as ten years ago the achievement of these goals seemed quite unrealistic. But because of the development of the techniques of recombinant DNA technology many of them have already been realized.

There are now two general approaches to mapping human chromosomes. The first, which owes its origin to the classical studies of T.H. Morgan and his colleagues on *Drosophila*, is genetic mapping, that is the use of linkage to assign the order of genes on particular chromosomes. The second, physical mapping, is more direct in that it entails the structural analysis of chromosomes with the objective of building up a map of their constituent genes. At its simplest level of resolution this involves chromosome banding, which was described in Chapter 2; the ultimate physical map would be a complete nucleotide sequence of the whole of the human genome. In practice gene hunting involves the combined use of both genetic and physical approaches.

In the sections that follow it will be convenient to describe the two approaches to human genome mapping separately and then to consider how, in practice, they are used together either to find genes or to produce chromosome maps.

● Genetic mapping

The principles of genetic linkage were outlined in Chapter 2. Genes are said to be linked if their loci are close together on the same chromosome and hence if they are passed on together rather than independently into individual gametes. If the chromosomal location of one of them is known then, by inference, the other can be assigned to the same area of the particular chromosome. In a medical context we are most often interested in finding a genetic marker to localize and hence isolate a gene for a particular disease.

To carry out linkage studies families are examined for both the presence of the particular marker and the disease or other trait that is being studied. If it turns out that the disease and marker loci are on separate chromosomes random assortment must occur, and hence the disease and the marker will be found as often together as they are apart in offspring. If, on the other hand, the two are close together independent assortment of this kind will not occur and they will stay together unless separated by a crossover at meiosis. As pointed out in Chapter 2, it is important to determine the phase of the linkage, i.e. whether the two markers are on the same chromosome or on the opposite members of a homologous chromosome pair. This can often be done in large families in which it is possible to study matings between compound heterozygotes for the two markers and normal individuals. If the two genes are on the same chromosome, that is linked in *cis* (see Chapter 2), they will appear together in the offspring; if they are on opposite pairs of homologous chromosomes, that is in *trans*, either one or the other will appear in the offspring, but never both. But whether the linkage is in *cis* or in *trans* it will be apparent that there is deviation from independent assortment of the two genes.

On average there are about 52 crossovers at meiosis, that is about one to six per chromosome depending on its length. If the marker and disease genes are unlinked the number of non-recombinants will equal the number of recombinants and the recombination fraction, that is the total number of recombinants divided by the total number of offspring, will be 50 per cent or 0.5. This figure reflects completely independent assortment. As the distance between the marker and the disease loci decreases there will be less chance of crossing-over and the number of recombinants will become fewer, i.e. the recombination fraction falls. It follows that this fraction, called θ, will vary from zero, indicating tight linkage, to 0.5, reflecting independent assortment. Linked loci are separated by a physical distance that is very small when the recombination fraction is close to zero, and at a greater distance when the recombination fraction is larger. Hence the recombination fraction can be taken as a measure of genetic distance. It follows that the primary object of genetic linkage analysis, between marker and disease loci for example, is to find out whether the recombination fraction is smaller than 0.5. Several methods have been devised to this end, the most common being the lod score.

In practice it is usually necessary to work out the most likely value of the recombination fraction by making assumptions about the phase of linkage and combining data from more than one family. The likelihood, or odds, is usually expressed as its logarithm; the $\log_{10}$ of the odds is called the lod score. Lod scores for different values of θ are calculated for each individual family and then added together. The sum of the lod scores is then plotted against various values for θ. This type of exercise results in a series of curves; the maximum likelihood estimate of θ is the value that corresponds to the peak of the curve (Fig. 36). A simple example of the calculation of a lod score from curves of this type is shown in the

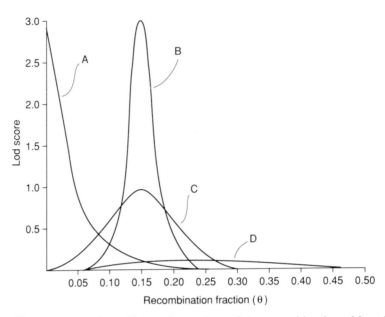

Figure 36. Lod scores plotted for various values of the recombination of fraction θ.
A High probability (1000:1) of very close linkage (θ <0.01), **B** high probability (1000:1)
that θ =0.15, **C** suggestion (10:1) of linkage, **D** no linkage. Modified from Emery (1984).

caption to Fig. 36. The 95 per cent probability limits of the maximum likely
estimate of θ can be estimated by subtracting 2.5 per cent of the total area under
the curve from each end. The area under the curve can be determined directly but
such calculations are extremely tedious and hence are usually carried out using a
computer program designed specifically for calculating lod scores, LIPED and
LINKAGE for example. A lod score of 3 indicates that the observed departure
from the expected segregation values, assuming linkage, would occur by chance
only once every 10^3 times. At this level of significance the alternate hypothesis,
that the two loci are linked, is acceptable.

It is apparent, therefore, that distance on genetic maps is a measure of
recombination frequency. Recombination is expressed in units called centimorgans (100 centimorgans = 1 Morgan). A recombination fraction of 0.1 (10 per
cent) indicates a map distance of 10 centimorgans. However, with increasing
distance between two genes the apparent recombination fraction falls because of
the occurrence of double crossovers. Furthermore, the frequency of autosomal
crossovers is not the same in females as in males, and varies between different
ends of the chromosomes; in general it is greater at the telomeric than the
centromeric ends. In relating physical maps to genetic maps all these factors need
to be taken into consideration. It has been calculated that the haploid genome is
of approximately 30 Morgans. Since the DNA that makes up the genome
contains approximately 3×10^9 base pairs (bp) one centimorgan is equivalent to

about 1 million bp. It seems likely that if a genetic linkage map could be constructed with a set of markers separated on average by one centimorgan, most genes would be located within a range of 100 000 to 10 million bp.

Until the advent of DNA technology the number of polymorphic marker traits for family linkage studies was limited. Among the most commonly employed were normal chromosome variants (heteromorphisms), blood groups, serum or red cell enzyme polymorphisms, and various immunogenetic markers. Although some progress was made using these systems it has only been over the last few years, following the appearance of DNA technology, that the linkage approach to mapping and isolating human genes has come into its own.

● DNA polymorphisms for genetic mapping

The advent of restriction enzyme technology suggested a completely new approach to defining potentially large numbers of marker loci. It always seemed likely that individuals would differ considerably in the structure of their DNA, particularly in regions that do not code for proteins and that are not involved in important regulatory functions. If this is the case there should be considerable variation between different persons in the pattern of restriction enzyme fragments generated after digestion of their DNA. Not surprisingly, perhaps, one of the early worries about the whole concept of restriction endonuclease analysis of human genes was the possibility that the potential frequency of such structural changes in DNA might give rise to far too much normal individual variability to make the analysis of genetic disorders feasible. As we shall see, it turns out that the amount of normal variation in structural loci is relatively small. On the other hand, there are harmless inherited variations in the structure of DNA throughout all the regions of the human genome that have been examined in detail.

It might help the reader if we digress briefly here to clarify our current (and perhaps rather loose) terminology in this field. It will be recalled that in an earlier chapter we defined a polymorphism, quoting E.B. Ford, as 'the existence in the same habitat at the same time of two or more distinct forms of the species . . .'. A good working extension of this definition is 'the occurrence of two or more alleles for a particular locus where at least two alleles appear with frequencies of more than 1 per cent' (Bodmer and Cavalli-Sforza 1976). The blood groups and haemoglobin variants are typical examples of polymorphic systems with multiple alleles. Variation in the structure of our DNA gives rise to base changes that have been called restriction fragment length polymorphisms (RFLPs), i.e. inherited differences in the size of DNA fragments produced when DNA is cut with specific restriction enzymes. Such RFLPs are not polymorphic in the sense of the Rh or HLA loci therefore. Nevertheless they provide a considerable degree of individual variation which is inherited according to Mendelian laws.

It follows that if we wish to study the inheritance of a gene for a product that we cannot identify, and there are RFLPs close enough to the gene, it should be possible to use them as markers to follow the inheritance of the particular gene through families. And if we know where the RFLP is, we should be able to find the adjacent gene. It is this notion that has revolutionized human genetics and is enabling us to find genes for human diseases before we know anything about their biochemical defect, and even before we have obtained specific probes with which to study them.

The molecular basis for the two main types of RFLPs is shown in Fig. 37. First, there are single base alterations or similar changes that either produce a new site of cleavage for a restriction enzyme or remove a previously existing one. Strictly speaking they are dimorphisms rather than polymorphisms. Thus, if we have a probe for a region of DNA close to one of these sites, different sized DNA fragments will be generated by the particular enzyme, depending on the presence or absence of the variant sequence. Second, there are so-called hypervariable regions (HVRs), parts of the genome that vary considerably in length and hence that generate many different sized restriction fragments.

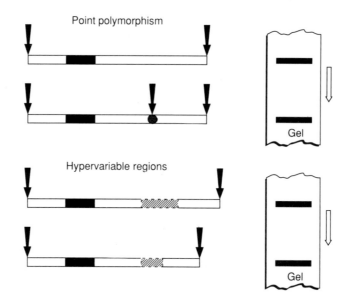

Figure 37. The different classes of restriction fragment length polymorphisms.

● Restriction fragment length polymorphisms due to single base changes

RFLPs due to single base alterations have been found within or near to almost all the human structural genes that have been analysed to date. The first detailed studies of this type of RFLP involved the εγδβ globin gene complex on chromosome 11 (see Chapter 3). The results showed a frequency of RFLPs of about one in every 500 bp, and suggested that they occur at random and are unlikely to have been subjected to any form of selection; in this sense they can be regarded as completely neutral mutations. Furthermore, they are inherited in a simple Mendelian fashion. Over the last few years a great deal has been learnt about the RFLPs in the human globin gene clusters. Since this information may well have important implications for our understanding of the arrangements of RFLPs elsewhere in the genome, it will repay us to look at these clusters in some detail.

Although more recent studies of the RFLPs in the β-like gene cluster have largely confirmed these early impressions, some revision has been necessary. In the 60 kb of DNA that make up the cluster there are at least thirteen sites that generate RFLPs (Fig. 38). Of these, seven are located in flanking DNA, three within introns, one in a pseudogene, and one in the coding part of the β globin gene. All the polymorphic sites for which sequence data are available result from single nucleotide substitutions. Nine of them are designated as 'public'; that is they occur in all racial groups and the frequency of the least common allele is greater than 5 per cent in every racial group studied. The remaining sites are called 'private' in that they are polymorphic in individuals of African origin but not in other racial groups.

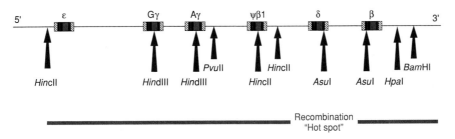

Figure 38. Restriction fragment length polymorphisms in the β globin gene cluster.

In general there is no difference in the frequency of the presence (+), or absence (−), of an RFLP between normal chromosomes and those that carry particular mutations of the β globin genes. There are however a few examples of so-called linkage disequilibrium between an RFLP and a β globin gene allele. For example, there is a strong association between the sickle cell gene and an *Hpa*I polymorphism in some American and West African Black populations, and an *Hinf*I site polymorphism is present in 70 per cent of normal chromosomes in American Blacks but only in 10 per cent of chromosomes carrying the sickle cell mutation. We shall return to describe these and other examples of linkage disequilibrium of this type in a later chapter; it must be emphasized that they are the exceptions rather than the rule.

How polymorphic can we expect a structural gene to be? A considerable amount of information about this important question has been collected for the human β globin gene over the last few years. Given that one per several hundred base pairs in the genome may vary between individuals, we would predict that there must be some neutral sequence variation within the β globin gene, which spans over 1600 bp. Are these changes relatively fixed, that is, are only a few sites polymorphic in most populations, or, alternatively, are the polymorphisms scattered throughout the gene and 'private' for various groups or families? It turns out that polymorphisms within the β globin gene are largely limited to specific nucleotide positions. Detailed examination of many genes from different populations has shown that the distribution of these normal variations are non-random and can be classified into specific patterns or frameworks. Many individuals are heterozygous for these normal variants and hence this provides an opportunity for identifying individual β globin genes on different chromosomes.

Another unexpected and potentially important observation about the pattern of RFLPs in the β globin gene family is that their distribution is not entirely random. Why should this surprise us? Suppose that a polymorphic site is found in 50 per cent of chromosomes examined in a particular population, and that a second site is present in 30 per cent of chromosomes in the same population. If the two sites are randomly associated, the probability of them both being present on a particular chromosome would be 50×30, i.e. 15 per cent; but if they are non-randomly associated, the probability of the presence of both will differ significantly from this figure. The pattern of polymorphic restriction sites in a particular region of a chromosome is called an RFLP haplotype. In fact, it turns out that there are only a few RFLP haplotypes in the β globin gene complex. The five polymorphic sites that are distributed over a 32 kb region 5' to the β globin gene are non-randomly associated such that three haplotypes account for 94 per cent of normal chromosomes in Greek, Italian, and Asian Indian populations. Similarly, the polymorphic sites that are distributed in an 18 kb region that extends 3' to the β globin gene are also non-randomly associated. Again, three haplotypes account for 90 per cent of normal chromosomes. Between these two regions there is 11 kb of DNA within which randomization of the 5' and 3' regions seems to occur (Fig. 38). It follows that there must be a higher rate of recombination in this region of the gene cluster.

The β thalassaemia mutations appear to have occurred relatively recently on the background of these RFLP haplotype arrangements, and in individual populations there is a strong correlation between the RFLP haplotype and a particular mutation. However, similar haplotypes are found in normal individuals and therefore the haplotype pattern cannot be used to predict the presence or absence of a β thalassaemia mutation in a particular individual. Furthermore, even within a population, the same mutation may occur in association with several different RFLP haplotypes. It remains to be seen whether there is something peculiar about the globin genes in this respect, or whether these rather complex RFLP relationships will be true for other human structural genes. I suspect that this will not always be the case. Much will depend on when mutations occurred in relation to the establishment of the RFLPs, and the subsequent degree of selection for a particular chromosome. We have still much to learn about the complex relationships between mutations and RFLP patterns.

Equally detailed studies of the distribution of RFLPs have also been carried out for the α globin gene cluster on chromosome 16. It turns out that this region of the genome is even more polymorphic than the β globin gene cluster. As well as many single point RFLPs this region also contains several hypervariable regions; we shall consider the latter later in this chapter. The distribution of single point RFLPs in the α globin gene cluster is also non-random and falls into a number of haplotypes, the frequency of which varies between different racial groups. Unlike the β gene cluster there is no evidence for a 'hot spot' for recombination in the α globin gene region. Many of the α thalassaemias, like the β thalassaemias, seem to have occurred on a particular RFLP haplotype which has then been selected along with the particular thalassaemia mutation. But, like the β thalassaemias, some forms of α thalassaemia occur on different haplotypes in different populations, indicating that the underlying mutation has occurred more than once during evolution.

What can be learnt from these rather complex properties of RFLPs in the globin gene clusters and, more important, do they have wider application to other human genes or gene clusters? Although the globin genes, because their mutations have come under such intense selection, may not be typical of other structural genes as regards the distribution of RFLP haplotypes and their relationship to inherited diseases, certain tentative conclusions can be drawn. First, and most important, is that there are RFLPs due to single nucleotide changes scattered throughout the gene cluster, both between and within structural genes. They provide an extremely valuable series of markers for following particular mutant genes through families. Thus it seems very likely that RFLP haplotypes will be definable for many genes and their flanking regions. Second, although occasionally there is strong linkage disequilibrium between a mutation and an RFLP, these are the exceptions rather than the rule. This probably only occurs if a mutant gene has come under strong selective pressure or has been widely disseminated from a single 'founder'. Finally, since the pattern of RFLPs in the β gene cluster is not entirely random, but appears to fall into several major classes at the 5′ and 3′ ends, separated by a region in which there has been a high degree of recombination, we may expect to find unusual combinations of RFLPs in other gene clusters if such 'hot spots' for recombination are common.

Clearly, therefore, single point RFLPs provide us with a valuable source of markers for tracking genes in individual families and for mapping studies and, at least in some cases, offer us the added bonus of being able to associate particular diseases with particular RFLP haplotypes. But how do we find single point RFLPs of this type?

In the case of the globin genes, or any other genes for which we are lucky enough to have a probe, the process of finding single point RFLPs is quite straightforward. Using probes for each individual gene and for regions in their immediate neighbourhood we simply analyse the restriction patterns by Southern blotting using a battery of different enzymes.

Of course we do not always have well-defined probes for structural loci or their immediate environment and in this case it is necessary to produce single or low copy DNA probes to detect RFLPs. To this end several approaches have been developed. One is to screen human DNA libraries with repetitive sequence DNA probes; occasionally a phage can be identified that contains no sequences of this type. These, presumed single sequence DNAs, can then be used directly as hybridization probes to search for RFLPs in genomic DNA by gene mapping. Ideally, probes selected in this way should represent about 15–20 kb of contiguous single copy DNA although in practice this is not always possible.

When setting out to find RFLPs it is helpful to concentrate on particular chromosomes. There are several ways in which this can be done. First, as we shall see later in this chapter, it is possible to isolate individual chromosomes using fluorescent-activated cell sorting. Once isolated, libraries can be made from the chromosome and screened for polymorphisms using unique sequence DNA probes. Another approach utilizes both somatic cell genetics and recombinant DNA technology. First, DNA from rodent/human hybrid cells is cloned in phage. The resulting phage are then screened for human DNA inserts by hybridization with labelled middle-repetitive human DNA. Since such sequences are interspersed through the human genome, and because interspecies hybridization does not occur under stringent conditions, it is often possible to identify phages carrying human DNA segments specific for the chromosome contained in the original hybrid cells. In this way it has been possible to obtain a collection of DNA fragments specific for regions of different human chromosomes. Using these, and a variety of other ingenious techniques, it has been possible to accumulate many hundreds of DNA probes, some of unknown location and others related to specific regions of chromosomes. These probes can be used together with a battery of restriction enzymes to search for single point RFLPs.

In general, polymorphisms seem to be relatively uncommon using most restriction enzymes, perhaps somewhere in the order of 1 per 200 sites. However, two enzymes, MspI and TaqI, show a higher frequency, somewhere in the order of 1 in 10 to 1 in 20 sites. This is because the particular sites that are identified by these enzymes include the CG dimer. The fact that mutations occur frequently at the sequence CpG probably reflects the frequent deamination of methyl cytosine to thymidine.

As shown in Fig. 39, a single point RFLP is reflected by two bands of more or less equal size on a restriction enzyme map, indicating that the particular individual is heterozygous for the RFLP. Once the polymorphism has been identified it is possible to carry out family studies to see whether it is linked to a mutant gene or other trait that is segregating within the family.

● Hypervariable regions

The frequency of heterozygosity for a particular marker system is a major factor in determining its usefulness for providing linkage information from family studies. Obviously the dimorphisms, i.e. the presence or absence of a cutting site generated by single point RFLPs which we have just described, are rather limited in this respect. On the other hand hypervariable regions of DNA (HVRs) yield

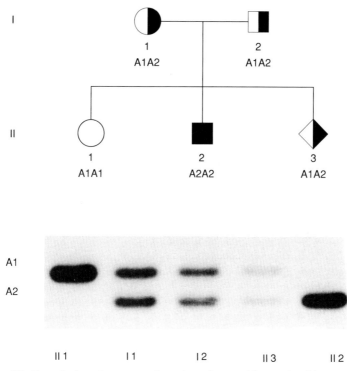

Figure 39. Restriction fragment length polymorphisms. In this example of the inheritance of a point polymorphism the family have an individual (II-2) with cystic fibrosis. Both parents are carriers. The RFLP A1/A2 is close to the CF gene and both parents are heterozygotes. The affected child (II-2) has received the A2 allele from both parents. The child II-1 is normal and has received the A1 allele from both parents. A fetus, II-3, is also heterozygous (A1/A2).

restriction fragments, the length of which varies widely within populations. These regions of DNA, to which no function has yet been attributed, are made up of short arrays, often GC-rich, which are repeated in tandem. It appears that it is the particular property of this structure that underlies the extraordinary variability in length of these sequences. These long homologous stretches of repetitive DNA are prone to recombination, probably through unequal exchange at meiosis or mitosis, or through slippage during DNA replication. These recombination events result in allelic differences in the number of repeated units present at HVR loci, and hence in length polymorphisms. It follows that the degree of heterozygosity at HVRs is very high, up to over 0.95 in some cases, and hence these regions may provide a great deal of information in genetic linkage studies.

The first HVR was discovered using an arbitrary DNA probe which generated fragments of more than 15 different lengths in a small sample of unrelated individuals. Subsequently similar regions were observed in relation to structural genes, including those for insulin, α globin, Harvey-*ras*, and myoglobin. It turns out that there are no less than five HVRs in the α globin gene cluster, one of which, the so-called 3′ HVR is extremely polymorphic (Fig. 40). Based on their molecular structure the more cumbersome title 'variable number of tandem repeats (VNTR) loci' has been used to describe single loci of this type. Because of their repeat structure these regions are also known as 'mini-satellite' DNA, and the probes that are used to define them as mini-satellite probes.

It is now apparent that some HVRs exist as families, the members of which are related by homology of a core unit of their tandem repeats and which are scattered throughout the genome. Furthermore, extensive experience suggests that the evolutionary instability that underlies the remarkable variability in lengths of these regions of DNA is not so great as to perturb segregation analysis, a fact that makes them extremely useful for linkage studies. These observations have been exploited in a particularly novel way by Alec Jeffreys. He was able to construct a DNA probe based on the sequence of a set of 33 bp tandem repeats that constitute an HVR in the myoglobin gene, which could detect by

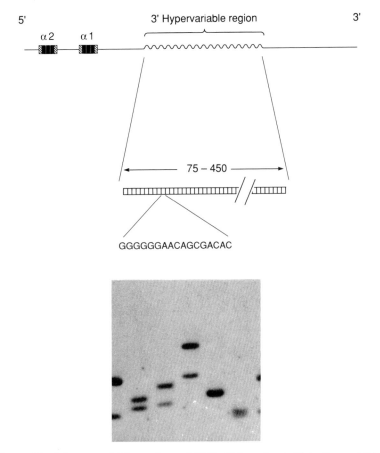

GGGGGGAACAGCGACAC

Figure 40. **A hypervariable region of DNA.** This region is 3′ to the α globin genes. It consists of variable numbers of tandem repeats. The gel shows the different patterns from a random group of individuals.

hybridization to genomic DNA a large number of loci containing tandem repeats of similar sequence. The restriction fragment pattern revealed by the sum of the HVR loci containing such related sequences, scattered throughout the whole of the human genome, constitutes a 'genetic fingerprint' which is completely unique to any one individual (Fig. 41). One of the practical problems of genetic fingerprinting of this type is that the number of loci that can be identified by partial homology to the tandem repeat sequence is quite enormous and this makes the interpretation of the resultant series of alleles particularly difficult. However, this difficulty can be overcome because the myoglobin HVR region that is used to develop such genetic fingerprints can also serve to screen DNA libraries and to identify clones representing unique (single copy) loci.

This general approach has been extended by making synthetic oligonucleotide probe sequences from several of the known hypervariable regions, as well as other candidate sequences, with which to probe human genomic libraries. In this way it has been possible to identify many other highly polymorphic genetic loci reflecting further families of HVRs.

In searching for HVRs some surprising findings have emerged. For example it

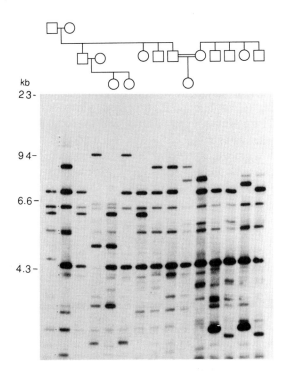

Figure 41. Genetic fingerprinting. The patterns are from the individuals shown in the pedigree; each member is above their respective track.

turns out that a sequence from the genome of the single-stranded bacteriophage, M13, detects a family of hypervariable sequences when used as a hybridization probe against human genomic DNA. This sequence is part of the phage gene III, which encodes a protein involved in the attachment to the bacterial F pilus in the process of infection, and which comprises a pair of CG-rich tandem repeats. The family of HVRs detected by the M13 tandem repeat is quite different from those detected by other mini-satellite probes. The frequency of band sharing between unrelated individuals of European descent is approximately 0.20 for bands larger than 2 kb, of which about 15 to 20 can be detected per individual.

The complexity of DNA fingerprinting makes it impossible to follow the inheritance of allele pairs, but within a very large pedigree a single band of a given size can, at least in the case of a preliminary analysis, be assumed to represent a single locus. However this is only an assumption and it may be inappropriate to carry out a lod score analysis on family data of this type which should therefore be regarded as a preliminary screening method for linkage. If a promising result turns up, that is if a band is found which segregates with a disease phenotype, it must be isolated and cloned to make a locus-specific probe which can be used to confirm or refute the particular linkage.

Although the development of probes for these different types of HVRs has provided us with a wealth of polymorphisms for mapping the genome and for 'finding' individual genes a word of caution is necessary. Recent work suggests that many of these loci are located near the tips (telomeric ends) of chromosomes. It is possible, therefore, that their overall usefulness for 'covering' the human genome with markers will be limited. Recently, however, an interspersed repeat with the sequence $(CA)^n$ has been identified which shows frequent length polymorphism. It turns out that there are some 50 000 copies (one every 60 kb) in the human genome. Length variables can be detected using oligonucleotide probes flanking the repeat sequences. Using such sequences, together with the polymerase chain reaction (see Chapter 3) it may be possible to move rapidly toward a genetic map. A particular attraction of this approach is that, unlike the other HVRs described earlier, these sequences occur on the X chromosome.

Although not of direct relevence to its value as a genetic marker, the discovery of all this repetitive DNA raises the intriguing question of why it is there at all. Mini-satellites are not confined to human DNA; similar sequences are found in other mammals, birds, plants, and fungi. As mentioned earlier, the first human HVR of this type was found to have a core sequence shared by several different mini-satellite families. It was noted that this sequence was similar to the crossover hotspot instigator (Chi) sequence of bacteriophage λ and *E. coli* which functions as a signal for homologous recombination. Could the human core sequence act as a recombination signal, or recombinator? This is an attractive hypothesis which has generated a great deal of work, and even more debate. But as more mini-satellite DNA sequences are unearthed, with differing core sequences, it is difficult to see how they can all subserve the role of recombination signals. Another explanation which, though less attractive from the functional viewpoint, seems equally plausible is that these regions of DNA are the products of the pecularities of local DNA structure. For example, the existence of multiple HVRs in the α globin gene complex may simply reflect the GC-rich structure of this region; frequent G-rich or C-rich duplications may, by further duplication and crossing-over, generate HVRs.

Regardless of how they have arisen, these highly polymorphic regions of DNA provide us with a very valuable source of linkage markers as we set out to map the human genome.

● Some genes that have been assigned by RFLP linkage

The first locus to be defined in this way was that for Duchenne muscular dystrophy. Human X-specific sequences were isolated from a genomic library constructed from X chromosomes purified by flow cytometry. X-specific clones were then assigned to regions of the chromosome by hybridization to somatic cell hybrid DNA or by *in situ* hybridization. Single copy probes were used to identify RFLPs to act as genetic markers for various X-linked diseases. One particular probe, RC8, showed a loose linkage to the locus for Duchenne muscular dystrophy. Not long after a number of other probes were defined that showed closer linkage. As we shall see later in this chapter these early studies have led to the discovery of the locus for Duchenne muscular dystrophy and to the elucidation of its cause.

It must be obvious by now that a certain amount of good luck is required to obtain a linkage for a particular gene using RFLPs in this way. This was certainly the case for another of the early success stories in this field, the finding of a genetic marker for Huntington's disease. Two large kindreds with many affected members were studied using twelve DNA probes, chosen because they contained no repetitive DNA sequences. One probe called G8, derived from a recombinant bacteriophage from a human gene library, was found to detect two invariant and several variable *Hind*III fragments in human genomic DNA. In fact it turned out that there were several polymorphic sites for this enzyme in relatively close proximity so that the frequency of recombination between them was negligible, that is they were inherited together as a unit or haploptype as defined earlier in this chapter for some of the RFLPs in the β globin gene cluster. The haplotypes were designated A, B, C, and D. In a large North American family the A haplotype was associated with Huntington's disease; in a Venezuelan pedigree it was the C haplotype. Subsequently a DNA probe (designated D4S10) was generated which was estimated to be four recombination units from the Huntington's disease gene and which was assigned to the terminal band of the short arm of chromosome 4. Over the last few years this probe has been used widely for predictive testing for Huntington's disease in many families.

The first disease locus to be assigned using HVR probes was that for adult polycystic disease of the kidney (APKD). Among many single point and HVR probes that were used to study several large Oxford kindreds with this condition, was included the one that identifies the highly polymorphic HVR region 3' to the α globin gene. Linkage between α globin and APKD was demonstrated and later confirmed in several other large kindreds from different populations. These results assigned the gene for APKD to the short arm of chromosome 16 close to the human α globin gene complex.

Once a linkage has been obtained between an RFLP and a locus for a particular disease or other trait it is essential to carry out large numbers of family studies, not only to confirm the linkage but also to determine whether there is genetic heterogeneity underlying the particular disorder. In other words, can mutations at more than one locus give rise to a particular clinical phenotype? Adult polycystic disease of the kidney is an interesting example of this problem. Although at first it appeared as though there was no heterogeneity, quite recently at least two families have been described with the phenotype of APKD in which there is good evidence that the genetic determinant is not linked to the α globin gene locus on chromosome 16. Perhaps this is not surprising. Long before molecular genetics came of age it was already apparent that some genetic diseases with identical phenotypes are due to mutations at different loci. For example, conventional blood group linkage studies carried out more than 20 years ago provided very clear evidence that hereditary elliptocytosis can result from mutations at at least two different loci, and we now know that three distinct loci are involved in the generation of this condition.

Over the last few years the list of loci for human single gene disorders which have been assigned by RFLP linkage analysis has increased dramatically. Some of these conditions are summarized in Table 17. As well as demonstrating genetic linkage it has often been possible to assign the particular RFLP to an individual chromosome using the techniques of somatic cell genetics as will be outlined later in this chapter.

● Progress in genetic mapping of the human genome

In their paper of 1980, which set out the theoretical basis for RFLP mapping, Botstein and his colleagues estimated that we might need only 150 different markers to link most of the important human genes to chromosomal regions containing RFLPs. Over the years since this seminal paper was published it has become apparent that this was rather an optimistic figure. In fact it now appears that hundreds of DNA probes for highly polymorphic sequences, scattered widely over the genome, will be required for a complete human linkage map.

Just how complete does our map need to be? A reasonable starting point might be a map of 10 centimorgans in which there is a greater than 90 per cent chance of being able to determine the approximate chromosomal location of any gene that we wish to find. Remarkable progress has been made over the last few years towards developing maps at this level of resolution. For example, Ray White and his colleagues at the University of Utah have reported the assignment of nearly 500 markers covering 17 chromosomes based on DNA from 59 different three-generation families. The markers on this map are separated on average by about

Table 17. *Examples of important disease loci that have been assigned by RFLP linkage*

Duchenne muscular dystrophy Xp21.3-p21.1
Huntington's disease 4p ter-16.3
Adult polycystic disease of the kidney 16p 13.3
Cystic fibrosis 7q31-q32
Familial polyposis coli 5q 21-q22
Retinoblastoma 13q14*
Neurofibromatosis (NF)
   NF1 17q11.2
   NF2 22q11-q13.1
Multiple endocrine neoplasia type 2a 10p11.2-q11.2
Spinal muscular atrophy 5q11.2-13.3
Hypophosphataemia Xp22.2-p22.1
Agammaglobulinaemia Xq21.33-q22
Severe combined immunodeficiency Xq13-q21.1
Charcot–Marie–Tooth disease Xq11-q13
Cleft palate Xq21.3-q.22
Spastic paraplegia Xq27-28
Friedreich's ataxia 9q13-q21.1
Familial schizophrenia? 5q11-13
Familial Alzheimer's disease? 21q21

---

*First assigned by other techniques.

10 centimorgans, that is about 10–20 million bp. A Boston team, based in Collaborative Research Incorporated, have produced an independent RFLP linkage map, consisting of 403 markers on average about 9 centimorgans apart. They believe that a new gene or marker on this map can be located relative to the existing markers in approximately 95 per cent of cases.

It is clear, therefore, that RFLPs are the key to finding our way to within a few million bases of a gene that we wish to find. Before describing how it is possible to find the actual genes following their approximate location by RFLP linkage it is necessary to consider, at least in outline, some of the methods for physical mapping that have been developed over recent years.

● Physical mapping techniques

Physical mapping of the human genome involves techniques of varying resolution that provide information ranging from the identity of individual chromosomes to the nucleotide sequence of specific regions of the chromosomes. The ultimate physical map would, of course, be the complete nucleotide sequence of the human genome.

At its simplest, physical mapping involves karyotyping to identify individual chromosomes, as outlined in Chapter 2. The use of fluorescent dyes as chromosome-specific stains has greatly facilitated accurate karyotyping. It turns out that each of the 24 different human chromosomes has a unique pattern of banding. Nearly 1000 distinct bands have been detected and it has been estimated that on average there are approximately 100 genes in a single band.

There are several low resolution techniques that are very useful for assigning genes to particular regions of chromosomes. These include somatic cell hybridization, *in situ* hybridization, and chromosome sorting.

● Low resolution mapping

Somatic cell hybridization

If human cells, fibroblasts for example, are mixed with rodent tumour cells grown in culture together with sendai virus, they tend to fuse together. Following fusion the chromosomes of each of the cells become mixed together and subsequently many of them are lost from the now hybrid cell; human chromosomes are preferentially lost compared with the rodent chromosomes. Furthermore, the human chromosomes are lost in a random fashion. Individual hybrid cells can then be propagated in culture and maintained as cell lines. Usually they contain between 8 and 12 human chromosomes in addition to a variable number of rodent chromosomes.

Human chromosomes can be identified in the hybrid cells and therefore it is possible to build up a panel of somatic cell hybrids containing specific chromosome combinations. The next step is to determine whether a particular gene is present or absent on the chromosomes of a particular hybrid line. Assignment of the gene can be carried out in several ways. For example, it may be possible to detect a specific gene product in hybrid cell lines and hence relate the gene to the chromosome that is unique to that line. Alternatively, if the gene has already been isolated by DNA cloning it can be used to identify complementary nucleotide sequences in DNA extracted from the somatic cell hybrids. A variety of other approaches can be used to identify individual genes using this technique.

In situ *hybridization*

This technique is used to identify the chromosomal location of genes directly. The principles of DNA hybridization were described in the previous chapter. *In situ* hybridization is carried out by using an appropriate probe, made either from cDNA or genomic DNA, to hybridize directly with complementary sequences on a particular chromosome. The probe is radiolabelled and applied under appropriate hybridizing conditions to standard chromosome spreads. If hybridization occurs the probe will bind to the DNA, and the rest of it can be washed off the slide. The hybridization signal is identified by autoradiography which shows a series of granules aggregating on the part of the chromosome to which the probe has hybridized (Fig. 42).

Several new technical advances promise to widen the scope of *in situ* hybridization. For example, the availability of non-radioactive probes should greatly improve resolution. But it is the development of competitive *in situ* suppression hybridization (CISH) together with increasingly sophisticated microscopy that promises to revolutionize the field of chromosomal analysis.

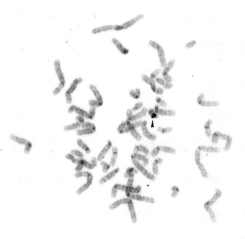

Figure 42. *In situ* hybridization using a radioactive gene probe. The probe is DW23, which binds specifically to the Y chromosome, as shown by arrow.

Essentially, CISH involves prehybridization with unlabelled DNA to reduce the background signals caused by interspersed repeat sequences. This allows the use of a variety of probes including cosmids and yeast artificial chromosomes. The resolution of the signal from *in situ* probes can be greatly increased by the use of dual or multichannel confocal fluorescence microscopy. By combining these new techniques it is possible to label entire chromosomes with chromosome-specific libraries, a pastime that is called chromosome painting. Added to all this is the recent observation that even better resolution can be obtained, perhaps down to as little as 25 kb, if interphase rather than metaphase chromosome preparations are used. It turns out that by using confocal, three-dimensional imaging it is possible to obtain particularly well-focused signals; the possibilities for mapping that are offered by these recent technical advances are quite remarkable.

Chromosome sorting

It is often useful to isolate individual human chromosomes for mapping or other purposes. This is achieved by flow cytometry and flow sorting. Fluorescent markers that bind to chromosomes are used in flow cytometry as the basis of separating chromosomes from one another. Because individual chromosomes differ in the degree to which they bind the fluorescent markers, it is possible to use this approach to physically separate at least some chromosomes from others. A dual-laser system of this type has been used successfully to separate all the human chromosomes, except numbers 10 and 11.

Other approaches to low resolution physical mapping

A variety of other approaches to obtaining approximate physical mapping of gene loci have been used. One involves measurement of gene dosage associated with various chromosomal aberrations. For example if a region of a particular chromosome is lost or duplicated the level of gene product can be used to provide a clue as to whether a particular gene is in the affected region. The chromosomal location of genes has also been sought by making use of the strong homology between human and mouse chromosomes. Some assignments have been made by studying the effects of radiation-induced gene segregation. Often several of these methods can be used together to define the location of a particular gene. We shall review their relative importance later on in this chapter.

● High resolution physical mapping

Several steps are involved in setting out to produce a high resolution physical map of part of the genome: isolation of chromosomal DNA; fragmentation of the DNA by restriction enzymes; the production of a library of cloned fragments; the ordering of the clones to reflect the original order of the particular fragments along the chromosome; and, finally, detailed restriction enzyme analysis and sequencing of individual clones.

We considered methods for the isolation, fragmentation, and cloning of DNA in the previous chapter. If we wish to establish that any two clones contain DNA fragments that normally lie next to each other in the genome it is first necessary to prepare a DNA library in such a way that it contains partially overlapping regions of chromosomal DNA. This involves treating the DNA with a frequent-cutting restriction enzyme under conditions in which the enzyme is not allowed to cut at all possible sites. By partially digesting DNA in this way, and by generating fragment sizes that are appropriate to our cloning vector, it is possible to produce a library of overlapping DNA segments. Until recently, cosmids were the most commonly used vectors for this purpose. As mentioned later, cosmids may be superseded by yeast cloning strategies in the future.

The next step in generating a physical map depends on precisely what we want it for. In clinical genetics we will often wish to map or even sequence a region of DNA starting from a cloned gene or, more importantly in the context of this chapter, to move from an RFLP marker to a gene that we are chasing. But whatever region we wish to analyse there will usually be a starting point. The idea therefore is to build up a series of overlapping phage or cosmid clones in order to define sequences distal to our starting point, which is our gene or RFLP marker. This is called *chromosome walking*. It begins by isolating a clone from an appropriate library that contains our starting point. Often the fragment is quite large and we can make life easier by isolating subfragments from one or other end of our first clone. After mapping and orientating our cloned DNA or subfragment, and so broadly defining its structure, we can then use it to identify other clones in our library that overlap with it. By restriction enzyme mapping or sequencing our new clone we can determine which part of it overlaps with the original clone and use it to search the library for another clone, and so on. If we have used cosmid clones we might expect to be able to cover about 20–40 kb at each step of our walk.

Although it is an extremely tedious pastime, chromosome walking has allowed the fine mapping and sequencing of quite large regions of DNA. However, this approach has serious problems, of which not the least important is that the walk may come to a grinding halt. This is because we may encounter regions of DNA that contain many repetitive sequences and are therefore very difficult to clone.

Thus chromosome walking is of limited value and other methods are required to traverse the vast lengths of DNA that need to be covered to link up RFLP markers with the genes that we are looking for. Over the last few years a great deal of work has gone into the development of methods to make this easier.

● Linking up genetic and physical maps; finding human genes

As we saw earlier, linkage analysis using one or other form of RFLP may land us close to a gene in which we are interested; but 'close' usually means about 1–5 centimorgans or more! In other words we may still be several million bases away from where we want to get to. In Fig. 43 the physical and genetic maps of the human genome are compared along with the various ways that are available for analysing DNA. It is apparent that Southern blotting, cloning, and even walking are not feasible for linking up regions of DNA which are so far apart. However, in the last few years methods have been developed that make it possible to deal with DNA fragments of millions of bases or more. In addition to these new fractionation techniques better ways have been found to help us to identify specific regions of DNA which are good candidates for containing functional genes or gene families.

● Pulsed-field gel electrophoresis (PFGE)

The gels that we have described so far can only separate DNA fragments of about 20 kb. Molecules of this size have linear dimensions comparable to the pore size

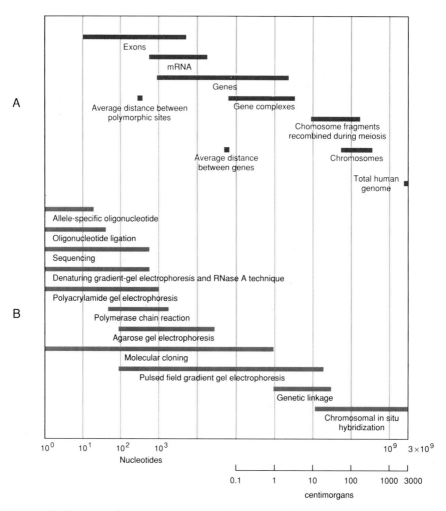

Figure 43. The size of the human genome in relationship to the various genetic and physical methods that are being applied to obtaining a map. **A** Ranges of informational units. **B** Techniques used in mapping. Modified from Landegren *et al.* (1988).

of the gel. On the other hand very large molecules, of 100–500 kb for example, are much larger or longer than the pores. However, even they can move into a gel by finding a path that involves many pores simultaneously. In this type of migration the forward force is proportional to the electric charge of the molecule, that is its length, and the drag due to friction is proportional to the number of pores through which the large molecule is passing, again being related to its length. The overall effect is that large molecules of different sizes move at the same rate and are not separated.

The principle of PFGE is periodically to change the orientation of the electric field. Every time this happens the large extended DNA molecules must reorientate and find a path through the gel matrix in another direction. This process is size dependent, that is very large molecules will take more time to reorientate than shorter ones. This remarkable phenomenon allows the resolution of DNA fragments of 100–1000 kb in size and, in some cases, even larger. The resultant gels can be blotted by standard methods (Fig. 44).

By performing a series of double digests it is possible to construct a long range restriction map of a chromosomal region. Of course this method also allows the identification of deletions and major chromosomal rearrangements.

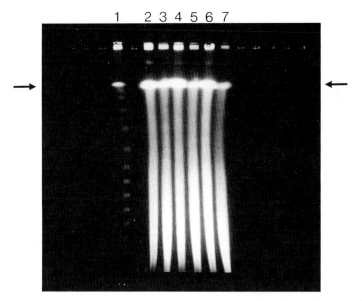

Figure 44. **Pulsed-field gel electrophoresis**. Lane 1 contains size markers in multiples of 48.5 kb. The lanes contain human DNA cut with different enzymes. The arrows show limit of resolution (600 kb). (Kindly prepared by Martin Bell.)

● Yeast cloning

The principles of yeast cloning were outlined in the previous chapter. It has been found that artificial yeast chromosomes allow stable propagation of human DNA fragments ranging in size from 100–700 kb. It should be possible, therefore, to clone a gene or a whole region of interest as one or a set of such large fragments which can then be mapped in detail or used to construct mini libraries.

● Jumping libraries

In the chromosome walking techniques that were discussed earlier every DNA fragment between our starting point and the gene that we are walking towards must be cloned and characterized. But if we are interested only in arriving at our destination why not get there by a series of 'jumps' that miss out these uninteresting regions in between. Such is the principle behind what are called jumping libraries.

The basic idea of a jumping library is illustrated in Fig. 45. Large DNA fragments are circularized so that the two extremities are brought together. If this is done in the presence of a selectable marker it should be possible to construct a library in which each clone contains nothing more than the two ends of the large DNA fragment from which it was derived. Several approaches have been used to construct libraries of this type. For example large DNA fragments have been obtained by partial digestion with an enzyme that cuts frequently. They are then sized by pulsed-field gel electrophoresis after which they are circularized and the ends cloned. Jumping libraries can be constructed starting at any location in the genome. In general about 3×10^6 clones are needed to have a high likelihood of being able to use the library from any given starting point. Smaller libraries can be constructed using enzymes that cut infrequently but this is only of value if the start of the jump is located near to a rare cutting site; this is rarely the case.

Although this method presents some formidable technical problems it has been used successfully; jumps of up to 500 kb have been achieved.

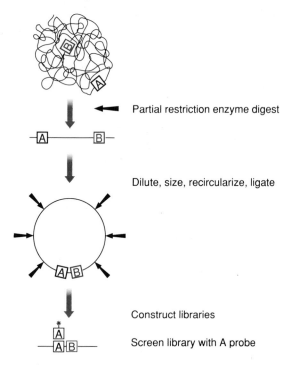

Partial restriction enzyme digest

Dilute, size, recircularize, ligate

Construct libraries

Screen library with A probe

Figure 45. The preparation of jumping library. The details of the various steps involved are described in the text.

● Using chromosome deletions for finding genes

If a single gene disorder is found in a patient with a chromosomal deletion it is reasonable to assume that the gene involved has been either completely or partially removed by the deletion. A number of ingenious techniques have been developed to try to find genes in this way and have led to the elucidation of the molecular basis for two important genetic diseases, Duchenne muscular dystrophy and chronic granulomatous disease.

The idea is to prepare libraries enriched for sequences that normally occupy the deleted region of DNA. Most of the approaches that have been developed for this purpose were based on the principle of DNA hybridization that we discussed in Chapter 3. They entail the reassociation of normal DNA in the presence of a large excess of DNA prepared from an individual with a particular deletion. Under these circumstances the sequences that reanneal together from the normal DNA but are not competed out will be those that lie in the deletion. A successful outcome depends on enhancing the rate of reassociation so that single copy sequences form hybrids. A number of methods have been developed to this end, one of the most useful being the PERT reaction, that is phenol-enhanced reassociation.

The most elegant application of this idea to date has been the isolation of sequences within the Duchenne muscular dystrophy locus on the X chromosome. This was facilitated by the identification of a patient with the disease who was found to have a deletion of about 6000 kb of the Xp21 region. The patient suffered from chronic granulomatous disease, and two other rare genetic diseases as well as muscular dystrophy. Hence it was assumed that these phenotypes are the result of loss of genes in the deleted region of DNA. Louis Kunkel and his colleagues from Boston isolated clones that lie within this deletion by a particularly ingenious competitive reannealing reaction. Essentially this involved taking normal human DNA from a cell line and cutting it into fragments with the enzyme *Mbo*I. The *Mbo*I fragments were mixed with a large excess of DNA from the patient with the deletion. The patient's DNA was fragmented by simple shearing, that is a process which leaves a variety of different broken ends. When the *Mbo*I and sheared fragments were mixed together and reannealed three types of hybrids were formed, normal with normal, abnormal with abnormal, and normal with abnormal. Since the abnormal DNA fragments were present in a large excess the only normal sequences that could reanneal together were those that were not 'competed out' by the abnormal sequences, that is those from the deletion region of DNA, present in the normal but not in the abnormal fragments. It was possible to select these hyrid molecules from the mixture because they had two *Mbo*I ends which could not be present in the hybrids between two stretches of sheared abnormal DNA or in mixed hybrids between normal and abnormal DNA. In fact *Mbo*I cuts DNA so that overlapping ends are generated which can be cloned directly into a plasmid vector cut with an appropriate restriction enzyme. In this way it was possible to enrich for the region of DNA that was deleted. Variations on this subtractive reassociation method have been used to define other regions of DNA involved in deletions.

Another approach to isolating genes that lie within deletions is to make use of messenger RNA extracted from the appropriate cells of patients with a deletion and from normal cells. Complementary DNA can be copied from these messenger RNAs and then the two are hybridized. The cDNA that does not hybridize should be that which has been derived from the normal cells and hence contains the sequences that are missing from the cell containing the deletion. By using a number of rounds of subtractive hybridization of this type it is possible to prepare cDNA which can then be labelled and used to identify DNA segments in normal genomic DNA containing the gene that is missing from the deleted DNA. This approach has been used to identify the gene that is involved in chronic granulomatous disease.

The value of using a cytogenic abnormality to find an important gene has been underlined again recently by the isolation of the gene for neurofibromatosis, type 1. The gene for this defect had been mapped genetically to 17q 11.2. By using data derived from two patients with this condition with balanced translocations involving this region, it was possible to further narrow the candidate interval, and by additional jumping techniques, a large gene was defined which contained the breakpoint of both these deletions. The function of these gene remains to be determined.

● Chromosome mediated gene transfer

As mentioned in Chapter 4 it is possible, using selectable markers, to transfer human chromosomes into mammalian recipient cells. This method can be scaled down to isolate small regions of chromosomes, so-called transgenomes, for detailed analysis. For example, it has been possible to augment regions of human chromosome 11p using the Harvey-*ras* oncogene as the appropriate marker. Similarly, attempts have been made to isolate the gene involved in cystic fibrosis; in this case the *Met* oncogene was used as a selectable marker for the appropriate region of chromosome 7. While this technique is quite useful it suffers from the disadvantage that the transfer procedure may be followed by rearrangements of DNA sequences or, even more troublesome, by the co-transfer of so-called non-syntenic DNA, i.e. sequences that do not reside on the same chromosome as the marker gene used in the somatic cell hybridization.

● Identifying regions of DNA as likely candidates for the gene of interest

In mapping the large pieces of DNA derived by these new methods it is helpful to have landmarks to direct us to functional genes. One particularly valuable development has been the identification of co-called HTF islands. These are regions of DNA in the human genome that are CpG-rich and yet are unmethylated. They are identified because they form a series of tiny fragments after digestion with the enzyme *Hpa*II, which only cuts unmethylated but not methylated sites; HTF stands for *Hpa*II-tiny-fragments. In fact many enzymes that cut infrequently have CpG in their recognition sites and are methylation-sensitive; the observation of a cluster of these sites is indicative of an HTF island.

It turns out that HTF islands mark the 5′ and 3′ ends of genes. Therefore they can be used to identify potential candidate genes in fragments of DNA obtained from appropriate chromosomal regions.

● Reverse genetics

There is still no adequate biochemical explanation for the clinical phenotypes of many single gene disorders. And often there are no animal models that mimic these diseases. Until the advent of recombinant DNA technology it always seemed as if the underlying cause of these conditions would remain an intractable problem. It is for the elucidation of the molecular pathology and pathophysiology of these disorders that the idea of reverse genetics has been developed.

In the previous sections we have seen how it may be possible to find the approximate location of a gene for a disorder of this type and then move along the chromosome until we reach the particular locus. Occasionally, we may be fortunate and come across a patient with the particular phenotype and find a chromosome deletion that may land us in the appropriate spot without having to go through this tedious process. Having found our gene in this way the next step is to sequence it and then try to make an educated guess as to its function by working out its probable amino acid sequence from the DNA sequence. This is the essence of reverse genetics (Fig. 46).

Although this idea is extremely attractive it has not been so easy to apply in practice. In fact it is now over five years since the locus for Huntington's disease was defined by RFLP linkage analysis, and yet the gene that is involved has still not been found. Indeed, until the last few months no genes had been identified after assignment by RFLP linkage analysis. Rather, the first success stories of reverse genetics relied on the chance finding of a patient with a deletion associated with a particular phenotype.

● Duchenne muscular dystrophy

The partial elucidation of the molecular basis for Duchenne muscular dystrophy (DMD) was the first successful application of reverse genetics. The initial clue to the localization of the DMD gene came from the observation of females affected with the disease who had balanced X/autosome translocations. Although the autosomal breakpoints were different in each case the X chromosome breaks lay within the region Xp21. This suggested that this region of the X chromosome might contain the DMD gene. Such localization was confirmed by linkage

Establish linkage

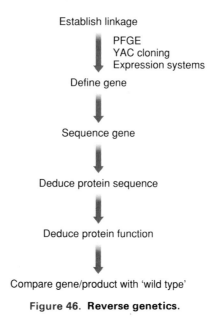

Figure 46. **Reverse genetics.**

studies using RFLPs flanking the Xp21 band. The RFLPs segregated in the same way in families with DMD and also in those with the milder condition, Becker muscular dystrophy. This suggested that the two phenotypes might result from mutations at the same locus.

Clones were isolated from within the DMD locus by genomic enrichment using DNA from a patient with a deletion within Xp21 who suffered from DMD, chronic granulomatous disease, retinitis pigmentosa, and another rare condition called the McLeod syndrome. The way in which clones were enriched for sequences in the deleted DNA was describe in an earlier section. One of six fragments derived from the Xp21 region (called pERT87) detected DNA deletions in a proportion of patients with DMD and was tightly linked to the disease in family studies. Approximately 200 kb of contiguous DNA in the pERT87 region, later called the DXS164 locus, was isolated by extensive chromosome walking. It turned out that breakpoints found in DMD patients were spread heterogeneously over the entire expanse of this region.

The next step was to search for RNA transcripts of the suspected DMD gene. To this end non-repetitive DNA segments within DXS164 were screened to see whether any of them were highly conserved across different species, a process called 'zoo blotting'. One particular region, located 70 kb distal to the original pERT87 clone, hybridized at high stringency with chicken as well as rodent and primate DNA. Sequencing of the homologous human and mouse segments disclosed an exon bounded by splicing signals. A probe against this region detected a large RNA species in human fetal muscle which was absent from several other tissues. Pulsed field gel electrophoresis of this 14 kb DMD mRNA covers a distance of at least 2.3 million bases, making this the largest gene complex so far defined. Antisera raised against expressed portions of the gene sequence cross-react with a 400 000 kD protein in adult and fetal muscle. This molecule has been called dystrophin, because its absence causes muscular dystrophy. Subsequent studies on the expression of the gene and its product showed that many patients with DMD do not produce any dystrophin at all, or very little, in their muscle cells whereas in the milder Becker muscular dystrophy some truncated protein products are produced. This suggests that Becker muscular dystrophy is due to the synthesis of lower molecular weight proteins which still retain some function in muscle. This finding does not hold for all cases however; the reason for the heterogeneity of clinical phenotypes associated with lesions of the DMD locus remains to be determined.

Dystrophin is estimated to correspond to only about 0.002 per cent of the total protein in a muscle cell, which probably explains why conventional biochemical techniques have been unable to demonstrate its absence in patients with muscular dystrophy. The molecule has domains that show homology with actin and spectrin. Recent immunological and messenger RNA analyses suggest that the DMD gene is expressed in both muscle and brain and that it is developmentally regulated in myogenic cells. But despite these studies the precise function of dystrophin remains to be determined.

The discovery of dystrophin by reverse genetics is a splendid vindication of the concept that genetic diseases of unknown aetiology can be tackled by first finding the gene and then working back to its product. Of course, finding the gene also enables us to proceed to determine the precise molecular pathology underlying the condition; we shall describe in more detail the types of molecular lesions that affect the DMD gene in the next chapter.

● Chronic granulomatous disease

Another and as yet incomplete success story in the field of reverse genetics is the determination of the gene involved in X-linked chronic granulomatous disease (CGD). This condition is characterized by defective phagocytic cell function and a marked susceptibility to infection. It has been known for a long time that the process of bacterial killing by macrophages and other phagocytic cells depends on superoxide generation by a membrane-bound NADPH-oxidase system. However, because of the considerable technical difficulties involved it was never possible to define the components of this system, at least until recently. Like Duchenne muscular dystrophy the gene for CGD was isolated by finding a patient with the condition who also had a deletion of the X chromosome, in fact the same deletion that was used to isolate the DMD gene.

The way in which the gene for CGD was defined by isolating its mRNA transcript was described earlier. When the predicted primary amino acid sequence derived from cDNA was compared with other proteins no significant homologies were noted, and in particular there was no obvious similarity to any of the cytochromes. Indeed, such homologies as were hinted at were more consistent with a membrane localization of the gene product. However, soon after this sequence was published two groups independently managed to purify the elusive neutrophil cytochrome b. It turned out that this molecule consists of a large glycosylated subunit of about 90 kd and a smaller, non-glycosylated polypeptide of 22 kd. Further studies demonstrated conclusively that the product of the CGD locus and the heavy chain of the neutrophil cytochrome b were one and the same. More recent studies have shown that this gene and the gene for the small subunit are expressed independently. Although the molecular pathology of the CGD gene is not yet worked out, and the precise functional interrelationship between the two subunits of cytochrome b remains unclear, it turns out that gamma interferon is able to increase the production of the large subunit of cytochrome b, at least in some patients with CGD. It is assumed, therefore, that these patients have mutations that permit the synthesis of some cytochrome b heavy chain, and that these lesions can be partly overcome by the stimulation of cytochrome b with interferon.

● Cystic fibrosis

The recent announcement of the probable isolation of the gene for cystic fibrosis (CF) is the final vindication of the 'new genetics', that is the notion that it is possible to obtain a linkage for a genetic disease of unknown cause, move along the chromosome, find the gene, sequence it and determine the molecular basis for the disease and, finally, define the gene product by reverse genetics.

First, using standard linkage markers it was found that the CF locus is on chromosome 7. The position on this chromosome was further defined by placing it between flanking markers called *MET* and *D7S8*, so defining a region of DNA of $1–2 \times 10^6$ bp. Subsequently further markers that mapped between *MET* and *D7S8* were found. Using these as starting points this large region of DNA was explored by the jumping techniques described earlier in this chapter. Ultimately a candidate gene was reached. This sequence was found to be highly conserved across species, a good indicator that it codes for something important! After considerable difficulty a complete sequence was obtained and found to differ between normal individuals and CF patients only by the deletion of a particular triplet that codes for phenylalanine in the CF DNA.

The protein sequence derived from the DNA sequence of the CF gene suggests that it is related to a family of ATP-dependent transport systems. The best characterized of this family are the bacterial transporters known as the periplasmic or binding-protein-dependent transport systems. Over 20 such systems are known, each specific for a different substrate, including amino acid, sugar, peptide, or inorganic ion. It turns out that the CF mutation is in an ATP binding domain. Since the viscid mucus that underlies the lung and gastrointestinal symptoms of CF may reflect a defect in chloride transport it seems likely that the basic molecular lesion has been found. In addition, it turns out that the transport system involved is also related to the multi-drug-resistance gene that is involved in resistance to cancer chemotherapy; the basic biological significance of these findings may be profound.

Since the first discovery of the CF gene, now known as the CF transmembrane conductance regulator (CFTR) gene, further work on its structure has been carried out and many groups have studied the prevalence and heterogeneity of its mutations in different populations. The CFTR gene is about 250 kb in length and contains 27 exons. It has two membrane-spanning domains, two ATP binding domains, and a region of unknown function which, since it may have some regulatory role, has been called the R domain. It turns out that the loss of the phenylalanine residue in the 10th exon of the CFTR gene occurs in about 70 per cent of CF chromosomes. Already a number of other mutations have been described including a frameshift in exon 11, nonsense mutations in exon 4 which includes the transmembrane domain, a number of different nonsense mutations involving exon 11 near the ATP-binding domain, and four different deletions or insertions, again involving the ATP-binding domains. Very recently a two nucleotide insertion in exon 13 has been found; this region includes the R domain. There is some early indication that, as judged by RFLP haplotype analysis, it may be possible to separate mutations that cause pancreatic insufficiency from those that are associated with normal pancreatic function.

These early success stories, and others that we will come across in later chapters, leave little doubt that at least in some cases it will be possible to work back from a gene to its product and hence to the molecular basis for a genetic disease; reverse genetics is possible.

● Future directions for genome mapping

In this brief account of the new approaches to gene hunting we have seen how the use of RFLPs has been unexpectedly successful in pin-pointing the chromosomal location of a number of genes for different diseases, the cause of which is unknown. We have also seen how, following these early successes, the field has slowed down because of our inability to move from RFLP markers to the genes that we are interested in. This has led to the development of new techniques which are starting to solve some of these problems. The success stories of muscular dystrophy, chronic granulomatous disease, and cystic fibrosis make it quite clear that once we have found individual genes that underlie diseases we should be able to define their products and hence the molecular basis for the particular illness. Hopefully, there will be other conditions like chronic granulomatous disease in which we will have the added bonus of developing a therapeutic strategy, even before we fully understand what is going on at the molecular level.

On the other hand, even allowing for the enormous strength of the newer techniques for working with large fragments of DNA, the difficulties of identifying individual genes as the basis for a particular genetic disorder should not be underestimated. These fragments may contain many structural genes and the central question is how do we identify the particular one that we are looking for. This question will arise again in a later chapter when we consider the use of RFLP linkage for the identification of genes that contribute towards common polygenic conditions. Undoubtedly many approaches will be required, some opportunistic, others relying on nothing but hard work.

Occasionally we may be able to make an educated guess at a likely candidate gene. For example, finding a linkage to one form of elliptocytosis and the Rh locus, and then discovering that an important red cell membrane protein, band 4.1, is close to the Rh locus, led to the elucidation of the molecular basis for one form of this condition. Subsequently it was discovered that a second type of elliptocytosis is linked to the Duffy blood group and, again, that the locus for the latter is close to that for α spectrin, another important red cell membrane protein. This in turn led to the definition of the molecular basis for a second type of elliptocytosis. Similarly, the finding that the form of diffuse cerebral sclerosis known as the Pelizaeus–Merzbacher syndrome is associated with an interstitial deletion at Xq22, together with the observation that the myelin proteolipid protein (PLP) gene is in this band, made the PLP gene a very likely candidate for the site of the mutation in this syndrome. In fact the PLP gene has been found to be altered in patients with this disorder; in one case a C→T transition, leading to a proline to serine substitution, has been demonstrated. There are several other examples where it was possible to go straight to a candidate gene in this way.

If our RFLP linkage simply leaves us with a long uncharted track of DNA with no obvious candidate genes in the region, how are we to proceed? Of course we might be lucky and find an obvious deletion of the region involved, by pulsed field gel electrophoresis for example, but this will not often be the case. A more general approach may be to use sequences generated from the approximate region that we are investigating in order to search for mRNA sequences in the particular tissue where the genetic defect is expressed, sweat glands or gut in the case of cystic fibrosis and the developing kidney in adult polycystic kidney disease, for example. Clearly, no one approach can be used to solve these difficult problems; the wide variety of different techniques that were needed finally to define the muscular dystrophy locus, even when there was a deletion to pin-point the region of DNA, emphasizes how much hard work will be involved in finding genes in this way.

Undoubtedly the future of chromosome mapping and the isolation of genes for diseases lies in the application of a number of different methods. It is interesting to reflect that, of the 1100 autosomal loci mapped by the end of 1988, nearly 100 had been assigned by two or more methods, and that somatic cell hybridization and *in situ* hybridization were by far the most productive techniques used. This observation, together with some indication of the wide range of methods applied are summarized in Table 18. It appears, therefore, that the future lies in improving our molecular technology while at the same time making full use of the wide range of methods of conventional somatic cell genetics and cytogenetics.

It is these early successes with RFLPs that have focused the attention of the world of human molecular biology on the idea of mapping the whole of the

Table 18. *Methods used to map autosomal loci (figures up to Nov. 1, 1987; modified from McKusick 1988)*

Method	No. of loci mapped
Somatic cell hybridization	747
In situ hybridization	337
Family linkage studies	314
Dosage effect	107
Chromosomal defects	80
Homology of synteny	66
RFLP	57
Radiation-induced segregation analysis	18
Others	94
Total (many by more than one method)	1820

human genome. As mentioned earlier, we are already fairly close to having a useful genetic map, and it is the strategies for physical mapping of the human genome that are now being widely discussed. The first step will be to analyse its overall organization by obtaining a complete set of overlapping clones, as mentioned earlier. This would provide a framework along which the regions defining products of particular interest could be identified long before the complete nucleotide sequence was determined. Some recent technical developments, described in Chapter 11, promise to make this feasible. Since the sequence of genetic regions of functional importance may constitute as little as one-tenth of the total genome, this goal may be achievable within the next ten or twenty years. Filling in the remainder will not be a very exciting pastime and may well have to wait until automation is much further advanced. We shall return to this topic in Chapter 11, and also to the vexed question of the level of priority that should be given the human genome sequencing projects.

● Further reading

Bodmer, W.F. and Cavalli-Sforza, L.L. (1976). *Genetics, evolution and man.* W.H. Freeman, San Francisco, CA.

Botstein, D., White, R.L., Skolnick, M. and Davies, R.W. (1980). Construction of a genetic linkage map in Man using restriction fragment length polymorphisms. *Am. J. Hum. Genet.*, **32**, 314–31.

Chamberlain, S., Shaw, J., Rowland, A., *et al.* (1988). Mapping of the mutation causing Friedreich's ataxia to human chromosome 9. *Nature*, **334**, 248–9.

Collins, F.S. (1988). Jumping libraries. In *Genome analysis*, (ed. K.E. Davies) IRL Press, Oxford.

Collins, F.S., Ponder, B.A.J., Seizinger, B.R., and Epstein, C.J. (1989). The von

Recklinghausen neurofibromatosis region on chromosome 17—genetic and physical maps come into focus. *Am. J. Hum. Genet.*, **44**, 1–5.

Davies, K.E. (ed.) (1986). *Human genetic diseases: A practical approach.* IRL Press, Oxford.

Davies, K.E. (ed.) (1988). *Genome analysis.* IRL Press, Oxford.

Davies, K.E. and Read, A.P. (1988). *Molecular basis of inherited disease.* IRL Press, Oxford.

Donis-Keller, H., Green, P., Helms, C., *et al.* (1987). A genetic linkage map of the human genome. *Cell*, **51**, 319–37.

Emanuel, B.S. (1988). Molecular cytogenetics: towards dissection of the contiguous gene syndromes. *Am. J. Hum. Gent.*, **43**, 575–8.

Gusella, J.F., Wexler, N.S., Conneally, P.M., *et al.* (1983). A polymorphic DNA marker genetically linked to Huntington's chorea. *Nature*, **306**, 234–8.

Hoffman, E.P., Brown, R.H. Jr., and Kunkel, L.M. (1987). Dystrophin: the protein product of the Duchenne muscular dystrophy locus. *Cell*, **51**, 919–28.

Jeffreys, A.J., Wilson, V., and Thein, S.L. (1985). Hypervariable 'minisatellite' regions in human DNA. *Nature*, **314**, 67–73.

Kerem, B.-T., Rommens, J.M., Buchanan, J.A., Markiewicz, D., Cox, T.K., Chakravarti, A., Buchwald, M., and Tsui, L.-C. (1989). Identification of the cystic fibrosis gene: genetic analysis. *Science*, **245**, 1073–80.

Koenig, M., Hoffman, E.P., Bertelson, C.J., Monaco, A.P., Feener, C., and Kunkel, L.M. (1987). Complete cloning of the Duchenne muscular dystrophy (DMD) cDNA and preliminary genomic organization of the DMD gene in normal and affected individuals. *Cell*, **50**, 509–17.

Landegren, U., Kaiser, R., Caskey, C.T., and Hood, L.H. (1988). DNA diagnosis—molecular techniques and automation. *Science*, **242**, 229–37.

Lander, E.S. and Botstein, D. (1986). Mapping complex genetic traits in humans: new strategies using a complete RFLP linkage map. *Cold Spring Harbor Symp. Quant. Biol.*, **51**, 49–62.

McKusick, V.A. (1988). *The morbid anatomy of the human genome.* Howard Hughes Medical Institute, Bethesda, MD.

Meissen, G.J., Myers, R.H., Mastromauro, C.A., *et al.* (1988). Predictive testing for Huntington's disease with use of a linked DNA marker. *New Engl. J. Med.*, **318**, 535–42.

Monaco, A.P. (1989). Dystrophin, the protein product of the Duchenne/Becker muscular dystrophy gene. *Trends Biochem.*, **14**, 412–15.

Nakamura, Y., Leppert, M., O'Connell, P., *et al.* (1987). Variable number of tandem repeat (VNTR) markers for human gene mapping. *Science*, **235**, 1616–22.

Olsen, M., Hood, L., Cantor, C., and Botstein, D. (1989). A common language for mapping the human genome. *Science*, **245**, 1434–5.

Patten, J.L., Johns, D.R., and Valle, D., *et al.* (1990). Mutation in a gene encoding the stimulatory G proteins of adenylate cyclase in Albright's hereditary osteodystrophy. *New England Journal of Medicine*, **322**, 1412–19.

Reeders, S.T., Breuning, M.H., Davies, K.E., *et al.* (1985). A highly polymorphic DNA marker linked to adult polycystic kidney disease on chromosome 16. *Nature*, **317**, 542–4.

Reeders, S.T., Germino, G.G., and Gillespie, G.A.J. (1989). Recent advances in the genetics of renal cystic disease. *Mol. Biol. Med.*, **6**, 81–6.

Riordan, J.R., Rommens, J.M., Kerem, B.-S., *et al.* (1989). Identifiation of the cystic fibrosis gene: cloning and characterization of complementary DNA. *Science*, **245**, 1066–73.

Robson, E.B. (1988). The human gene map. *Phil. Trans. R. Soc. Lond. B.*, **319**, 229–37.

Rommens, J.M., Iannuzzi, M.C., Kerem, B.-S., *et al.* (1989). Identification of the cystic fibrosis gene: chromosome walking and jumping. *Science*, **245**, 1059–65.

Southern, E.M. (1988). Prospects for a complete molecular map of the human genome. *Phil. Trans. R. Soc. Lond. B.*, **319**, 299–307.

Tsui, L.-C. (1989). Tracing the mutations in cystic fibrosis by means of closely linked DNA markers. *Am. J. Hum. Genet.*, **44**, 303–6.

US Congress, Office of Technology Assessment (1988). *Mapping our genes—The genomic project: How big, how fast?* US Government Printing Office, Washington, DC.

Wallace, M.R., *et al.* (1990). Type 1 neurofibromatosis gene: identification of a large transcript disrupted in three NF1 patients. *Science*, **249**, 181–6.

White, M.B., Amos, J., Hsu, J.M.C., *et al.* (1990). A frame-shift mutation in the cystic fibrosis gene. *Nature*, **334**, 665–7.

White, R., Leppert, M., O'Connell, P., *et al.* (1985). Construction of human genetic linkage maps. I. Progress and perspectives. *Cold Spring Harbor Symp. Quant. Biol.*, **51**, 29–38.

Wyman, A.R. and White, R. (1980). A highly polymorphic locus in human DNA. *Proc. Natl. Acad. Sci. USA*, **77**, 6754–8.

The molecular pathology of single gene disorders

6

In 1945 a conversation took place on an overnight train between Denver and Chicago which was to have far-reaching consequences for human genetics. The participants were Linus Pauling, the distinguished protein chemist, and William Castle, the haematologist from Boston whose earlier work had played a major role in leading to an understanding of the cause of pernicious anaemia. Castle told Pauling that he and his colleagues had noticed that, in the deoxygenated state, the cells of patients with sickle cell anaemia show birefringence in polarized light. This, he suggested, might mean that the haemoglobin of these cells is undergoing some kind of molecular alignment or orientation. Pauling realized that this might be telling us that the defect in sickle cell anaemia is within the haemoglobin molecule and he suggeted to one of his young colleagues, Harvey Itano, that this could be an interesting research project. How right he was! In 1949 Pauling, Itano, and their colleagues announced that the haemoglobin of patients with sickle cell anaemia has a different rate of migration in an electric field to that of normal individuals. This, they reasoned, must mean that the net charges of the two molecules are different and hence that there must be a difference in their amino acid constitution. Hence Pauling and his colleagues invented the term 'molecular disease' to describe sickle cell anaemia.

The confirmation of these predictions came in 1956 when Vernon Ingram found that sickle cell haemoglobin differs from normal haemoglobin by a single amino acid substitution, valine for glutamic acid. At about the same time it was found that this substitution involves one of the pair of globin peptide chains that constitute adult haemoglobin. This finding provided direct evidence in support of the one-gene-one-enzyme (or in this case peptide chain) concept, intimated in his Croonian Lectures in 1908 by Archibald Garrod and later put on a solid experimental footing by the classical studies on *Neurospora* of Beadle and Tatum.

It was these seminal findings that led to the widespread use of electrophoresis, that is the study of the movement of proteins in an electrical field, as an analytical tool for examining human proteins, both in health and disease. It soon became apparent that nearly all of them are remarkably polymorphic and that at least some of this variability is reflected in defective function and hence in disease.

However, as information relating the structural variability of proteins to disease slowly amassed it became apparent that many genetic disorders are not due to the production of a structurally abnormal protein but, rather, are the result of a reduced output of a particular protein. This led to the notion that these diseases are caused by mutations that interfere with the regulation of the rate of protein synthesis. Little further progress was made until it became possible to apply the methods of recombinant DNA technology to study the fine structure of human genes, as outlined in previous chapters.

As we have seen, in the late 1970s methods became available for isolating mRNA, for producing gene probes, and for cloning and sequencing human genes. These new tools were soon applied to the study of single gene disorders, notably the thalassaemias and other genetic diseases of haemoglobin production. It was no accident that these conditions were among the first to be studied in detail by the new tools of molecular biology. After all, much was known about their genetic transmission and many of them had already been defined as being due to single amino acid substitutions in one or other of the globin chains of haemoglobin. It was already apparent that the thalassaemias were a ready-made model for defining disorders due to a reduced rate of production of a protein, in this case either the α or β chains of haemoglobin. In the relatively short time since the first globin genes were sequenced a great deal has been learnt about the molecular pathology of monogenic diseases. Indeed, it seems likely that we already have a relatively complete picture of the repertoire of the types of underlying molecular lesions.

It turns out that the majority of these conditions result from simple mutations that involve structural genes and interfere with their transcription or with the processing or translation of their products. The 'old' theories, that disorders resulting from a reduced output of a protein or enzyme are due to regulatory mutations, have had to be revised; most of these conditions can be explained satisfactorily by point mutations or deletions that modify the output from a mutant locus.

● Types and levels of abnormal gene expression

In an earlier chapter we saw how gene action is reflected by a regulated flow of information reflecting the transcription of structural genes into messenger RNA (mRNA) precursors, a complicated series of steps involving processing of the large precursor molecules into definitive mRNAs and, finally, cytoplasmic translation of mRNA into a protein product. Although the mutations that underlie single gene disorders must be present in the DNA of the structural gene involved, they may manifest themselves at any of these levels (Fig. 47). That is, there may be a reduced rate of transcription of a gene, a variety of abnormalities involving the processing of mRNA precursors, defects of initiation, translation, or termination of the synthesis of the protein product on the cytoplasmic mRNA template, or an abnormality in the structure of the gene product.

By and large, mutations that produce disease are manifest in two ways. First, a single base substitution or more subtle rearrangement of a gene may alter the structure of the mRNA such that an abnormal protein product is synthesized. If this alters the charge on the protein molecule it will be reflected by a change in its electrophoretic pattern. However, it should be remembered that many amino acid substitutions are neutral, that is they do not change the net charge of the

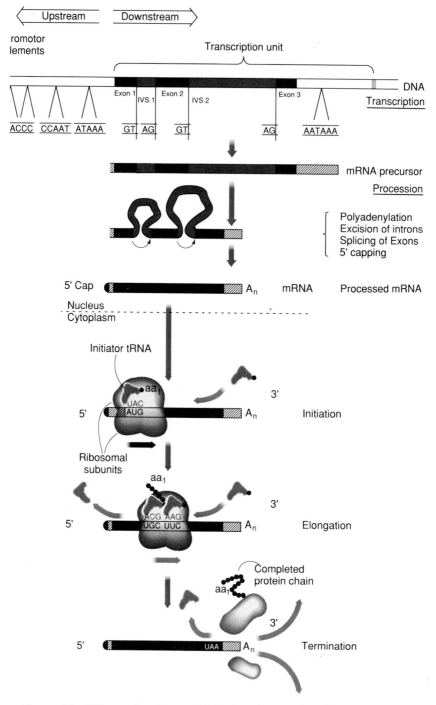

Figure 47. **Different levels at which the phenotypic effects of mutations are mediated.**

protein and therefore cannot be detected by electrophoresis. But, regardless of the type of substitution, if it changes the function or stability of the protein it usually results in an abnormal phenotype. The second group of mutations are those that cause a reduction or absence of a particular protein product. It is now apparent that this latter class of disorders may result from mutations that involve transcription or processing of mRNA or that act at the translational level by interfering with initiation, elongation, or termination.

Table 19. *Types of mutations that underlie single gene disorders*

Reduced output of gene product	Synthesis of an abnormal gene product
Transcription	Mis-sense mutations (point mutations)
Insertions	Fusion genes
Deletion or partial deletion	Insertions
Promotor box mutations	Deletions
Other regulatory mutations	Elongated products
Processing of messenger RNA	Chain termination mutations
Mutations involving splicing	Frameshift mutations
PolyA addition site mutations	Defective post-translational modification
Translation	
Mutations involving initiation, elongation, or termination	

Unfortunately no biological classifications are entirely satisfactory. For example, it turns out that some disorders that appear to result from defective synthesis of a particular protein are actually caused by the production of a structurally abnormal protein which is so unstable that its level in the cell is markedly reduced; in some cases there may be no detectable protein product at all. And as we shall see later, structural abnormalities of proteins may have even more subtle effects on their final level in the cell. An overall classification of the major molecular mechanisms that underlie monogenic diseases together with some well-characterized examples is shown in Table 19.

In the sections that follow we shall consider examples of each of these different types of mutations. Because they were the first to be characterized we shall start with the protein variants that result from point mutations or more subtle rearrangements of their genes. We shall then consider the more heterogeneous basis for disorders that result from a reduced output of a protein.

● Monogenic disorders resulting from the synthesis of an abnormal protein

The majority of monogenic disorders that result from the synthesis of a structurally abnormal protein reflect single base mutations in the parent genes.

There are a few examples of structural variants that are caused by much more extensive defects of genes, in particular major rearrangements that lead to the formation of fusion genes that code for novel protein products. Originally these mutations were defined by the standard methods of protein chemistry. More recently it has been possible to deduce the structural changes in proteins from analysis of their parent genes.

● Point mutations producing abnormal protein products

Much of our early knowledge about the protean manifestations of single base substitutions and other mutations on human gene function was derived from the abnormal haemoglobin field. In the following sections I shall describe the different structural haemoglobin variants that result from single base mis-sense substitutions, or more subtle changes, and some examples of other single gene disorders that have arisen by similar mechanisms.

● General considerations

The genetic control of the structure of human haemoglobin was described in Chapter 3. The inherited disorders of haemoglobin fall into three groups. First there are the structural haemoglobin variants. Second, there are the thalassaemias, which are characterized by a reduced rate of production of either the α or β globin chains and which are therefore divided into the α and β thalassaemias. Finally, there is a clinically unimportant group of conditions in which there is a defect in the normal switch from fetal to adult haemoglobin production, hereditary persistence of fetal haemoglobin.

Over 400 human structural haemoglobin variants have been described, of which 95 per cent are due to single amino acid substitutions in the α or β globin chains. All of those identified so far are consistent with a single base substitution in the corresponding triplet codon of the globin gene DNA and, of course, in its corresponding mRNA sequence. For descriptive purposes it is usual to describe the nucleotide sequence changes created in the transcription product of a gene, that is its mRNA. This custom will be adhered to throughout this chapter though it should be remembered that this change will be the result of a corresponding base change in the DNA sequence of the particular structural gene.

In describing the haemoglobin variants it should be remembered that originally they were named by letters of the alphabet, but because these were soon used up it became customary to designate them by their place of discovery. This convention is now used to name many other protein variants, prothrombin Barcelona or fibrinogen Baltimore, for example. It must be admitted, however, that usage is not entirely consistent. Names of abnormal haemoglobins range from the exotic (haemoglobin Aida), through the chauvinistic (haemoglobin Bart's or Brigham) or parochial (haemoglobin Riverdale–Bronx), to the patriotic (haemoglobin Abraham Lincoln) and even the poetic (haemoglobin Constant Spring). The position of the mutation is described by numbering from the amino-terminal end, i.e. β6 is the sixth amino acid residue along the β chain.

As we have seen, most haemoglobin variants reflect single base changes in the α or β globin chain genes. For example, haemoglobins Rainier (β145 Tyr→Cys), Bethesda (β145 Tyr→His) and Fort Gordon (β145 Tyr→Asp) can all be explained by a different single base substitution in the triplet UAU, which codes for tyrosine at position 145 in the normal β globin chain gene. A few variants have been found that have amino acid replacements at two different sites on the same globin chain. Three of these involve the haemoglobin S substitution (β6 Glu→ Val). These variants could have arisen by one of two mechanisms; a new mutation on a variant (β^S) gene or a crossover between two variant genes.

It can be calculated that there are 2583 potential single base substitutions for the 141 residues of the α chain and the 146 residues of the β chain. Of these, 1690 would result in an amino acid replacement, but only a third would cause a change in charge which would allow the abnormal haemoglobin to be identified by electrophoresis. Remarkably, about 45 per cent of these potential variants have already been discovered.

As we saw in Chapter 3, the genetic code shows ambiguity of nucleotide sequences; several different codons can code for any particular amino acid. Interestingly, there are several abnormal haemoglobins, of which the structure suggests that there is limited ambiguity of the nucleotide sequence of the codons for the human globin genes. For example, haemoglobins Koln and San Diego result from the replacement of valine by methionine at positions 98 and 109 in the β globin gene, respectively. There is only one codon for methionine, AUG, but there are four possible codons for valine, GUG, GUA, GUC, or GUU. The methionine codon AUG could only derive from a single base substitution in one of the four possible valine codons, GUG, in which the first G is substituted by A. There are similar examples that suggest there is only limited mRNA codon ambiguity. In fact it turns out that most, if not all, individuals share a unique nucleotide sequence for their β globin genes, with little or no variability in the nucleotide sequence at the third position of various codons. Although subsequent sequence analysis of globin genes and their messenger RNAs have shown some individual variability it is, as was mentioned in the previous chapter, remarkably small. It is not yet known whether this rule applies to all human structural genes.

● Consequences of point mutations for protein structure

Most point mutations do not alter the structure of a protein except for a single amino acid substitution. Although this may profoundly alter the function of the protein its overall structure only differs from the 'wild-type' protein by the single amino acid replacement. There are exceptions, however. Occasionally, substitutions may involve the chain termination or initiation codons, or may scramble the genetic code such that either elongated or shortened peptide chain products are produced. Again, the best studied examples that we have so far are from the haemoglobin field.

Elongated peptide chains

Some human haemoglobin variants are characterized by elongation of either the α or β globin chains. These extended gene products result from one of three different mechanisms; base substitutions in the chain termination codon, frameshift mutations, or the preservation of the initiator methionine residue.

The first abnormal haemoglobin with an elongated subunit to be characterized was haemoglobin Constant Spring (named after a suburb of Kingston, Jamaica, the home of the first family to have the variant sequenced). The α chain of this variant is elongated at its C-terminus by an additional 31 amino acid residues. The fact that the elongated portion does not resemble any part of the normal α chain sequence suggested that it had not arisen from a crossover between two adjacent α genes. In fact it results from a single base mutation in the α chain termination codon, UAA to CAA which is the codon for glutamine. This substitution leads to the insertion of glutamine instead of the α globin chain terminating at its usual position at 141. The additional residues attached to the C-terminal end mean that the α globin mRNA continues to be translated through a region that is not normally utilized until another in-phase stop codon is reached (Fig. 48). The result is an α chain with 31 additional residues at the C-terminal end.

The notion that single base substitutions in a chain termination codon can give rise to an elongated α chain has interesting implications. It was predicted, and soon confirmed, that other variants might exist, with different substitutions in the chain termination codon but with identical residues in their elongated C-terminal ends (Fig. 48). For example, haemoglobin Icaria has an identical structure to

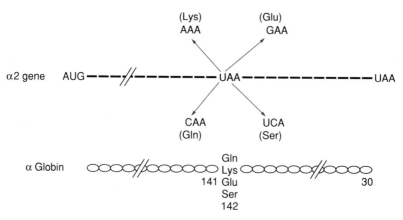

Figure 48. The α globin chain termination mutants.

haemoglobin Constant Spring except that position 142 contains lysine instead of glutamine; this reflects the change UAA→AAA rather than UAA→CAA. In fact a family of elongated α globin chain variants has been discovered, all of which result from single base substitutions in the α chain termination codon UAA (Fig. 48). The α chain termination mutations are all produced at a reduced rate, and give rise to the phenotype of α thalassaemia. We shall return to this topic later.

Another mechanism for producing an elongated peptide chain was worked out after the discovery of a variant called haemoglobin Wayne. This also has an elongated α chain, in this case identical to normal α chains up to residue 138, after which it differs by having a unique sequence of eight amino acids, thus extending beyond the length of the α chain by five residues. The mechanism that underlies this variant is illustrated in Fig. 49. A deletion of one base, either C at codon 138 or A at codon 139, results in a frameshift, i.e. a single base is lost and the reading frame of the genetic code is completely altered beyond this point. As shown in Fig. 49 the α chain termination codon UAA is thrown out of phase, and translation thus continues until an in-phase termination codon is encountered. There are several other haemoglobin variants in which elongated chains result from frameshifts of this type.

Yet another haemoglobin variant has been discovered, called Grady, in which there is an elongated α chain. In this case there appears to have been internal duplication of part of the sequence of the α globin gene. Between positions 118 and 119 there is the sequence Glu-Phe-Thr which is preceded by an identical sequence, indicating a simple internal duplication. It seems likely that this has

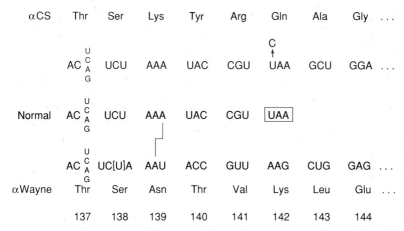

Figure 49. **The mechanism of production of the elongated α chain variants, haemoglobins Constant Spring and Wayne.** In the case of haemoglobin Constant Spring there has been a single base change in the chain termination codon. In the case of haemoglobin Wayne it is assumed that there has been loss of one of the bases of the codon which normally codes for serine at position 138. This has resulted in a frame shift such that the sequence of the α chain is elongated up to residue 146 after which it is terminated by the generation of a chain termination codon UAG.

resulted from abnormal and unequal crossing-over between either allelic α chain genes or between different α chain loci. We shall return to the mechanisms of insertions later in this chapter.

So far, we have considered haemoglobin variants with elongated globin chains that are either extended at their C-terminal ends or in which there has been an internal insertion. However, it turns out that there is another family of variants that are elongated at their amino-terminal end. For example, haemoglobin Long Island differs from haemoglobin A in two respects; the second position in the β chain contains proline instead of histidine, and there is a methionine residue at the N-terminal end of the β chain next to valine which is the usual first residue in this chain; the amino-terminal sequence is thus Met-Val-Pro-Leu instead of the normal Val-His-Leu. Other variants of this type have been discovered. It seems likely that they reflect a defect in processing of newly synthesized globin chains due to a single amino acid substitution near the amino-terminal end.

As we saw in Chapter 3, methionine is the first residue to be incorporated into a growing peptide chain. Normally, during translation of the nascent polypeptide this residue is cleaved, leaving valine as the amino-terminal residue in the case of both the α and β chains of haemoglobin. In haemoglobin Long Island the substitution of proline for histidine in the second position in the chain somehow interferes with this cleavage mechanism so that this variant has both a proline at position 3 in the β chain and an abnormal methionine preceding the usual amino-terminal valine residue.

Shortened gene products

Some haemoglobin variants have shortened globin chains; one or several adjacent amino acids are missing from the abnormal chains and the remainder of the subunit is normal. It seems likely that they arose from a deletion of one or more intact codons; if an entire codon is lost the reading frame will remain in phase and the remainder of the amino acid sequence will not vary from normal. Analysis of the nucleotide sequence of β globin mRNA in regions in which these deletions have occurred has shown that there is a reiterated nucleotide sequence, from two to eight bases in length. This suggests that these deletion mutants have resulted from misalignment of these sequences during meiosis, with non-homologous crossing-over such that a variable sized segment of the gene corresponding to the lost residues is deleted.

Fusion variants

The first example of this kind of protein was haemoglobin Lepore. (To save readers a fruitless search through their atlases it is worth mentioning *en passant* that Lepore is the family name of the first patient to be found with this variant.) Haemoglobin Lepore has normal α chains combined with abnormal non-α chains that have a particularly novel sequence; the first 50–80 amino acids have the normal amino-terminal sequence of δ chains, whereas the last 60–90 residues have the normal C-terminal amino acid sequences of β chains. The Lepore non-α chain is thus a δβ fusion product; that is a hybrid made up of normal δ and β chain sequences. It is likely that the fusion gene has arisen from non-homologous crossing-over between part of the δ chain locus on one chromosome and part of the β chain locus on the complementary chromosome, as shown in Fig. 50. It follows that an event of this type should also generate a chromosome containing an 'anti-Lepore' locus which, in addition to carrying normal δ and β loci, contains a βδ fusion gene, i.e. the mirror image of the Lepore gene. In fact a number of 'anti-Lepore' haemoglobin variants of this type have been found.

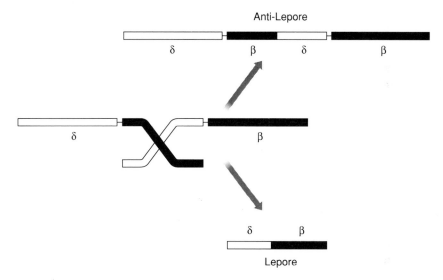

Figure 50. The generation of haemoglobin Lepore and its anti-Lepore counterpart by unequal crossing over.

There is a family of human haemoglobin variants due to the production of fusion chain genes of this type. Presumably this will be a general phenomenon wherever there are gene families with linked loci with rather similar structures that can undergo non-homologous crossovers. We shall return to this theme later in the chapter when we consider α thalassaemia.

An elegant example of this type of mechanism for the production of individual variability is the molecular pathology of red–green colour blindness. The genes that control colour vision consist of two linked clusters which are involved with the synthesis of red and green pigments and which lie on the X chromosome, and another set for the blue pigment which is on an autosome. It has been found that the X-linked form of red–green colour blindness results from an unequal crossing-over event with the production of varying numbers of genes for the red and green pigments; Lepore-like fusion genes are generated in the process. We shall consider in a later section how variation in the number of structural genes brought about by unequal crossing-over can modify the function of a family of genes.

● Structural protein variants as the cause of disease

Over the years since Pauling's discovery that sickle cell disease results from a structural variation in haemoglobin the methods of electrophoretic separation of proteins have been greatly improved and refined. At the same time techniques for the purification and analysis of the structure of proteins have become extremely powerful. These advances have led to the identification of variations in protein structure as the basis of many human diseases. It is not possible, given the constraints of space, to describe each of these in detail. Some examples are summarized in Table 20.

The main question that always arises when a single-base amino acid substitution is found in the gene product of a patient with a particular genetic disorder is how does the alteration in protein structure give rise to the particular clinical phenotype. And of course, single gene disorders represent only the tip of the iceberg of human variability. An equally important question for human biology is how much our individual variability, within what appears to be the normal range, can be ascribed to heritable alterations in protein structure. We shall return to this question when we consider the problems of polygenic disease in the next chapter. Here we shall examine a few examples of how structural changes in proteins are related to human diseases.

● Structure–function relationships for variant proteins resulting from mutations of structural genes

The results of single amino acid substitutions in proteins or their subunits vary depending on the type of amino acid that is substituted and the site of the substitution in the particular protein. It should be emphasized that many amino acid substitutions have no effect on function or stability; only a handful of the 400 or more human haemoglobin variants cause any clinical disability.

The primary amino acid sequence of a protein or its subunits determines the way that it assumes its secondary structure, an α helix or a β pleated sheet for example. Some amino acid substitutions can shift the equilibrium between α helix and a random coil in a particular part of a protein. The effect is to cause abnormalities of tertiary structure and to reduce the overall stability of the protein or its subunit. For example, proline cannot participate in an α helix except as one of the initial three residues. Thus proline substitutions, or the substitution of proline by another amino acid, can sometimes seriously disrupt helical conformation and result in protein instability.

Many proteins are folded into a complex tertiary configuration, so that most of the charged amino acids such as lysine, arginine, glutamic acid, and aspartic acid

Table 20. *Some examples of how mutations that alter protein structure cause disease (see text for details)*

Modification of allosteric properties
  Haemoglobin variants with increased or reduced oxygen binding leading to polycythaemia or methaemoglobinaemia
Reduced stability
  Unstable haemoglobin variants—haemolytic anaemia
  Spectrin variants—haemolytic anaemia
  Collagen variants—skeletal disorder
Impaired polymerization
  Fibrinogen variants—abnormal bleeding
Impaired secretion. Intracellular accumulation—
  α_1 antitrypsin deficiency (PI-Z), liver failure
Altered substrate affinity
  Antithrombin III variants—thrombosis

Defective receptor function
  Synthesis, transport, failure to bind, failure to cluster
    LDL receptor—hypercholesterolaemia
Failure of signalling
  Insulin receptor—diabetes
  Vitamin D receptor—vitamin D-resistant ricketts
  Growth hormone receptor—dwarfism
Defective photoreceptor function
  Rhodopsin—retinitis pigmentosa
Defective post-translational modification
  Hyperproinsulinaemia—diabetes
  Christmas disease (factor IX deficiency)—bleeding
Modification of active sites of enzymes
  Mutations involving active sites of lysosomal hydrolases—storage diseases

are found on the surface of the molecule, allowing their ionized groups to be in contact with water. On the other hand, residues orientated towards the interior of the molecule have non-polar groups; thus the inside of the molecule is stabilized by hydrophobic interactions. The substitution of a charged for an uncharged residue can disrupt these important interactions and also lead to molecular instability.

Finally, some amino acid substitutions alter the function of a protein without interfering with its gross structure or stability. As we shall see as we examine the examples that follow, this can occur in a wide variety of ways.

Structural haemoglobin variants

Studies of the abnormal human haemoglobin variants that cause diseases have provided a wealth of examples of abnormal structure–function relationships for protein variants.

The commonest abnormal haemoglobin, sickle cell haemoglobin, results from the substitution of valine for glutamic acid at the 6th position in the β globin chain. This change somehow stabilizes haemoglobin molecules in the deoxy configuration such that long linear stacks are formed which cause sickling of the red blood cells. This in turn leads to their premature destruction in the circulation and to the blockage of small vessels with damage to the tissues that they supply.

There is a family of unstable haemoglobin variants which cause haemolytic anaemia. The instability results from several different molecular mechanisms. Some involve amino acid substitutions in the vicinity of the haem pocket, a hydrophobic crevice in the surface of the α and β subunits of haemoglobin in which lies the haem molecule. Amino acid substitutions in this pocket decrease the stability of haem-globin linkage, alter the shape of the subunit, and hence lead to molecular instability (Fig. 51). Other substitutions, particularly proline, cause disruption of the secondary structure of subunits, as outlined above. A third group of unstable haemoglobins are caused by substitutions in the interior of the subnit. Finally, there are several unstable haemoglobins that result from deletions of groups of amino acids and lead to instability of subunits, or elongation of globin chains which may also cause instability, in this case by adding a hydrophobic segment to the C-terminal end of the affected chains. All these variants tend to precipitate in red cells in the circulation, causing them to become rigid and hence leading to their premature destruction.

Another group of haemoglobin variants result in hereditary polycythaemia, a condition characterized by an abnormally high haemoglobin level and an increased red cell count. In this case the amino acid substitutions interfere with the normal steric changes that occur during oxygen delivery, and leave the haemoglobin molecules 'fixed' in the oxy configuration. This leads to inefficient tissue oxygenation, erythropoietin production by the kidney, and hence polycythaemia. The oxygen affinity of haemoglobin also varies according to the intracellular level of 2,3-diphosphoglycerate, a molecule that binds specifically to certain residues in the space between the β globin chains in the de-oxy

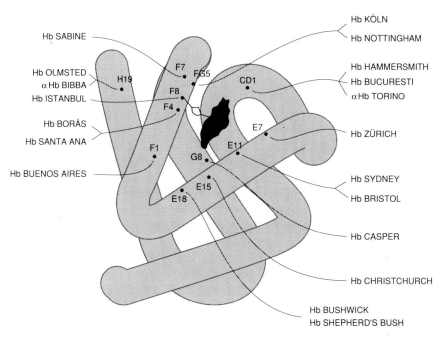

Figure 51. Unstable haemoglobin variants due to amino acid substitutions in the region of the haem pocket.

configuration and so modifies the oxygen affinity of the molecule. Amino acid substitutions that weaken these interactions also produce high-affinity haemoglobin variants.

There is a family of abnormal haemoglobins associated with congenital cyanosis (a blue tinge to the skin and mucous membranes) due to methaemoglobinaemia. In this condition the iron atom of haemoglobin is permanently in the oxidized (Fe^{3+}) state and hence cannot transport oxygen. The iron atom of the haem group of haemoglobin is normally linked to a histidine residue in the haem pocket. Another histidine residue is situated on the opposite side of the pocket, the place where oxygen normally binds. It turns out that most of the haemoglobin variants associated with permanent methaemoglobinaemia involve the substitution of a tyrosine residue for either one or other of the haem-related histidine residues. It seems likely that the phenolic groups of the substituted tyrosine residues are able to form a covalent link with the haem iron, stabilizing the atom in the oxidized state.

These examples of the molecular pathology of the structural haemoglobin variants provide an elegant picture of how single amino acid substitutions may profoundly alter the stability or function of a protein.

The abnormal fibrinogens

Fibrinogen is an important protein of the blood clotting system. Under the action of the enzyme thrombin it can be converted to insoluble fibrin which forms the scaffolding of a blood clot. However, this is a dynamic process and fibrin is also susceptible to enzymatic degradation by plasmin, part of the fail-safe system to prevent unwanted clotting. The mutations of the fibrinogen molecule provide an interesting example of how different structural changes in specific sites of a complex protein can produce widely different clinical disorders.

Fibrinogen consists of three pairs of peptide chains, αA, βB, and γ, which are linked together by disulphide bonds. Thrombin catalyses removal of the A peptide from the α chain and the B peptide from the β chain, thus exposing charged polymerization sites in specific domains of fibrin. These charged regions are able to bind to oppositely charged regions of adjacent fibrinogen molecules leading to the production of an elongated, staggered fibrin polymer. The loose clot formed in this way is then stabilized by the formation of further covalent bonds by the action of a blood clotting factor called factor XIII. During the degradation of fibrin, plasminogen binds to the molecule and cleaves each of the three chains at selective sites to release a variety of degradation products.

Many fibrinogen variants have been found on routine analysis and in some cases they are associated with abnormal fibrinogen function; the clinical disorders that result from abnormal fibrinogens are called the dysfibrinogenaemias. The variants are named, like the haemoglobins, by their place of discovery.

Some forms of dysfibrinogenaemia are characterized by abnormal bleeding. The most severe is associated with fibrinogen Detroit I, which has an arginine to serine substitution in the α chain causing delayed release of fibrinopeptide A and hence impaired polymerization of fibrin. Similarly, fibrinogen Pontoise has an amino acid substitution in the middle of the β chain which produces a new carbohydrate attachment site. Again this seems to interfere with polymerization. On the other hand, some fibrinogen variants lead to an increased risk of thrombosis. For example, fibrinogen New York has a deletion of amino acids 9 through 72 in the β chain. This variant does not bind plasminogen and hence interferes with plasmin generation and clot dissolution. At least four different fibrinogen variants have been found to cause defective wound healing. For example, fibrinogen Paris has a γ chain with 22 additional residues at its C-terminal end. It probably results from a frameshift mutation similar to those described earlier for some of the haemoglobin variants.

Some of the asymptomatic dysfibrinogenaemias, which have been recognized by prolonged blood clotting times, also show some interesting structure/function relationships. For example fibrinogen Lille, which has an aspartic acid substituted by asparagine at position 7 in the α chain, shows defective fibrinopeptide release in the test tube but, surprisingly, this does not cause excessive bleeding.

A particularly interesting observation concerns the relationship between abnormal fibrinogens and repeated spontaneous abortion. Two variants, Metz and Bethesda, show a clear association with this phenomenon; normal clotting factors are, of course, necessary for the formation and maintenance of the placenta. Fibrinogen Metz is characterized by defective fibrinopeptide release resulting from an arginine to cysteine substitution at position 16 in the Aα chain.

The other well-defined fibrinogen disorder is afibrinogenaemia, i.e. the lack of any demonstrable fibrinogen. Surprisingly many affected patients do not have a particularly severe bleeding disorder. The molecular basis for this condition is not yet worked out; the gene appears to be intact and it may well have a similar molecular pathology to the thalassaemias described later in this chapter.

The abnormal fibrinogens, like the haemoglobin variants, provide an elegant example of how amino acid substitutions at different positions in proteins can produce completely different clinical phenotypes.

Serpins

The serpins are a superfamily of glycoproteins, most of which are inhibitors of serine proteinases. The family includes such important enzymes as α_1-antitrypsin, anti-thrombin, anti-plasmin, and a heparin co-factor which, like anti-thrombin, is involved in inhibiting coagulation. Although the molecular pathology of these enzymes has not yet been worked out in such detail as the haemoglobin system there is little doubt about the medical importance of inherited abnormalities of members of this glycoprotein family.

The main inhibitor of trypsin in serum is called α_1-antitrypsin. This important enzyme also inhibits chymotrypsin, collagenase, elastase, and some leucocyte proteases, and plays an important role in neutralizing the harmful effects of these enzymes. Although less widely studied than haemoglobin or fibrinogen it is becoming apparent that α_1-antitrypsin is the product of a highly polymorphic gene locus. Currently, about 75 alleles have been recognized at this locus, which is called PI (protease inhibitor). The common or wild-type form of α_1-antitrypsin is called PI-M. The rare variants have been given letter designations, which run alphabetically from anode to cathode on electrophoresis.

There are two important alleles associated with liver or lung disease, called PI-Z and PI-S. These variants differ from PI-M by single amino acid substitutions; in the case of PI-Z a glutamic acid is replaced by a lysine and in PI-S a different glutamic acid is replaced by valine. It is not yet certain why these substitutions cause a reduced output of the gene products or how the associated clinical phenotypes are mediated. In the case of the homozygous PI-Z the level of α_1 antitrypsin in the serum is markedly reduced. This condition is associated with the development of severe emphysema and it is thought that this may result from the effects of excessive activity of elastase derived from neutrophils in the pulmonary circulation.

It has been found that α_1 antitrypsin aggregates in the liver cells of PI-Z homozygotes. The defective production of α_1 antitrypsin in such individuals appears to result from a post-translational defect occurring at the level of the rought endoplasmic reticulum of α_1 antitrypsin-producing cells. The latter have normal levels of α_1 antitrypsin mRNA but show a marked reduction in the secretion of the enzyme together with its cellular accumulation. Crystallographic studies have shown that the substituted glutamic acid normally forms a salt-like bridge with a nearby lysine residue. It is possible that this helps newly synthesized α_1 antitrypsin to fold into the appropriate tertiary configuration. It has been suggested that the inability to form this salt bridge consequent on the PI-Z mutation results in the accumulation of the enzyme, that is the lysine substitution impedes the normal intracellular processing of α_1 antitrypsin.

A rare variant of PI, PI Pittsburg, has an arginine residue instead of a methionine at position 358; this molecule no longer inhibits elastase but, remarkably, inhibits thrombin which is the enzyme required to convert fibrinogen to fibrin in the production of a blood clot. Hence its deficiency leads to a severe haemorrhagic tendency in heterozygotes.

Another member of the serpin family which is receiving increasing attention is anti-thrombin III (AT III). This is a single chain glycoprotein of 432 amino acids and is the major inhibitor of several proteases in the coagulation pathway, including thrombin. Under normal conditions the inhibitory effect is relatively slow but is greatly accelerated in the presence of heparin. As might be expected a deficiency or ineffective activity of anti-thrombin III leads to an increased tendency to thrombosis.

It turns out that anti-thrombin III deficiency can result from the defective production of the protein or from the synthesis of a functionally abnormal molecule. Structural studies have shown that the heparin binding domains of AT III are encoded by exons 2 and 3 of the gene while the active centre is coded by exon 6. At least twelve structural variants of AT III have been identified, ten of which involve exon 2 mutations and lead to defective heparin binding; the other two are point mutations in exon 6 and directly involve the active site of the enzyme.

Mutations that result in defective receptor activity

There is increasing evidence that point mutations may have profound effects on receptor function. One of the most elegant stories in this field is the elucidation of the mutations involving different regions of the low density lipoprotein (LDL) receptor gene, which lead to a breakdown of the control of cholesterol metabolism and to the clinical picture of monogenic hypercholesterolaemia and premature vascular disease.

The low density lipoprotein receptor is a cell surface glycoprotein which is synthesized in the rough endoplasmic reticulum as a precursor. The receptor has a complicated life-style which involves it travelling to the Golgi complex and thence to the cell surface where it interacts with two plasma cholesterol-binding proteins, apo B and apo E. The receptors then undergo a remarkable recyling process (see Fig. 71, page 204), during which they first appear on the cell surface in coated pits. Within a few minutes of their formation the pits invaginate to form endocytic vesicles. Multiple vesicles fuse to create larger sacs called endosomes. When the the pH of the endosome falls below 6.4 the low density lipoprotein dissociates from the receptor which then returns to the surface; each receptor makes one round trip about every ten minutes in a continuous fashion, whether or not it is occupied by low density lipoprotein.

Monogenic hypercholesterolaemia can result from a variety of mutations of the LDL receptor gene (Fig. 52). At least some of the molecular defects are characterized by a marked reduction in the rate of receptor synthesis and are due to mechanisms that will be described later in this chapter; in some cases no receptors are synthesized at all. A second class of mutations result in a reduced rate of transportation from the endoplasmic reticulum to the Golgi apparatus. A third class is characterized by normal synthesis but failure to bind low density lipoprotein; several of these mutations involve amino acid substitutions in the cysteine-rich LDL binding domain. Finally, there is a class of mutations in which the receptors reach the cell surface and bind low density lipoprotein but fail to cluster in coated pits. All the mutations producing the latter abnormality involve the cytoplasmic tail of the receptor which protrudes into the cell cytoplasm; in one case a tyrosine to cysteine substitution in the middle of the cytoplasmic tail domain is involved.

Another receptor in which mutations have been identified to profoundly alter function is that for insulin. The insulin receptor is a plasma membrane glycoprotein consisting of two α subunits which bind insulin, and two β subunits which have tyrosine-specific protein kinase activity. When insulin is bound to the α subunits the tyrosine kinase activity of the β subunits is stimulated and this in turn leads to autophosphorylation of the receptor, conformational changes in the β subunit, and activation of the receptor kinase towards other intracellular substrates. This leads to rapid phosphorylation and dephosphorylation of intermediary substrates on serine residues, activation of secondary mediators of insulin action, modulation of enzyme activity, and a variety of other changes in gene expression.

There are two rare clinical syndromes characterized by extreme resistance to insulin. The first, or type A syndrome, occurs in women with androgen excess and

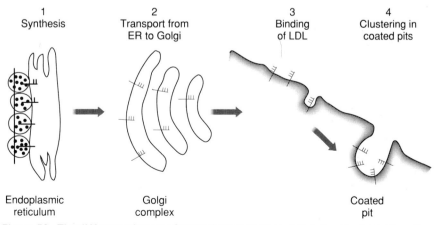

| 1 | 2 | 3 | 4 |
| Synthesis | Transport from ER to Golgi | Binding of LDL | Clustering in coated pits |

| Endoplasmic reticulum | Golgi complex | | Coated pit |

Figure 52. The different classes of mutations that disrupt the structure and function of the LDL receptor and cause familial hypercholesterolaemia.

menstrual abnormalities often associated with polycystic ovaries. The second, which has the rather exotic name leprechaunism, is seen in children who also have elfin faces, hirsutism, thick skin, and diminished body fat. One individual with the type A syndrome has been found to have a point mutation in the β subunit which results in the substitution of serine for tryptophan in the kinase domain; two other different mutations have been found in the same domain. Interestingly, these mutations have usually been found in heterozygotes and therefore the genetic defect occurs on cells with mixed populations of normal and mutant receptors. Remarkably, the presence of the mutant receptor appears to have a negative effect on the activity of the normal receptor.

Another type of defective receptor function due to a point mutation is exemplified by a rare disorder characterized by the development of rickets because of an inherited resistance to vitamin D. As mentioned in Chapter 3, steroid hormones bind to receptors that interact directly with DNA. At least some DNA binding proteins have a so-called 'zinc finger' motif (see Chapter 3). Recent studies of the vitamin D receptor genes of patients with vitamin D-resistant rickets have demonstrated single amino acid substitutions in the first or second zinc finger regions of the receptor; presumably these substitutions interfere with DNA binding and hence with receptor function. Recently, single amino acid substitutions involving the growth hormone receptor have been found in patients with Laron dwarfism, a condition characterized by resistance to growth hormone.

These remarkable studies emphasize the many ways in which receptor function may be interfered with by point mutations.

Photoreceptor mutations and blindness

Quite recently another very elegant example of structure/function relations for point mutations that alter the structure of gene products has been unearthed. Retinitis pigmentosa is the name given to a heterogeneous set of inherited defects, all of which lead to blindness. Since many of these conditions affect only the retina or associated retinal pigment it always seemed likely that the genes that are involved would be those that are expressed only in the retina or which play an important role in its function. It turns out that one form of autosomally dominant retinitis pigmentosa results from a single amino acid substitution in the rhodopsin molecule.

Rhodopsin is the photoreceptor in the rod cells of the retina. It consists of an integral membrane protein called opsin attached to a vitamin A derived chromophore, 11-*cis* retinal. The opsin peptide chain spans the lipid bilayer and forms a complex three dimensional array which forms the binding site for the chromophore. After absorption of light, rhodopsin is activated and triggers a cascade of reactions that decrease the second messenger cGMP concentration in the cell. This, in turn, elicits hyperpolarization of the cell's plasma membrane which is the neurophysiological visual signal.

It turns out that a single base transversion, C to A, which results in the change of a proline to a histidine residue at position 23 in the opsin molecule so alters its configuration that it causes the retinal degeneration characteristic of retinitis pigmentosa. Interestingly the proline at position 23 is conserved in all vertebrate opsins and in other related signal receptors such as the β-adrenergic receptor.

Amino acid substitutions involving post-translational modification of protein

Some proteins undergo post-translational modification of their structure. Several point mutations that interfere with this process have been described.

Insulin consists of two dissimilar peptide chains, A and B, linked by two disulphide bonds. However, unlike many other proteins that consist of structurally distinct subunits, insulin is under the control of a single gene locus; chains A and B are derived from a one-chain precursor, pre-pro-insulin. Pre-pro-insulin is converted to pro-insulin by cleavage of a signal sequence. Pro-insulin is converted to insulin by the enzymatic removal of a segment that connects the amino-terminal end of the A chain to the carboxyl-terminal end of the B chain, called the C peptide. There is a well-characterized condition called familial hyperproinsulinaemia which results from mutations that involve the cleavage sites connecting the A chains to the C peptide. For example the substitution of an arginine residue at position 65 causes the C peptide to remain joined to the insulin A chain.

Another example of a defect in post-translational modification is a mutation responsible for one form of the bleeding disorder Christmas disease. This condition, which is similar to haemophilia, is characterized by a lifelong bleeding tendency due to the deficiency of a blood-clotting factor called factor IX. Factor IX is synthesized as a precursor which is probably cleaved proteolytically in at least two positions, during which a pre-peptide and a pro-peptide region are removed. One type of Christmas disease results from a single amino acid substitution at position -4 in the pro-peptide region; an arginine residue is replaced by a glutamine residue. This change results in the production of a stable, longer protein with 18 additional amino acids attached to the N-terminal pro-peptide regions. This observation suggests that during the normal maturation of factor IX a signal peptidase cleaves the peptide bond between amino acids -18 and -19, generating an unstable profactor IX intermediate; further proteolytic processing to the mature factor IX molecule must depend on the presence of the normal arginine residue at position 4. Interestingly, this arginine residue is not unique to the factor IX precursor but is also found in factor X and prothrombin, and in many other sequences processed by site-specific trypsin-like enzymes, C3, C4, and C5 of the complement system, and tissue plasminogen activator, for example.

As mentioned earlier, there is a family of abnormal haemoglobins with elongated globin chains, including some with additional residues at the N-terminal end. These variants also offer some interesting insights into post-translational modification of proteins. The amino-terminal methionine residue, the translation product of the AUG initiation codon, is present only transiently in the nascent peptide chains of most proteins. One variant, haemoglobin Long Island, has a methionine residue at the end of the β globin chain; the third residue is proline instead of histidine. It seems likely that this amino acid substitution causes either a structural or a charge difference in the nascent β globin chain which interferes with the methionine-aminopeptidase mechanism or causes a change in the secondary structure of the mRNA of sufficient magnitude to impair the removal of the amino-terminal methionine residue.

Recent studies on methylmalonic acidaemia (MMA) provide another elegant example of this type of defect. This condition is highly heterogeneous, but one form results from a deficiency of the enzyme methylmalonyl CoA mutase (MCM). This is a vitamin B_{12}-dependent enzyme which is involved in the degradation of various branch chain amino acids, and odd chain fatty acids towards the Krebs cycle. Infants with a deficiency of MCM present in the first few days of life with metabolic acidosis, selective aminoacidaemia, and hypoglycaemia. MCM is a mitochondrial enzyme which is encoded by a nuclear gene. After synthesis on cytoplasmic ribosomes as a propeptide containing a mitochondrial targeting sequence, the enzyme is transported to the mitochondria where it recognizes a specific receptor and is cleaved during the process of transport into the mitochondrial matrix. One type of this disorder results from a nonsense mutation (see later section) within the mitrochondrial leader sequence. The result is that truncated proteins are formed which cannot be transported to the mitochondria and which are unstable in the cytoplasm.

Amino acid substitutions in complex proteins; genetic disorders of collagen

Collagen accounts for about 25 per cent of total body protein. It is essential for the integrity of bone, dentine, tendon, blood vessels, cornea, heart valves, and many other tissues. The genetic disorders of collagen, though rare, constitute a wide spectrum of conditions ranging from lethal deforming disorders to mild conditions such as the floppy mitral valve syndrome. They include such well-defined disorders as osteogenesis imperfecta (brittle bone syndrome), Ehlers–Danlos syndrome, and Marfan's disease. They will probably turn out to encompass a number of other skeletal conditions such as achondroplasia.

There are three types of collagen, I, II, and III. Type I collagen occurs in all tissues except cartilage and the vitreous of the eye. The major stress-bearing structures such as tendons, bone, and ligaments are particularly rich in this variety. Type II collagen occurs in cartilage and in the vitreous of the eye. Type III collagen is found in most tissues except bone and dentine, and reaches its highest concentration in pliable tissue such as skin, gut, and blood vessel walls. The main functional domain of collagen is a triple helix formed by hydrogen bonding between three subunits, called α chains. The characteristics of the three types of collagen, including their different types of α chains, molecular configurations, and their individual genes and chromosome assignments are summarized in Table 21. The amino acid sequence of the α chains is very unusual. The most striking feature is the presence of glycine at every third residue which, since it has no side chain, can pack into the middle of the helix. The sequence of an α-chain helical domain can be written $(Gly-X-Y)_n$, where $n = 3380 \pm 2$ for all three

Table 21. *The major fibrillar collagens*

Collagen type	Subunits	Structural gene locus	Chromosomal assignment (human)	Known molecular configurations
I	α1(I)	COL 1 A1	17q21-q22	$(\alpha1(1)_2\alpha2(1)$ and
	α2(1)	COL 1 A2	7q22	$(\alpha1(1))_3$
II	α1(11)	COL 2 A1	12q13	$(\alpha1(11))_3$
III	α1(111)	COL 3 A1	2q23	$(\alpha1(111))_3$

fibrillar collagens. X is often proline and Y hydroxyproline. At both ends of the helix there are short domains called telopeptides containing lysine residues through which adjacent helices are cross-linked by covalent bonds. The organization of the genes that control the different α chains of collagen is quite remarkable. The 4.5 kb of coding sequences in all four chains are dispersed in 51 exons through a total gene length of 38 kb.

Over the last few years it has become apparent that at least some genetic disorders of collagen result from either amino acid substitutions in critical regions of the collagen molecule or from similarly sited deletions. The mutations that involve collagen offer a particularly interesting problem in relating structure to function. The first mutation to be defined for a collagen disorder was a deletion of 84 amino acids in the α1(I) chain of collagen from a case of lethal osteogenesis imperfecta. Although neither parent was available for examination the most likely explanation for this observation is that the deletion occurred in one of the parental germ-lines. Since the other α1(I) allele was apparently normal, how is it that this deletion resulted in a lethal bone disease? As shown in Table 21, type I molecules contain two α1(I) chains and receive, presumably, contributions from both alleles. Thus one mutant allele would generate populations of molecules containing 0, 1, or 2 mutant α1(I) chains. If we assume random pairing of the α1(I) chains these molecules will occur in ratios of 1:2:1. Thus three out of four molecules would contain at least one mutant chain and only a quarter would be normal.

Another patient with lethal osteogenesis imperfecta has been found to have a mutation of the α1(I) chain, in this case the substitution of glycine with cysteine. This substitution might, by steric hindrance, prevent the formation of several interchain hydrogen bonds required for stability of the molecule. Again neither parent carried the mutant allele. Abnormalities of the α2(I) chain have also been found in osteogenesis imperfecta and in Marfan's disease. In one case a short deletion of the α2(I) chain was observed. Despite the apparent severity of this lesion the affected patient survived, presumably because he formed trimers of α1(I) which are effective although not perfect substitutes for the authentic type 1 molecules, i.e. α1(I)2(I).

Based on these observations two main types of mutations of collagen have been proposed—included and excluded. In the first, the mutation leads to the incorporation of an abnormal chain into a collagen molecule which is then abnormal. This serves to amplify the mutant allele by absorbing the products of normal genes into molecules which are then destroyed, a phenomenon that has been called protein suicide. In the second class, a mutation disrupts the structure to such an extent as to prevent incorporation of the product of the mutant allele into collagen molecules. Thus even though these mutations have such a catastrophic effect on protein structure, because they are excluded from collagen molecules the associated phenotype is less severe than in the included class; only normal molecules will be produced, albeit in a reduced amount. These concepts are illustrated in Fig. 53.

There are over 100 disorders of growth that appear to result from abnormalities of the growth plate or resting cartilage. The major elements of cartilage are type II collagen, chondroitin sulphate, proteoglycan, link protein, and hyaluronic acid. It is apparent from the recent successes in this field that it should soon be possible to analyse the complex molecular mechanisms that underlie these distressing conditions.

Amino acid substitutions that cause accumulation of abnormal metabolites

Many metabolic activities require the production and subsequent degradation of a wide variety of metabolites. These processes are enzymatically controlled and many enzymes are involved in both the synthetic and degradative pathways. There is a group of conditions, known collectively as the storage disorders, which result from genetic abnormalities of enzymes in the degradation pathways. The modest decrease of enzyme activity that occurs in heterozygotes is not usually sufficient to cause the pathological accumulation of storage material. Thus most of these disorders are inherited in an autosomal recessive fashion. Occasionally they are sex-linked.

Most storage diseases are due to deficiencies of lysosomal hydrolases. These enzymes have a number of features in common. First, they have a signal sequence that plays a critical role in their synthesis and targeting to lysosomes, cellular organelles in which degradative activities occur. Most of these enzymes are glycoproteins and the attachment of the carbohydrate is a function of certain critical sequences in their constituent peptide chains. After they have crossed the endoplasmic reticulum they undergo glycosylation of selected asparagine residues, after which a preformed oligosaccharide is transferred to the nascent peptide chain. Some of the sugars are then excised after which the glycoprotein moves to the Golgi apparatus of the cell where further complex modification occurs under the sequential action of two further enzymes. The end result of this complex processing is the production of a specific recognition signal which is required for binding to specific receptors that target the enzyme to the correct location in the lysosomal membrane. These complicated pathways are open to a wide variety of genetic defects; most of them involve the protein part of the

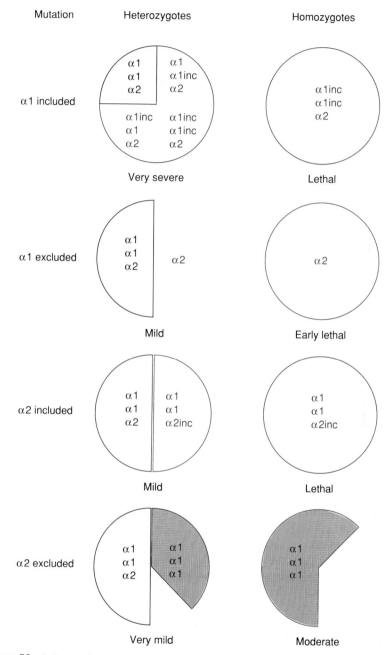

Figure 53. Schematic representation of the effects of *included* (inc) and *excluded* (exc) mutants. The circles represent the total output of type 1 collagen molecules or chains produced by the presence in the genome of one (heterozygous) or two (homozygous) mutant genes at each locus predicted by assuming random association of allelic products. Black segments or half circles indicate normal collagen; red, abnormal collagen. Incomplete circles indicate quantitative reduction. Modified from Sykes (1985).

particular enzyme. However, a condition called I cell disease has been described in which a deficiency of a particular phosphotransferase results in defective function of several different glycohydrolases.

The end result of these mutations is the accumulation of a variety of metabolic by-products, usually within the reticuloendothelial cells of different organs, particularly the brain, liver, and spleen. Although many of these diseases are turning out to result from defects in the rate of enzyme production due to mutations similar to those described in the thalassaemias in the next section, a few are due to amino acid substitutions, Tay Sachs disease in Ashkenazi Jews and Gaucher's disease for example.

Tay Sachs disease is one of a family of inherited disorders called the gangliosidoses which are characterized by excessive accumulation of glycolipids in the tissues. In its most severe form it is associated with progressive weakness, lack of muscle tone, and blindness occurring within the first year of life. The enzymic hydrolysis of lipids is carried out by two lysosomal glycoproteins, hexosaminidase A and an activator protein called G_{m2}. It turns out that hexosaminidase A consists of two subunits, α, and β, which are encoded on different chromosomes. Defects in any of these three loci may give rise to a defect in lysosomal metabolism. Molecular studies have revealed considerable genetic heterogeneity within these diseases. While some of them undoubtedly result from defects in mRNA transcription others are turning out to result from point mutations and amino acid substitutions. For example, some cases of Tay Sachs disease result from the substitution of arginine by histidine in the catalytic site of hexosaminidase A.

Similar molecular heterogeneity underlies the different types of Gaucher disease, a disorder in which there is accumulation of a substance called glucosylceramide in the lysosomes of reticuloendothelial cells. The gene for the enzyme that is defective in this disorder, glucocerebrosidase, has been cloned and mapped to chromosome 1q21. A number of mutations have been found in association with different phenotypes of Gaucher disease. For example the substitution of proline for leucine at residue 444 destroys the α helical structure of the protein. A second substitution, serine for asparagine at position 370, is also likely to alter the configuration of the enzyme, with drastic results on its function.

Another interesting example of the accumulation of abnormal metabolites due to a structural alteration in a protein is the rare disorder familial amyloidotic polyneuropathy (FAP). In this condition an amyloid-like substance accumulates in the peripheral nervous system. This gives rise to distal loss of sensation and also to disorders of autonomic function including postural hypotension, abnormal sweating, impotence, and gastrointestinal dysfunction. The pathological feature is the deposition of amyloid fibrils in the peripheral nerves, heart, and kidneys, but not in the brain.

It has been found that FAP results from a single amino acid substitution in a protein called transthyretin, formerly known as pre-albumin. Transthyretin is the transport protein for the thyroid hormone, thyroxine, and also for vitamin A. In Japanese, Portuguese, and Swedish families with FAP there is a substitution of methionine for valine at position 30 in transthyretin; in Jewish populations the disorder results from the substitution of glycine for threonine at position 49. The abnormal transthyretin circulates in plasma from early life although often the disease dose not present until much later. It is presumed that the amino acid substitution causes the accumulation of protein in peripheral nerves although the actual mechanism remains to be elucidated. This disease has interesting similarities to Alzheimer's disease, a much commoner condition that we will consider in the next chapter.

Mutations that involve membrane proteins

The maintenance of the shape and mobility of cells is of major importance for their normal function. The human red blood cell is a good example. Consider its lifestyle. It survives for about 120 days in the circulation during which time it is subjected to enormous stresses and strains. One moment it is being ejected under high pressure from the heart into large blood vessels, seconds later it is dragged along the microcirculation through orifices which are considerably less than its own diameter, and its only rest periods are spent in the osmotically unfavourable backwaters of the spleen. As well as maintaining its flexibility it has to survive in an unfriendly environment in which there is a high level of sodium and low level of potassium. And if this were not enough it is constantly being bombarded with noxious oxidants which tend to damage both membrane and haemoglobin. The end point of this precarious existence is the final indignity of being eaten by a macrophage.

The membrane of the red cell is constructed rather like a sandwich which is composed of a bilayer of lipids and integral membrane proteins joined to an underlying protein skeleton. The skeleton consists of a meshwork of tetramers and oligomers of a protein called spectrin cross-linked by two other proteins called 4.1 and actin. It is joined to the membrane by interactions of spectrin with ankrin and probably by further interactions between protein 4.1 and another surface protein called glycophorin. The skeleton is the major determinant of the shape, strength, and flexibility of the cells and also helps to regulate the organization of lipids and mobility of the integral proteins.

There are several inherited disorders of the red cell membrane; all of them are phenotypically and genetically heterogeneous. One condition, hereditary elliptocytosis, is characterized by the production of oval rather than round red cells. In some cases the disorder is completely innocuous whereas in others there is shortened red cell survival and haemolytic anaemia. In recent years considerable attention has been directed towards analysis of inherited changes in the structure of spectrin in these disorders. Spectrin is the main skeleton protein and is made up of two large polypeptide chains, α and β, which are structurally similar but functionally distinct. The gene for α spectrin is located on chromosome 1 and that for β spectrin on chromosome 14. It turns out that, rather like the unstable haemoglobin variants, proline substitutions may have a profound effect on the function and stability of spectrin molecules. For example, the substitution in the α chain of proline for leucine at residue 254, or of proline for glutamine at residue 465 leads to abnormal spectrin structure and, ultimately, to the elliptocytic shape and abnormal membrane properties characteristic of the red cells of one type of hereditary elliptocytosis. In addition, a number of defects in the structure of protein 4.1 have been described in patients with elliptocytosis. In one such case it appears that there has been an insertion of 34 amino acids at the border of the region of protein 4.1 where spectrin and actin interact with each other. In addition, defective production of protein 4.1 has been described; the mechanisms again appear to be heterogeneous and will be considered in a later section.

Another relatively common inherited disorder of the red cell membrane is characterized by the production of spherical rather than biconcave red cells. This condition, called hereditary spherocytosis, is genetically heterogeneous and may be inherited as either an autosomal dominant or recessive condition. It is now clear that erythrocyte membranes from patients with the dominant form of the condition are deficient in spectrin and that the degree of deficiency correlates well with the severity of the disease and with the degree of spherocytosis. The precise mechanism for the spectrin deficiency remains to be determined.

There seems little doubt, therefore, that there will be a wide range of single gene disorders involving these critical membrane proteins and that some of them will result from structural alterations. Because of the difficulty in isolating and purifying these large proteins, it is likely that further progress will follow the cloning and sequencing of their particular genes to try to determine the nature of the underlying amino acid substitutions. This will be a very rewarding area for trying to understand the relationship between structure and function for the complex protein interactions that underlie the integrity of cell membranes.

● Structure/function relationships for protein variants; summary

In this short survey we have seen how single amino acid substitutions or more subtle variations in protein structure may profoundly alter their function. So far only a few systems, in particular haemoglobin, LDL and other receptors, serpins, and fibrinogen have been worked out in sufficient detail to provide precise information about how variation in the primary structure of a protein can modify its function. It should be remembered that many proteins show heterogeneity in their structure, much of which appears to be harmless. In fact there is probably a spectrum from such 'normal' variability, through extremely mild alterations in function, to structural changes that cause a serious disability. We shall return to the problem of the significance of inherited functional variability in proteins when we consider polygenic inheritance and polygenic disease in the next chapter.

● Molecular lesions that result in the production of reduced amounts of gene products

Many genetic disorders are caused by a reduced output of an enzyme or other type of protein; in some cases no product can be detected. Such protein as is produced is structurally normal. Although it used to be thought that these conditions would result from mutations of regulatory loci recent work has shown that this is rarely the case. In fact the majority of them seem to result from simple *cis*-acting mutations that involve structural genes or sequences in their flanking regions or adjacent areas of DNA (Table 22).

The most spectacular progress in our understanding of the molecular pathology of this class of disorders comes from studies of the thalassaemias, the commonest genetic diseases of mankind. As described in Chapter 2, this heterogeneous group of conditions is characterized by a reduced rate of synthesis of one or more pairs of the globin chains of adult haemoglobin. The commonest types are α and β thalassaemia, which are characterized by defective α or β globin chain synthesis respectively. This leads to imbalanced globin chain production; most of the clinical and haematological manifestations can be ascribed to the deleterious effects of the globin subunits that are produced in excess, α chains in β thalassaemia and β chains in α thalassaemia (Fig. 54).

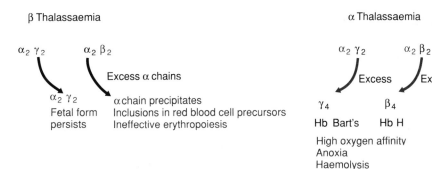

Normal

$\alpha_2 \gamma_2$ $\alpha_2 \beta_2$

Hb F   Hb A

β Thalassaemia α Thalassaemia

$\alpha_2 \gamma_2$ $\alpha_2 \beta_2$ $\alpha_2 \gamma_2$ $\alpha_2 \beta_2$

          Excess α chains   Excess   Excess

$\alpha_2 \gamma_2$ α chain precipitates γ_4 β_4
Fetal form   Inclusions in red blood cell precursors   Hb Bart's   Hb H
persists   Ineffective erythropoiesis

                                      High oxygen affinity
                                      Anoxia
                                      Haemolysis

Figure 54. The α and β thalassaemias.

The genetic control of haemoglobin and the arrangement of the different globin genes was described in Chapter 3 and is summarized in Fig. 11 (page 57). There are two α globin genes per haploid genome, but only one β globin gene. The α thalassaemias are classified into α^+ thalassaemia, in which there is reduced α chain production, usually representing the output of only one of the pair of linked α globin genes, and α^0 thalassaemia in which the output of both genes is defective (Fig. 55). The β thalassaemias are similarly classified; in β^+ thalassaemia there is a reduced output of β globin chains while in β^0 thalassaemia no globin chains are synthesized.

Sequence analyses of the α and β globin genes of patients with α or β

Table 22. *Examples of the molecular basis of monogenic disorders characterized by defective synthesis of a gene product*

Transcription
Deletions
α and β thalassaemia. Duchenne muscular dystrophy. Haemophilia A and B.
Cystic fibrosis. Lesch-Nyhan syndrome. Hypercholesterolaemia. AT III deficiency.
Growth hormone deficiency. Osteogenesis imperfecta
Insertions
Haemoglobin variants. Haemophilia. Lipoprotein lipase deficiency. Marfan's syndrome
Hypercholesterolaemia
Inversions
δβ thalassaemia. Apo A-I deficiency. Haemophilia
Fusion genes
δβ thalassaemia. Red/green colour blindness
Point mutations in upstream promotor elements
β thalassaemia
Duplications
Hypercholesterolaemia

Messenger RNA processing
Splice junction
α and β thalassaemia. Phenylketonuria. Porphyria (acute)

Cryptic splice sites in introns
  β thalassaemia
Consensus sequence mutations
  β thalassaemia
Cryptic splice sites in exons
  β thalassaemia
PolyA signal site mutations
  α and β thalassaemia

Translation
Initiation codon
  α and β thalassaemia. Pseudohypoparathyroidism. Retinal degeneration
Nonsense mutations
  β thalassaemia. Haemophilia A and **B**. Lesch-Nyhan syndrome. Hypercholesterolaemia. 21 hydroxylase deficiency. Protein C deficiency. OTC deficiency. Porphyria (acute). Methylmalonic acidaemia. Many others
Frameshift mutations
  β thalassaemia. Haemophilia. Abnormal fibrinogens. Duchenne muscular dystrophy. Many others
Termination codon
  α thalassaemia

Unstable proteins due to mis-sense mutations
  α and β thalassaemia. Elliptocytosis. Many others

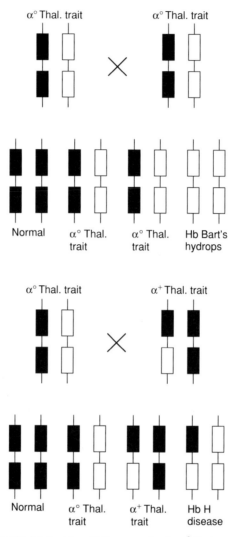

Figure 55. **The genetic basis of α thalassaemia**. In α⁰ thalassaemia no α chains are produced whereas in α⁺ thalassaemia there is some output from the affected chromosome. The shaded blocks represent normal α globin genes; the open blocks represent α globin genes that are deleted or otherwise inactivated.

thalassaemia have provided a remarkable picture of the repertoire of human molecular pathology; indeed they have probably shown us most of the mutations that can involve structural genes. In the sections that follow we shall examine the different mechanisms that underlie these conditions and other genetic disorders that are characterized by a reduced output of a particular gene product.

Although all these disorders result from mutations of the structural genes, the resulting defects are manifest at the levels of transcription, mRNA processing, translation, or post-translational stability.

● Mutations that cause defective transcription

Gene deletions and variation in gene number

There are many examples of partial or complete deletions of genes as the basis for inherited diseases. Furthermore, we are starting to learn how they may have arisen. One field that has been particularly productive in this respect is the analysis of the α thalassaemias.

As shown in Figs 11 and 55 there are two closely linked α globin genes on chromosome 16. In many forms of $α^+$ thalassaemia there is a deletion involving this chromosome which leaves a single functional α gene. In most types of $α°$ thalassaemia both α globin genes are lost (Figs 55 and 56). The most likely mechanism for the production of a chromosome with a single α globin gene is non-homologous crossing-over between the two α globin gene loci after mispairing of homologous chromosomes during meiosis. Duplicated loci like the α genes have arisen by a reduplication event which is mirrored by regions of homology in the flanking regions of the particular genes involved. In the case of the α globin genes these regions are called X, Y, and Z (Fig. 57). It turns out that several different crossovers have occurred within these 'homology boxes', resulting in specific types of $α^+$ thalassaemia. If these ideas are correct, the reciprocal product of the crossover event, a chromosome carrying three α globin gene loci, should be observed (Fig. 57). In fact such cases have been found in every human population studied so far. Similar mechanisms are almost certainly involved in the generation of variable numbers of γ globin genes on chromosome 11; individuals with one, three, or even four γ genes per haploid genome (on one of a pair of chromosomes) have been found.

There are other mechanisms for the production of gene deletions. Recent work on the deletions that cause $α°$ thalassaemia and on those that involve the β globin gene cluster and give rise to the phenotype of δβ thalassaemia or hereditary persistence of fetal haemoglobin (HPFH) (Fig. 58) have shown that some of the breakpoints involve sequences with characteristics of *Alu*I repeats. The *Alu*I family, so-called because of the presence of a recognition site for this restriction endonuclease in the centre of the consensus sequence, constitutes a series of repeats of about 300 nucleotides which occur some 300 000–500 000 times throughout the human genome. These units, although they have a high degree of homology, have no known function despite the fact that at least some of them are transcribed. It is possible that deletions may follow a legitimate recombination event between two *Alu*I sequences, either by chromosome misalignment or the production of a loop structure on a single chromosome (Fig. 59).

In addition to the deletions involving the α or β globin gene cluster there are other examples that appear to have involved *Alu-Alu* recombination, notably one

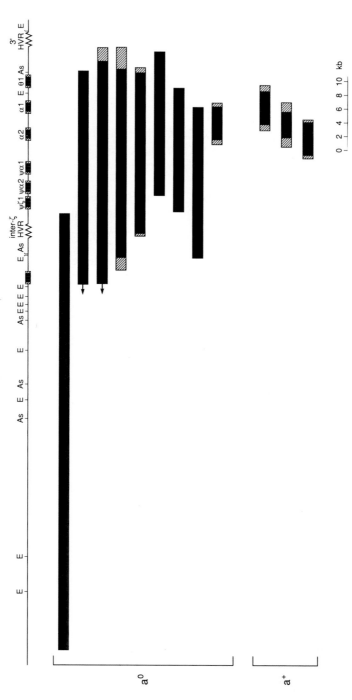

Figure 56. **Some of the deletions of the α globin gene complex that give rise to α^0 and α^+ thalassaemia.** The normal α globin genes together with hypervariable regions (HVR) and restriction enzyme sites in the flanking regions are shown at the top of the figure.

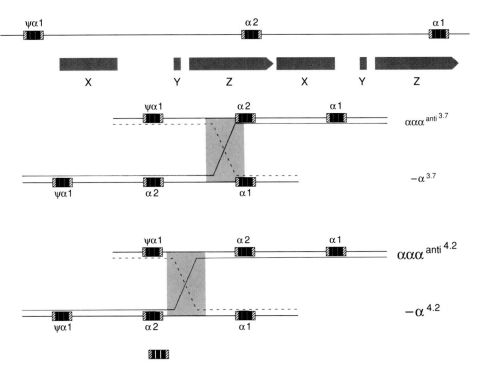

Figure 57. Crossovers which give rise to the two common forms of α⁺ thalassaemia. The X, Y, and Z boxes are regions of homology. The two Z boxes are 3.7 kb apart and unequal crossing over gives rise to a chromosome with a single α gene and one with three α genes. Similarly, the X boxes, which are 4.2 kb apart provides a site for crossing over which gives the same arrangements although associated with a deletion of 4.2 instead of 3.7 kb.

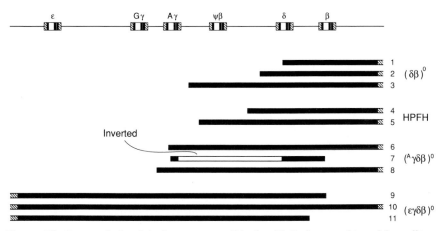

Figure 58. Some of the deletions responsible for δβ thalassaemia and hereditary persistence of fetal haemoglobin (HPFH). $(\delta\beta)^0$ indicates no output of these gene products as the result of the deletion. Two other forms of thalassaemia are produced by longer deletions that remove either the $^A\gamma$, δ, and β genes, or the ε, γ, δ, and β genes.

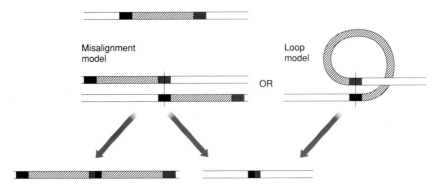

Figure 59. Two possible models for the generation of deletions by recombination between homologous sequences of DNA. This mis-alignment model would also give rise to a chromosome with duplication of these regions.

involving the LDL receptor. It is possible that because of their high degree of homology the *Alu* repetitive sequences serve as 'hot spots' for recombination. On the other hand at least some of the long deletions of the α and β globin gene clusters involve non-related sequences, that is they are examples of illegitimate recombination.

Another interesting feature of deletions of the α and β globin gene clusters is that in many cases they are of similar length, even though they involve different points along the genome. A novel mechanism explaining these observations proposes that the deletions are generated by the loss of chromatin loops at different stages of DNA replication as chromatin moves through specific attachment sites on the nuclear matrix; following breakage the two ends of the DNA become reunited with the loss of a loop. Recent evidence in favour of this notion has come from the study of an α° thalassaemia deletion in which the gap across the deletion appears to have been 'filled-in' by a DNA sequence that is found normally at least 34 kb upstream from the site of the deletion. This could only have happened if the deletion had involved a large loop of DNA which brought the 'filler' sequence into the observed site and orientation (Fig. 60).

Other genetic disorders result from gene deletions. They are found commonly in haemophilia, Christmas disease, Lesch–Nyhan syndrome, and Duchenne muscular dystrophy (DMD). They vary in size from small intragenic deletions to enormous lesions that remove the whole of these large genes. For example, one deletion found in a haemophiliac child removes the whole of the factor VIII gene; this was found to be a *de novo* mutation since it was not present in the boy's mother. Deletions have also been found in some, though not all, cases of genetic growth hormone deficiency and antithrombin III deficiency.

The phenotypes associated with deletions should be quite straightforward; the gene is lost and there can be no product. Although this is usually the case, it is turning out that deletions can have more suble effects. For example, several of the deletions that involve the α and β globin gene cluster (Figs 56 and 58) end many

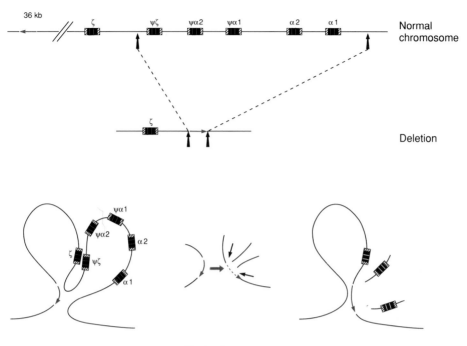

Mechanism

Figure 60. Evidence for looping out of DNA as the basis for a gene deletion. The deletion involves the α gene cluster with removal of the region between the arrows. Sequence analysis reveals that there is a short sequence of DNA bridging the ends of the deletion which is normally found 36 kb upstream from the complex. It is suggested that this region has been brought into the deletion in an inverted orientation by the formation of a loop structure as shown; the deletion has been caused by a break across the base of the loop.

kilobases upstream from the α and β globin genes. Yet in these cases these genes are either non-functional or their output is greatly reduced. Whether this reflects the removal of critical upstream regulatory sequences, a topic that we shall return to later in this chapter, or whether they have a more general effect in disrupting the functional domains of these genes, remains to be seen.

The phenotypes associated with deletions of the DMD locus on the X chromosome have also come under intense study in recent years. At least 50 per cent of deletions associated with DMD and the milder Becker muscular dystrophy (BMD) arise near the centre of the gene and extend towards the 3' end. The 3' ends of these deletions are very heterogeneous suggesting that the DNA sequences responsible lie within the common intron where the deletions originate. A start has been made in trying to relate the size and extent of these deletions to the associated clinical phenotype. We shall return to this question in a later section.

Fusion genes

Another interesting and important result of chromosomal misalignment and abnormal crossing-over is the production of fusion genes which code for hybrid proteins. The first and best studied example is haemoglobin Lepore, which, as we saw earlier, has normal α chains combined with non-α chains which have the N-terminal amino acid sequence of δ chains of haemoglobin A₂ and the C-terminal sequence of β chains of haemoglobin A. This variant appears to have arisen through non-homologous crossing-over between part of the β locus on one chromosome and part of the δ locus on the complementary chromosome (see Fig. 50, page 147). Such an event should give rise to two abnormal chromosomes, one with a Lepore gene and the other with its opposite counterpart, an anti-Lepore gene. In fact both these arrangements have been found in a number of patients (see page 147). A similar mechanism seems to have been involved in the production of one of the sialoglycoproteins of the red cell surface.

Another elegant example of the generation of variation in gene number and the production of fusion genes comes from studies on the molecular genetics of colour vision and colour blindness. Human colour vision is based on three light-sensitive pigments. The genes for the red and green pigments show 96 per cent identity and lie in a tandem array on the X chromosome on which there is a single red pigment gene and variable numbers of green pigment genes; the blue pigment gene shows less homology and is on an autosome. Many of the different forms of red/green colour blindness appear to have resulted from unequal crossing-over between the red and green pigment genes with the production of varying numbers of different fusion genes (Fig. 61).

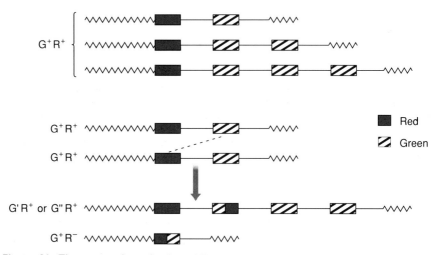

Figure 61. The generation of colour-blindness by unequal recombination between red and green pigment genes with the formation of fusion genes.

Inversions

The term 'inversion' signifies that a region of DNA is back-to-front with respect to its normal orientation in the genome. The first example of a human gene inversion was found in a patient with the phenotype of δβ thalassaemia, a mild inherited anaemia in which there is no δ or β globin chain production from the affected chromosome (Fig. 58). The inversion involves a region of DNA between the δ and γ globin genes; there is also a small deletion at each end of the inversion. A highly speculative model has been proposed, whereby an inversion of this type is generated by interactions between two chromosomal loops (Fig. 62).

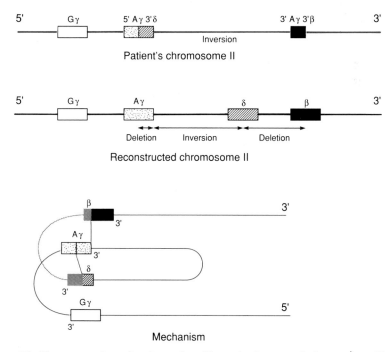

Figure 62. The generation of an inversion. The region between the human ^γ and δ genes is inverted with small deletions at each end of the inversion. The patient's chromosome is shown together with a reconstruction suggesting the events that led to the inversion. The most likely mechanism is the formation of loops which have brought the four globin genes into apposition, abnormal crossing over, and the generation of small deletions together with an inversion as shown.

Insertions

As mentioned earlier in this chapter, there are several structural haemoglobin variants with elongated α or β chains due to insertions of triplet codons within the exons of the α or β globin chain genes such that the code remains in sequence. Hence normal α or β chains are produced with additional amino acid residues inserted at different positions along their length. The molecular mechanisms involved are described on page 145.

Recently it has been found that another monogenic disorder, lipoprotein lipase deficiency, results from gene insertions. Lipoprotein lipase (LPL) plays an important role in triacylglycerol metabolism. The clinical syndrome of LPL deficiency is characterized by abdominal pain, enlargement of the liver and spleen, the development of xanthomas, and the presence of creamy plasma due an increased level of chylomicrons. It turns out that this condition is quite heterogeneous at the molecular level. Analysis of the LPL gene has revealed that several cases result from insertions whereas at least one results from a deletion. Major rearrangements account for about 25 per cent of the mutations of this gene, with a single unique insertion being the most common. Whether the molecular mechanism is the same as that proposed for the insertions observed in the haemoglobin genes remains to be determined, as does the way in which the insertion leads to a reduced output of the gene product.

Quite recently a novel mechanism for the generation of an insertion has been found which is totally different from that causing insertions in the globin and LPL genes. It involves the factor VIII locus and is the first example of a human gene insertion associated with an L1 sequence. The latter belongs to a family of long interspersed, repetitive elements present in approximately 10^5 copies throughout the genome. L1 elements have A-rich 3′ ends and two long open reading frames called orf-1 and orf-2, the second of which encodes a potential peptide with homology to reverse transcriptase. This structure suggests that L1 sequences may function as non-viral retrotransposons. Transposons are a variety of transposable genetic elements that occur in both prokaryotes and eukaryotes. They are flanked by inverted repeat sequences, which in turn are flanked by direct repeats, and often possess genes in addition to those required for their insertion. They are, in effect, elements that are probably involved in moving genes from place to place within the genome. From studies of two unrelated patients it turns out that an L1 sequence has been integrated into an exon of the factor VIII gene. Both insertions contain 3′ portions of the L1 sequence, including the polyA tract, and create target duplications of at least 12 nucleotides in the factor VIII gene. How often the insertion has occurred of L1 sequences involving retro-transposition of DNA sequences through RNA intermediates into new locations in the human genome is not yet clear. But this may represent a novel mechanism for producing genetic disease.

It turns out, therefore, that insertions are a fairly common cause of human molecular pathology. Recent work suggests that several varieties of the Lesch–Nyhan syndrome are due to inserts in the HGPRT gene, and one form of Marfan's syndrome may be associated with an insert in the COLA2 gene.

Promotor box mutations

Several forms of β thalassaemia have been described in which point mutations were found 'upstream' from the β globin gene (Fig. 63) either within or adjacent

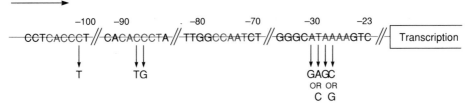

Figure 63. Mutations of the promotor regions of the β globin gene.

to the promotor boxes described in Chapter 3. These mutations are associated with a variable reduction in output from the adjacent β globin chain loci. Their existence emphasizes the importance of these highly conserved regions of DNA and confirms their proposed promotor function.

● Defective processing of messenger RNA

As described in Chapter 3, the primary mRNA transcript has to be processed by the removal of introns, joining together of exons, and by polyadenylation. Work in the thalassaemia field has provided a wealth of examples of molecular pathology involving these complex processes.

Splice junction mutations

We have already discussed how normal splicing of mRNA is dependent on the presence of GT and AG dinucleotides at the 5′ and 3′ intron-exon junctions. There are seven examples of different β° thalassaemia mutations in which a single base substitution in one of these critical sites completely abolishes β globin chain production; no normal mRNA is produced (Fig. 64). These findings underline the critical importance of these sequences for normal splicing. A similar type of lesion is responsible for the form of phenylketonuria that is common in some north European populations.

Cryptic splice sites in introns

There are much more subtle abnormalities of mRNA processing due to point mutations. Several examples are listed in Table 22. Single base substitutions within introns may result in preferential alternative splicing of the precursor β mRNA molecules at the site of the mutation. For example, a common form of β thalassaemia that occurs in the Mediterranean population results from a single nucleotide substitution, G→A, at position 110 of the first intervening sequence (IVS1) of the β globin gene. This change produces an AG sequence that happens to be preceded by a stretch of pyrimidines and thus forms a functional 3′ acceptor consensus sequence. About 80 per cent of the processed mRNA is the result of

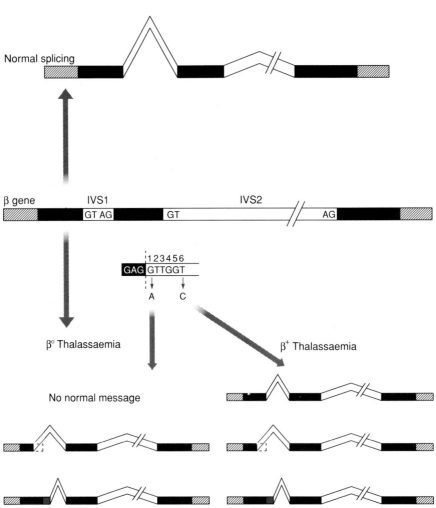

Figure 64. Splice junction mutations. The normal splicing mechanism is shown above. The exons are represented as black boxes and the introns are unshaded. Below are shown the results of two different base substitutions, either at the splice junction or in the consensus sequence near the junction. The first involves the invariant donor GT sequence; no normally spliced β globin mRNA (dotted lines) is produced. Two abnormally spliced mRNA molecules are synthesized by splicing into sites which are not normally utilized. The T→C substitution at the 6th position produces an alternate splicing site so that some normal mRNA and several different species of abnormal mRNA are produced. This leads to the phenotype of β⁺ thalassaemia.

splicing into this site rather than the normal 3′ IVS1 AG (Fig. 65). The mRNA produced as the result of the abnormal splicing contains intron sequences and is therefore useless as a template for globin chain synthesis. Because this site is used preferentially, more abnormal than normal mRNA is produced and therefore there is a severe deficiency of β chain production.

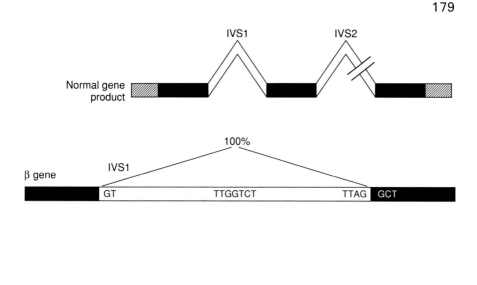

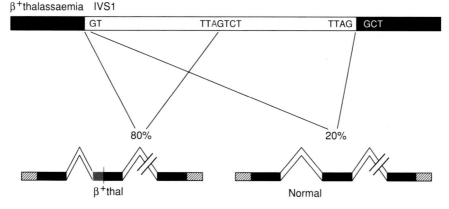

Figure 65. A mutation in the first intron of the β globin gene. The G→A substitution at position 110 in the first intron of the β globin gene produces a new acceptor site. Eighty per cent of the time this site is used for splicing with the production of an abnormal messenger RNA which contains intron sequences; 20 per cent of normal messenger RNA is produced. This leads to the clinical picture of severe β⁺ thalassaemia in which only 20 per cent of normal chain production occurs.

Consensus sequence mutations

As mentioned in Chapter 3, in additional to the GT/AG junctional sequences there are highly conserved sequences at the boundaries between introns and exons that must also be involved in splicing of mRNA.

Several forms of β thalassaemia have been described which result from the production of alternative splicing sites within these consensus sequences. For example, there are two varieties that are caused by single base changes at nucleotide positions 5 or 6 at the 5′ end of the first intervening sequence (Fig. 64).

Splicing occurs both at the normal site and at the new sites generated by these base changes. The effects of these point mutations are remarkably subtle. Some of those at position 5 cause a severe defect of β chain production, while that at position 6 is associated with an extremely mild phenotype. Several other types of thalassaemia have been described in which point mutations in the second intervening sequence cause alternative splicing sites and hence abnormal β globin mRNA molecules.

Cryptic splice sites in exons

Perhaps even more remarkable is the fact that mutations have been found in exons of the globin genes that seem to activate 'cryptic' splice sites. One of these is particularly interesting because it is also associated with the production of a structural haemoglobin variant, haemoglobin E. This variant has a substitution of lysine for glutamic acid at position 26. This results from the codon change GAG→AAG (Fig. 66). The latter seems to activate a 'cryptic' splice site which competes with the normal 5′ splice site and leads to a reduced output of β globin chains. This may be why haemoglobin E is associated with a β thalassaemic blood picture.

Several other single gene disorders sometimes result from splice junction mutations. They include phenylketonuria, haemophilia, and Christmas disease (factor IX deficiency). One variety of Christmas disease results from a deletion of an entire exon of the factor IX gene. Despite this, an abnormal gene product is produced, presumably by linking the remaining exons together during mRNA processing.

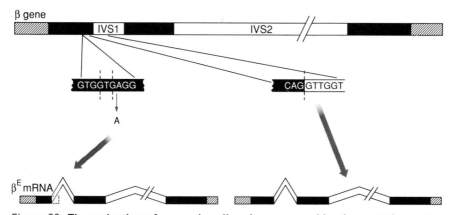

Figure 66. The activation of a cryptic splice site generated by the mutation which gives rise to haemoglobin E. There is a sequence in the first exon which is similar to the concensus sequence at the exon I/IVS I junction. The G→A substitution which causes haemoglobin E activates this cryptic splice site which is then utilized at a low level. Thus there is some abnormal mRNA produced which lacks exon sequences and contains a premature stop codon; also the splicing of normal β globin mRNA is retarded. This is the reason why haemoglobin E is produced at a relatively low level and causes a mild thalassaemia phenotype.

PolyA signal site mutations

Finally, polyadenylation signal site mutations also interfere with the normal processing of mRNA. For example, the single base change AATAAA→AATAAT, which is found in the α globin genes of patients with α thalassaemia in the Middle East and Mediterranean region, drastically reduces the production of α globin chains from the α2 globin gene. Instead of the normal cutting and polyadenylation of the mRNA precursor a long molecule is produced which does not appear in the cytoplasm. A small amount of polyadenylated mRNA is produced, but the overall effect is to almost entirely inactivate the affected globin gene. It is also possible that this mutation may in some way interfere with the termination of globin gene transcription. A single base change in the polyadenylation signal sequence also has been observed in the β globin gene as the basis for one type of β thalassaemia.

Recently a polyadenylation signal mutation was found in the gene for arylsulphatase in persons with a subclinical deficiency of the enzyme, a condition called pseudodeficiency.

● Mutations that interfere with translation

Initiation codon mutations

Several mutations have been observed in patients with α thalassaemia which involve either the initiation codon itself or the sequences immediately adjacent to it. As would be expected no α chains are produced from the affected α globin gene.

Recently, another novel mutation involving initiation of protein synthesis has been described. This involves the G proteins, the products of a large gene family that bind guanine nucleotides and which we have already met in Chapter 3 and will encounter again when we discuss the action of certain oncogenes. Each G protein consists of three distinct subunits called α, β, and γ. It is the α subunit that actually binds and hydrolyses GTP. The cell surface receptors that are coupled to G proteins receive a diverse series of signals including information from photons of light, neurotransmitters, and hormones. The first disease in which a G protein abnormality was found was a condition called pseudohypoparathyroidism, so called because patients with this disorder have hypocalcaemia and hypophosphataemia which are found in ordinary hypoparathyroidism but in this case result from resistance to parathyroid hormone rather than from its deficiency. It is already clear that this is a heterogeneous condition. One form has been found in a family with the features of pseudohypoparathyroidism associated with a reduced function of G protein activity. It turned out that this resulted from a mutation in the Gα gene which was characterized as a change in the initiator codon, ATG to GTG. It is believed that a defect in the α subunit of the stimulatory G protein of adenylate cyclase, which is necessary for the action of parathyroid and other hormones that use cyclic AMP as an intracellular second messenger is responsible for the clinical manifestations of hormone resistance in these patients.

Another rare condition which seems to be due to an initiation codon mutation is a form of chorioretinal degeneration which appears to be due to a deficiency of ornithine-δ-aminotransferase. In one family this has been traced to an ATG–ATA transition in the initiation codon of the gene that controls this enzyme.

Nonsense mutations

A number of point mutations have been found which cause scrambling of the genetic code and hence make it impossible for the translation of a normal gene product. Again many of these examples come from the thalassaemia field although similar lesions have been observed in many other disorders including haemophilia, Christmas disease, the Lesch–Nyhan syndrome, monogenic hypercholesterolaemia, 21 hydroxylase deficiency, and protein C deficiency.

The first mutation of this kind to be identified, in a Chinese patient, was a substitution of codon 17 of the β globin mRNA, AAG→UAG, which changes a lysine codon to a premature termination codon and causes β° thalassaemia. A similar type of mutation is commonly found in Mediterranean patients with β thalassaemia, in this case an alteration in codon 39, CAG→UAG; CAG codes for glutamine in the normal β globin chain. Clearly, if there is a chain termination codon in the middle of the mRNA, translation will cease prematurely with the production of a shortened and physiologically useless peptide fragment (Fig. 67).

Frameshift mutations

Another way in which the genetic code can be scrambled is by the generation of a so-called frameshift mutation, which is the basis of at least seven different forms of β thalassaemia, some cases of haemophilia and Christmas disease, and several other single gene disorders. Since proteins are encoded by a triplet code the loss or insertion of one, two, or four nucleotides in the coding region of a gene will throw the reading frame out of sequence. The result is that a completely anomalous amino acid sequence is added to a normally initiated globin chain. Sometimes the altered base sequence generates a new termination codon leading to premature termination of translation of the abnormal mRNA (Fig. 68). If the altered mRNA can be translated there is a complete change of sequence after the site of the frameshift mutation. As mentioned earlier, several human haemoglo-

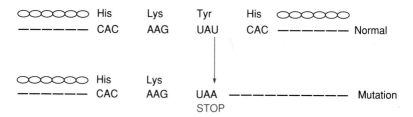

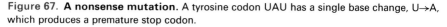

Figure 67. **A nonsense mutation.** A tyrosine codon UAU has a single base change, U→A, which produces a premature stop codon.

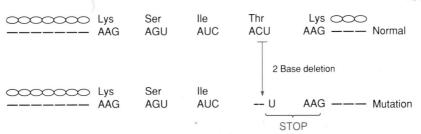

Figure 68. A frameshift mutation. Two bases have been deleted from a threonine codon, ACU. This leaves a U which now links up with the next two bases of the next lysine codon to produce UAA, which is a stop codon.

bin variants with an elongated α or β chain result from frameshift mutations; in this case the normal stop codon is thrown out of sequence and the scrambled mRNA is translated until another stop codon is produced, so leading to an elongated translation product (see page 145). Some fibrinogen variants result from frameshift mutations of this type.

Termination codon mutations

The termination codon mutations were described earlier in this chapter (page 144). So far they have been observed only in the α globin genes. The base alteration results in the insertion of an amino acid instead of chain termination. Messenger RNA sequence that is not normally utilized is then translated until another in-phase stop codon is reached. The result is an elongated but stable α chain (see Fig. 48, page 144).

A problem that has worried us since we deduced the nature of these mutations many years before DNA sequencing was available is why these elongated α chains are produced so inefficiently that the stop codon mutations are all associated with the clinical phenotype of α thalassaemia. There is nothing wrong with the translation of these long mRNAs. Rather it appears that the actual process of translating the additional 3′ mRNA sequences somehow destabilized the α globin mRNA.

● Unstable protein products

As mentioned earlier in this chapter, some monogenic disorders are characterized by the absence of a gene product due to the synthesis of a highly unstable polypeptide which is degraded immediately after synthesis. Again, the best examples come from the haemoglobin field. In some cases very small amounts of unstable globin chain can be demonstrated by *in vitro* radioactive labelling studies; but in others no product can be identified and the molecular pathology can be deduced only by sequencing the appropriate gene and making an educated guess as to the likely effect of the amino acid substitution that would follow the base change.

Recent studies along these lines have provided insights into how subtle differences in the length of abnormal translation products may change a recessive to a dominant phenotype. Most β thalassaemia carriers, even if they have β⁰ thalassaemia mutations, are symptomless and simply have hypochromic red cells which reflect underhaemoglobinization due to the lack of activity of one of the pairs of β globin genes. However, it has been known for some years that some individuals who are heterozygous for β thalassaemia have severe anaemia with enlarged spleens. It was always difficult to understand how this could be; how could a heterozygote be worse off than having no β globin genes produced from one locus? The anaemia of thalassaemia is due to globin chain imbalance and therefore it seemed reasonable to suspect that this dominant form of β thalassaemia must, in some way, reflect the presence of a greater degree of imbalanced globin chain production than is usually the case in β⁰ thalassaemia heterozygotes. As mentioned earlier many forms of β⁰ thalassaemia result from nonsense or frameshift mutations which result in the production of truncated β globin chains. Presumably these, together with the excess of α chains that are produced as the result of one defective β globin chain locus in heterozygotes, are destroyed by proteolysis in the red cell precursor. It turns out however that if the premature stop point is in the third exon, or if there is a frameshift mutation in this region that produces an elongated variant, there is a greater degree of globin chain precipitation. This is made up of excess α chains together with haem-containing β chains. Since haem is inserted round about residue 90 it appears that these longer truncated gene products that bind haem form a stable precipitate; the shorter products that do not contain haem are easily digested. Thus recessiveness or dominance in β thalassaemia is a subtle reflection of the length and properties of the truncated globin chains that are synthesized due to mutations at different points along the β globin gene.

● Mutations that are 'distant' from structural genes

As we have seen, most of the mutations that interfere with the production of peptide chains involve either the structural genes themselves or important regulatory sequences in their immediate flanking regions. However, a few exceptions have been encountered. For example, as mentioned earlier, deletions have been found in the α or β globin gene complex which lie upstream from the α or β globin genes and yet appear to switch them off (see Figs 56 and 58). In one case, involving the α globin genes, the deletion ends about 16 kb upstream from the structural genes yet the latter are down regulated. Until recently it was not clear how this effect is mediated. It might involve major alterations of the functional domains of these genes such that critical regulatory sequences involved in their normal expression are lost.

Recently a so-called dominant control region (DCR) has been identified upstream from the β-like globin gene cluster which may be required for activation of the entire multi-gene complex. It is possible that the loss of this region causes loss of β gene function in individuals with long deletions of the complexes that remove the DCR but leave the β genes intact (Fig. 58). An α globin DCR has also been identified, together with several deletions that involve this sequence and inactivate the α globin genes on the same chromosome.

There is some evidence, again from the globin field, that unlinked genes may have effects on structural genes. For example, there is one type of hereditary persistence of fetal haemoglobin in which the genetic determinant appears to segregate quite independently from the globin gene clusters. Whether this represents a true regulatory gene mutation remains to be determined, however; the bulk of monogenic disorders seem to result from simple *cis*-acting mutations that involve the structural genes or their immediate environment.

● Phenotype/genotype relationships for mutations that alter the output of structural genes

● Modification of phenotypes associated with genetic deletions

Although it is still early days a start has been made in trying to relate the molecular lesions (outlined in the previous sections) to their associated clinical phenotypes. As might be expected, deletions completely remove or inactivate structural genes. Thus the α° and β° thalassaemias are characterized by an absence of adult haemoglobin production and, usually, with a severe clinical phenotype. Similarly, the large deletions that involve the factor VIII or IX genes cause severe forms of haemophilia or Christmas disease.

The situation with the deletions involving the locus that directs the production of dystrophin on the X chromosome is more complicated, however. As mentioned earlier, dystrophin was discovered by reverse genetics by deriving its amino acid sequence from the nucleotide sequence of the gene that is deleted in patients with Duchenne muscular dystrophy (DMD). There are two main varieties of muscular dystrophy that seem to result from mutations of this locus. First, there is typical DMD, which is characterized by severe muscle weakness starting early in life. Second, there is a milder condition called Becker muscular dystrophy (BMD). It has been possible, by preparing antibodies to dystrophin, to examine the relationship between the clinical phenotypes of DMD and BMD and the abundance and size of dystrophin. This work suggests that where there is a major deficiency of dystrophin there is a more severe clinical phenotype, while patients with BMD may have qualitative abnormalities of the protein. These studies have been supported by structural analyses of the dystrophin locus. Many of the deletions in DMD patients were found to result in frameshifts with stop codons immediately downstream of the deletion, which would give rise to a severely truncated form of dystrophin. In contrast, the deletions that give rise to BMD are such that a small but potentially functional form of dystrophin could be produced. These correlations are not absolutely consistent, however, and at least one case of BMD has been reported in a patient with an intragenic deletion spanning approximately one-third of the entire DMD gene. No doubt these studies will be extended over the next few years and provide us with an extremely valuable model for understanding structure/function relationships consequent on different sized deletions or other mutations of very large genes.

Surprisingly, however, even when a gene is completely deleted there may be some variation in the clinical phenotype. For example, β° thalassaemia is not always severe. There is increasing evidence that such variability in expression may result from inherited differences in ability to produce the γ chains of fetal haemoglobin and hence to compensate for defective β chain production. Similar phenotypic heterogeneity has been observed in patients with deletions of the LDL receptor gene. As mentioned below, it is becoming apparent that much of this type of clinical variability is a reflection of phenotypic modification by the products of other gene loci with related functions.

● Modification of phenotypes by mutations that involve the regulation of transcription or messenger RNA processing

Mutations that involve splicing of upstream regulatory boxes are associated with a wide variety of clinical phenotypes. Some of them cause a very small reduction in the output from the affected locus and therefore are associated with a very mild clinical phenotype. For example, most of the β thalassaemias that are due to mutations in or near the upstream regulatory boxes have a mild phenotype. Interestingly, there is a recent description of a point mutation at position -101 which is completely 'silent' in heterozygotes. In compound heterozygotes in which the other β thalassaemia mutation is more severe there is a moderate degree of anaemia.

There is, of course, enormous potential for variability in expression of the mutations that involve splicing of mRNA. If a point mutation opens up a new splice site the resulting phenotype will depend on how often splicing occurs at the abnormal site compared with a normal splice site. We saw earlier in this chapter how subtle these effects can be when we considered the mutations that occur in the first six bases of the first intron of the β globin gene. No doubt as we learn more about the molecular pathology of single gene disorders we shall be able to describe phenotypes ranging from almost normal to lethal based on the precise site and action of point mutations of this type.

● Modification of phenotype by genetic variability at other loci

The thalassaemia field has also provided us with some elegant examples of how the phenotype of single gene disorders may be modified by the action of other genes. For example, some patients who are homozygotes or compound heterozygotes for different β thalassaemia mutations have an unusually mild clinical course. The major cause of the severe anaemia of β thalassaemia is an imbalance of globin chain synthesis; the excess α chains consequent on defective β chain production precipitate and damage the developing red cell precursors in the bone marrow and the red blood cells in the peripheral circulation. It follows, therefore, that anything that reduces the magnitude of the excess of α chains should ameliorate the condition. Some of the ways in which this can occur are illustrated in Fig. 69. Obviously, a milder defect in β chain synthesis is one. Another, and at first not so obvious, is the co-inheritance of α thalassaemia. This 'experiment of nature' clearly demonstrates the importance of globin chain imbalance in this disorder. Patients who inherit one or more α thalassaemia determinants together with β thalassaemia have a much milder phenotype because they have less globin chain imbalance. Similarly, as mentioned earlier, there are a number of mutations that seem to increase γ chain production in patients with β thalassaemia. Since α chains combine with γ chains to produce fetal haemoglobin this also leads to less globin chain imbalance and a milder phenotype. In clinical practice, population studies suggest that most of the variability in the phenotype of β thalassaemia can be explained by these three mechanisms (see Fig. 69).

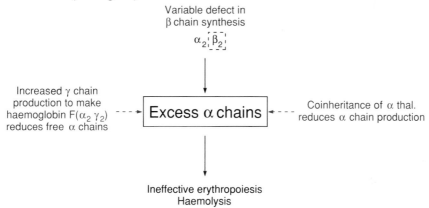

Figure 69. The various genetic mechanisms which may modify the phenotype of β thalassaemia.

There is growing evidence that the phenotype of other monogenic disorders can be modified by the action of genes with related function. Individuals who are homozygous for mutations at the LDL receptor locus usually succumb to a heart attack in early life. On the other hand, heterozygotes may have heart attacks by the age of 40 or they may remain unaffected. Very recently, at least some of this heterogeneity has been found to reflect polymorphisms in other proteins that affect cholesterol levels. Doubtless many more examples of phenotypic modification by the action of genes with related functions will be found.

● X chromosome inactivation or somatic mosaicism as a modifier of
   phenotype

In Chapter 2 we saw how one X chromosome is inactivated very early during fetal development. Since this is a random process, and because it occurs so early during development, there is considerable variability in the pattern of inactivation. In females who are heterozygous for a genetic defect on the X chromosome about 50 per cent of the red cells express the defect and 50 per cent are normal. However, because inactivation is random, there may by chance be many more cells that carry the mutation giving a phenotype very similar to that of a hemizygous affected male. Somatic mosaicism may also modify the clinical phenotype. For example, mildly affected parents of children with lethal osteogenesis imperfecta have been found to be mosaic for mutations of type 1 procollagen. It is likely that such new mutations occurred during the parents' embryonic development such that only a proportion of the cells in their different tissues were involved. If the offspring happened to inherit germ cells carrying the mutation, they would have a much more severe disease.

● Modification of phenotype by parental imprinting

There is increasing evidence that the clinical phenotype of single gene disorders, and some of the more complex genetic conditions that we shall encounter in later chapters, may be modified depending on whether they are inherited on the paternal or maternal chromosomes. For example the early onset of symptoms of Huntington's disease and spinocerebellar ataxia appears to be associated with paternal transmission, whereas the more severe variety of neurofibromatosis I, or the early onset of neurofibromatosis II, is found in cases of maternal transmission.

How is this remarkable epigenetic effect mediated? The mechanism is not yet understood in detail although it appears that different states of methylation of the parental chromosomes may be involved. Regardless of the precise molecular basis for this extraordinary phenomenon, it is becoming apparent that imprinting of this type may have profound phenotypic effects, involving changes from recessive to dominant inheritance in some cases. We shall return to this topic in a later chapter when we consider some of the rare inherited forms of cancer.

● Unusual phenotypes associated with cytoplasmic inheritance

So far in this chapter we have considered the molecular pathology of single gene disorders that are carried in our nuclear DNA. However, there is increasing evidence that some genetic diseases result from inherited abnormalities of mitochondrial DNA. Because of the patterns of inheritance of our mitochondria these disorders have certain phenotypic peculiarities.

Each human mitochondrion contains several copies of an identical circular genome, 16 569 bp in length, that includes some of the subunits of the electron transport chain at the inner mitochondrial membrane together with components of ATP synthase. All mitochondrial DNA is maternally derived. Mutations of the mitochondrial genome have been implicated in a few diseases to date, the mitochondrial myopathies and Leber's optic neuropathy, for example.

The mitochondrial myopathies are a group of disorders characterized by muscle weakness and multisystem disease. They are often associated with defects in the electron transport chain and are usually maternally inherited. Several molecular defects have been found in mitochondrial DNA in these conditions. For example, nine patients with mitochondrial myopathy were found to be heteroplasmic (that is to have both normal and abnormal mitochondria); the abnormal mitochondrial DNA contained a 2–7 kb deletion which was found in muscle cells but not in other body tissues. In other cases of mitochondrial myopathy duplications of mitochondrial DNA have been found. The reason for the apparent tissue specificity of these lesions is not clear. There is some recent evidence that it may reflect tissue-specific expression of certain genes involved in the regulation of oxidative phosphorylation. Deletions have also been found in a form of encephalomyopathy called the Kearns–Sayre syndrome.

In Leber's optic neuropathy an arginine to histidine substitution has been found at codon 340 in the NADH dehydrogenase subunit gene. In this case the mutation was found to be homoplasmic, that is it occurred in all mitochondria. On the other hand the mutation is not always associated with the clinical picture of Leber's disease and therefore another factor may be required for its phenotypic expression. Point mutations have been found recently in a form of myoclonic epilepsy associated with ragged red muscle fibres.

It is not yet clear how these mitochondrial mutations arose and clearly there is scope for enormous phenotypic variation depending on the tissue distribution of the mutant mitochondria and whether they are heteroplasmic or homoplasmic.

● The heterogeneity of monogenic disease

In this chapter we have seen that monogenic disease is highly heterogeneous at the molecular level and how it is starting to be possible to understand the remarkable variability in clinical phenotypes by analysing these diseases at the molecular level.

The different form of thalassaemia result from over 100 different mutations of the α and β globin genes. As pointed out in the previous chapter RFLP haplotype analysis has suggested that these mutations have occurred independently in different populations and then reached their current high frequencies by selection. Detailed analysis of the mutations in different parts of the world has shown that most populations have two or three common mutations and a varying number of rare ones. It follows, that with the exception of isolated populations or those in which cousin marriage is the norm, most severely affected patients are compound heterozygotes for two different molecular forms of α or β thalassaemia.

We have already seen how many of the common X-linked disorders result from new mutations and therefore it is not surprising that they are turning out to be extremely heterogeneous at the molecular level. Studies of the molecular defect in Duchenne muscular dystrophy, Lesch–Nyhan syndrome and in haemophilia A and B have demonstrated a wide range of different mutations similar to those that have been found in the thalassaemias.

Recent work on the molecular basis of cystic fibrosis is also disclosing remarkable molecular heterogeneity. While about 60–70 per cent of chromosomes that have been analysed in north European and American populations show the loss of the phenylalanine residue at position 508 there is already evidence for remarkable heterogeneity among the rest of the mutations that have been discovered. These include mis-sense and nonsense mutations, frameshifts, and deletions or insertions, all involving the ATP-binding or transmembrane domains of the CFTR gene. RFLP haplotype analysis suggests a common origin for the position 508 mutation and other specific haplotype relationships for some of the more recently described mutations. As mentioned in earlier chapters it seems likely that the cystic fibrosis gene has come under some kind of selection in north Europeans although until its function is better understood it will be very difficult to make a guess as to what the pressures may have been.

In Chapter 2 we discussed the potential heterogeneity of dominant disorders and suggested that these might be more homogeneous. Although there is very little information available yet, recent data about the mutations of the LDL receptor that produce familial hypercholesterolaemia are interesting and unexpected. So far, between 30 and 40 different mutations of this gene have been described including insertions, deletions, nonsense and mis-sense lesions, and frameshifts. The ways in which these interfere with receptor structure and function were outlined earlier in this chapter. It turns out that in nearly every American family that has been studied there is a different mutation. Globally the position is slightly less heterogeneous. About 70 per cent of French Canadians with the condition have the same deletion and in South Africa two particular mutations predominate suggesting that perhaps these were brought into the country by the original Dutch settlers. Similarly, a particular nonsense mutation predominates in Lebanese, while in Finns over 50 per cent have the same deletion at the end of the LDL receptor gene. Monogenic hypercholesterolaemia does not have any major effect on reproductive fitness and the finding of the remarkable heterogeneity of molecular defects in the American population is particularly interesting.

Clearly much remains to be learnt about the population genetics of human disease at the molecular level and how different mutations have been disseminated. But from a practical point of view it is quite clear that if we are to use DNA technology in diagnostic and preventative genetics we will have to develop screening systems which take into account the extraordinary diversity of mutations that underlie monogeneic disease.

● Summary

It appears that we already have a good idea of the repertoire of the types of mutations that are involved in single gene disorders. It is also possible to start to understand how these molecular lesions give rise to such varied clinical phenotypes and how the interactions of other genes may modify their clinical expression. These monogenic disorders represent one extreme of genetic diversity. It follows, therefore, that the scope for variability associated with less profound effects on function must be quite enormous. In the next chapter we shall consider the much more difficult question of how such variability at a number of gene loci might interact to produce susceptibility or resistance to common diseases.

● Further reading

Amselem, S., Duquesnoy, P., Altree, O., *et al.* (1989). Laron dwarfism and mutations of the growth hormone-receptor gene. *New Engl. J. Med.*, **321**, 989–95.

Boswell, D.R. and Carrell, R.W. (1989). Genetic engineering and the serpins. *BioEssays*, **8**, 83–7.

Byers, P. (1989). Molecular heterogeneity of the chondrodysplasias. *Am. J. Hum. Genet.*, **45**, 1–4.

Carrell, R.W., Aulak, K.S., and Owen, M.C. (1989). The molecular pathology of the serpins. *Mol. Biol. Med.*, **6**, 35–42.

Crabtree, G.R. (1987). The molecular biology of fibrinogen. In *The molecular basis of blood diseases*, (ed. G. Stamatoyannopoulos, A.W. Nienhuis, P. Leder, and P.W. Majerus), pp. 631–61. W.B. Saunders, Philadelphia, PA.

Davies, K.E. (1985). Molecular genetics of the human X chromosome. *J. Med. Genet.*, **22**, 243–9.

Davies, K.E. (1986). *Human genetic diseases: A practical approach.* IRL Press, Oxford.

Davies, K.E. and Read, A.P. (1988). *Molecular basis of inherited disease.* IRL Press, Oxford.

Davies, K. E. and Robson, K.J.H. (1987). Molecular analysis of human monogenic diseases. *BioEssays*, **6**, 247–53.

DiLella, A.G., Marvit, J., Kidsky, A.S., Guttler, F., and Woo, S.L.C. (1986). Tight linkage between a splicing mutation and a specific DNA haplotype in phenylketonuria. *Nature*, **322**, 799–803.

DiLella, A.G. and Woo, S.L.C. (1987). Molecular basis of phenylketonuria and its clinical applications. *Mol. Biol. Med.*, **4**, 183–92.

Dinauer, M.C., Orkin, S.H., Brown, R., Jesaitios, A.J., and Parkos, C.A. (1987). The glycoprotein encoded by the X-linked chronic granulomatous disease locus is a component of the neutrophil cytochrome *b* locus. *Nature*, **327**, 717–20.

Dryja, T.P., McGee, T.L., Reichel, E., *et al.* (1990). A point mutation of the rhodopsin gene in one form of retinitis pigmentosa. *Nature*, **343**, 364–6.

Higgs, D.R., Vickers, M.A., Wilkie, A.O.M., Pretorius, I.-M., Jarman, A.P., and Weatherall, D.J. (1989). A review of the molecular genetics of the human α-globin gene cluster. *Blood*, **73**, 1081–104.

Hoffman, E.P., Brown, R.H., and Kunkel, L.M. (1987). Dystrophin: the protein product of the Duchenne muscular dystrophy locus. *Cell*, **51**, 919–28.

Koenig, M., Hoffman, E.P., Bertelson, C.J., Monaco, A.P., Feener, C., and Kunkel, L.M. (1987). Complete cloning of the Duchenne muscular dystrophy (DMD) cDNA and preliminary genomic organization of the DMD gene in normal and affected individuals. *Cell*, **50**, 509–17.

Lander, E.S. and Lodish, H. (1990). Mitochondrial disease: gene mapping and gene therapy. *Cell*, **61**, 925–6.

Ledley, F.D. (1990). Perspectives on methylmalonic acidaemia resulting from molecular cloning of methylmalonyl CoA mutase. *BioEssays*, **12**, 335–40.

Love, D.R. and Davies, K.E. (1989). Duchenne muscular dystrophy: the gene and the protein. *Mol. Biol. Med.*, **6**, 7–17.

Monaco, A.P. (1989). Dystrophin, the protein product of the Duchenne/Becker muscular dystrophy gene. *Trends Biochem.*, **14**, 412–15.

Nathans, J., Thomas, D., and Hogness, D.S. (1986). Molecular genetics of human color vision: the genes encoding blue, green, and red pigments. *Science*, **232**, 193–202.

Nienhuis, A.W., Anagnou, N.P., and Ley, T.J. (1984). Review: Advances in thalassemia research. *Blood*, **63**, 738–58.

Orkin, S.H. (1987). Disorders of hemoglobin synthesis: the thalassemias. In *The molecular basis of blood diseases*, (ed. G. Stamatoyannopoulos, A.W. Nienhuis, P. Leder, and P.W. Majerus), pp. 106–26. W.B. Saunders, Philadelphia, PA.

Orkin, S.H. (1989). X-linked chronic granulomatous disease: more than two years later. *Mol. Biol. Med.*, **6**, 1–5.

Perutz, M.F. (1987). Molecular anatomy, physiology, and pathology of hemoglobin. In *The molecular basis of blood diseases*, (ed. G. Stamatoyannopoulos, A.W. Nienhuis, P. Leder, and P.W. Majerus), pp. 127–78. W.B. Saunders, Philadelphia, PA.

Reik, W. (1989). Genomic imprinting and genetic disorders in man. *Trends Genet.*, **5**, 331–6.

Riordan, J.R., Rommens, J.M., Kerem, B.S. *et al.* (1989). Identification of the cystic fibrosis gene: cloning and characterization of complementary DNA. *Science*, **245**, 1066–73.

Sykes, B. (1985). The molecular genetics of collagen. *BioEssays*, **3**, 112–17.

Sykes, B. (1989). Inherited collagen disorders. *Mol. Biol. Med.*, **6**, 19–26.

Teahan, C., Rowe, P., Parker, P., Totty, N., and Segal, A.W. (1987). The X-linked chronic granulomatous disease gene codes for the β-chain of cytochrome b_{-245}. *Nature*, **327**, 720–1.

Thein, S.L., Hesketh, C., Taylor, P., *et al.* (1990). Molecular basis for dominantly inherited inclusion body β-thalassemia. *Proc. Natl. Acad. Sci. USA.*, **87**, 3924–28.

Thein, S.L. and Weatherell, D.J. (1988). The thalassaemias. In *Recent advances in haematology*, **5**, (ed. A.V. Hoffbrand), pp. 43–74. Churchill Livingstone, Edinburgh.

Wallace, D.C. (1989). Mitochondrial DNA mutations and neuromuscular disease. *Trends Genet.*, **5**, 9–13.

Wallace, D.C., Singh, G., Lott, M.T., Hodge, J.A., Schurr, T.G., Lezza, A.M.S., Elsas, L.J. II, and Nikoskelainen, E.K. (1988). Mitochondrial DNA mutations associated with Leber's hereditary optic neuropathy. *Science*, **242**, 1427–30.

Wallace, G.A., Starman, B.J., Zinn, A.B., and Byers, P.H. (1990). Variable expression of osteogenesis imperfecta in a nuclear family is explained by somatic mosaicism for a lethal point mutation in the α(1) gene (COL1A1) of type 1 collagen in a parent. *Am. J. Hum. Genet.*, **46**, 1034–40.

Weatherall, D.J. and Clegg, J.B. (1981). *The thalassaemia syndromes*, 3rd edn. Blackwell Scientific, Oxford.

Woo, S.L.C., Lidsky, A.S., Guttler, F., Chandra, T., and Robson, K.J.H. (1983). Cloned human phenylalanine hydroxylase gene allows prenatal diagnosis and carrier detection of classical phenylketonuria. *Nature*, **306**, 151–5.

Molecular genetics
and common diseases

7

While the phenotypes of the single gene disorders that we considered in the previous chapter may be modified to some degree by the action of other genes and environmental factors, they result predominantly from the deleterious effect of the mutant gene. On the other hand, while our genetic make-up may make us prone to infections or even to careless behaviour, an attack of pneumonia or being knocked over by a bus are events in which the environment plays a predominant role. When we come to some of the major public health problems of western society such as heart disease, stroke, hypertension, diabetes, cancer, psychiatric illnesses, and rheumatism things become much more complicated. These conditions tend to run in families and, as was pointed out in Chapter 2, twin studies have shown that many of them have a strong genetic component. On the other hand their occurrence cannot be traced through families in a way suggesting the action of a single mutant gene. Furthermore, epidemiological studies tell us that environmental factors such as diet, smoking, alcohol intake, and many of the other good things of life, play a major role in their pathogenesis. It appears, therefore, that these disorders are caused by the interaction of environmental factors with several genes at different loci, each with an additive effect. Hitherto it has been very difficult to try to define the individual genes in these polygenic systems. The advent of recombinant DNA technology now offers a new and promising approach to this difficult problem.

Why do we wish to define the genes that might be important in the development of a heart attack or a major psychiatric illness? Do we really want to know that our newborn baby is likely to have a heart attack at the age of 45 or become demented at 60? Questions like this, and similarly confused thinking about the motivation for being curious about the genetics of common diseases, are asked all too commonly and are tending to bring this potentially important aspect of the new genetics into disrepute.

The answer is, of course, that we are not anxious to know whether a newborn baby is likely to drop dead at the age of 40 unless we can do something useful to prevent it happening. The major reason for wishing to define the genes that constitute these polygenic systems is to find out what their products do and how they differ in their function from those of individuals who are not at increased risk for these conditions. Although we have made enormous progress in the symptomatic treatment of these common diseases we still know virtually nothing about their underlying cause. If we can unravel the biochemical basis of their genetic component it is very likely that we will begin to understand why they occur and hence, hopefully, how either to prevent or manage them much more effectively. For example, if we could define one or more of the genes that are involved in the pathogenesis of schizophrenia, and if we could identify the products and their function we should have made a major inroad into starting to understand the biochemical basis of this common and distressing condition.

● General approaches to the analysis of the molecular basis for polygenic disease

Although there are many ways in which we might tackle this difficult problem they fall into two broad categories. First, there is the 'candidate gene' approach. In other words we attempt to make an educated guess as to which genes might be involved in a particular disease. For example, in the case of diabetes it is easy to draw up a list of possibilities; insulin and its receptor, other hormones and their receptors involved in glucose metabolism, insulin-like growth factors, and so on. If we are fortunate enough to have probes for the genes for these particular proteins, and we can identify appropriate RFLPs, we could then use them in family studies to see if any particular RFLPs segregate with the disorder. If so it is likely that the particular gene that we are marking is involved in its pathogenesis. The second approach is even more daunting. Here we simply amass families with as many affected invididuals as possible and go on a 'blind hunt' with batteries of probes for single point RFLPs or hypervariable regions and hope that we will strike lucky and obtain a linkage.

Whichever approach we take we also have to decide on the kind of families to study. Again there are two main ways to tackle the problem. First, we can try to find large multiple-generation families in which there are individuals with the particular disorder that we wish to study. Alternatively, we can use what is called the 'sib-pair' method. This entails looking for polymorphisms of particular candidate genes or random RFLPs to see if they tend to segregate in affected sibships compared to non-affected siblings.

It will be apparent that whichever of these approaches is pursued the difficulties are formidable. Many of the diseases in which we are particularly interested, coronary thrombosis, hypertension, diabetes, and so on, occur only in middle age or later. Already we are in trouble. Obtaining multiple generation families is extremely difficult and we will often be forced to use sib-pair analysis. And there will be considerable ascertainment problems. It is quite possible that we will carry out our sib-pair analysis today, and score for high blood pressure or a previous heart attack, and tomorrow one or more of the 'normal' siblings will have a heart attack or develop high blood pressure. Of course we can make allowances for incorrect ascertainment of this type, but unless our linkage data are extremely strong this problem will make it very difficult to locate the genes that we are looking for. And, of course, unless we have picked a candidate gene we will be in the same position as we were when RFLP linkage analysis landed us a few million bases from our single gene disorders of unknown cause; we are left with a long and difficult hunt to try to find the genes that are of interest to us.

Regardless of the way we decide to search for some of the important genes that make up the polygenic systems that underlie common diseases it is important not to underestimate the mathematical difficulties that we will encounter. Research into methods for analysis of continuous variation resulting from the action of multiple genes has, hitherto, relied primarily on biometrical approaches that set out to analyse phenotypic distributions and then to attempt to estimate the statistical effects of the different genes involved. Although this field has been productive it has been bedevilled by difficulties, not the least of which is the complexity of the mathematical models that describe multi-locus systems, together with the many assumptions that have to be made to reduce some of the mathematical treatments to manageable dimensions.

So far most of the work that has been carried out in the field of polygenic disease and DNA polymorphisms has made use of the standard lod or location score analyses described in Chapter 4. Clearly we shall need to improve the efficiency of these techniques as we move into the analysis of more complex genetic systems. As pointed out by Lander and Botstein, once we have a reasonable genetic map of the human genome with appropriate RFLPs it will be more efficient to search for individual genes by what is called 'interval mapping', that is testing the hypothesis that a particular trait maps in the middle of the interval between an adjacent pair of RFLPs compared with the hypothesis that is unlinked to the interval. But as we progress in the study of polygenic systems we shall run into a number of difficulties including genetic heterogeneity, incomplete penetrance, genetic predisposition, gene interaction, and so on. Quite recently the method of interval mapping has been modified for the analysis of quantitative trait loci (QTL). Essentially this approach reduces the confounding effects of recombination between marker loci and QTL, exploits efficiently the information from RFLP linkage data, and provides greater precision than was previously obtainable. The method depends on the choice of a particularly stringent threshold for a significant lod score to reduce the probability of false positives. The results are depicted as QTL likelihood maps, a highly informative format to summarize large amounts of information. Likelihood maps represent the probability that one or more QTL lie at a particular point of the genome. Lander and Botstein have described how mapping efficiency may be increased by selective genotyping of only extreme progeny, that is individuals that tend to provide the most linkage information, and by progeny testing to reduce the confounding effects of environmental variants. A full description of these highly sophisticated mathematical treatments of family data is beyond the scope of this book and will be found in a recent publication by Lander and Botstein. Although at the time of writing the application of these new mathematical treatments has been confined largely to the tomato breading fraternity, a long way from heart attacks, they show great promise for the analysis of polygenic disease.

As might have been predicted, most progress to date in the field of polygenic disease has been made in conditions such as autoimmune disease or cancer where there were good candidates genes to work with. But even where there were not, some preliminary information has been obtained. In the sections that follow we will examine a few of the conditions that seem to offer promise for this extremely important application of the new genetics.

● Diabetes

Diabetes mellitus is one of the most important diseases of western society. Even though the different forms of the condition can be controlled with insulin, drugs, or diet it is still a major cause of morbidity and mortality because of the long-term complications, particularly those involving the cardiovascular system, kidneys, and eyes.

Diabetes is usually classified as either insulin-dependent (IDDM, or type 1) or non-insulin-dependent (NIDDM, or type 2). As we saw in Chapter 2, twin studies have suggested that inherited factors play an important role in both types although they appear to be of much greater significance in type 2 diabetes. Diabetes is a good place to start when considering the applications of recombinant DNA technology to the study of common polygenic diseases; there is no lack of candidate genes and because the disease is so common large pedigrees are relatively easy to obtain.

The insulin gene itself, together with that for the insulin receptor, were among the first candidates to be studied even though it always seemed unlikely that the common forms of diabetes would be due to lesions at these loci. The insulin gene is situated on the short arm of chromosome 11, band 15. Within the 45 000 bp segment of this chromosome, which includes the insulin gene, there are several short interspersed middle-repetitive sequences of the *Alu* family and, approximately 360 bases upstream from the start of the insulin gene itself, there is a hypervariable region (HVR) with sequence homology to HVRs near the human α globin chain genes. Variation in the size of the alleles generated in this region is due to different numbers of tandem repeats of a family of 14–15 bp oligonucleotides. The gene itself is 1430 bp long and contains two introns. The insulin receptor is an integral membrane protein composed of two α and two β subunits. The α subunit contains the insulin binding site and is linked to the amino-terminal portion of the β subunit by a disulphide bond. The receptor is anchored in the plasma membrane through a single membrane-spanning region in the β subunit. The α and β subunits are generated by proteolytic processing of a single chain precursor.

While a few rare cases of diabetes have been found to be due to mutations that alter the structure of insulin or its receptor (see Chapter 6) it is now clear that neither of the common forms of diabetes result from lesions of this type. Extensive population studies have suggested that there is linkage disequilibrium between different alleles in the HVR near the insulin gene and both type 1 and type 2 diabetes. In other words, particular length polymorphisms in the hypervariable region appear to have been found in association with these forms of diabetes more often than can be explained by chance alone. However, these data are bedevilled by differences in the frequency of hypervariable alleles between races and by the fact that at least some of the results are not consistent between different studies. If the data are telling us anything, it is unlikely that they are pointing towards the insulin gene or its environs being involved directly in either type of diabetes. Rather they suggest that there might be a gene close to that for insulin which is modifying the phenotype towards susceptibility or resistance to diabetes.

It seems very likely that type 1 diabetes is an autoimmune disease. There appears to be immune destruction of the pancreas, against which circulating autoantibodies can be demonstrated. It has been known for some time that there is a strong association between IDDM and particular haplotypes of the HLA-DR gene family. More recently, attention has centred on the DR (class II) genes.

The structure of the class II gene complex was outlined in Chapter 3. It contains three subregions, DP, DQ, and DR, each of which contains at least one expressed α and β chain gene. This is a highly polymorphic system which has been defined by the use of class II specific antibodies, the ability of T cells to recognize and proliferate in response to foreign class II molecules (the mixed lymphocyte reaction or MLR) and, most recently, by RFLP analysis and direct gene sequencing. The class II gene family is illustrated in Fig. 17 (Chapter 3), which also shows the loci involved in regulating gene products that are identified in these different ways and the extent to which they are polymorphic. The reader should not underestimate the complexity of this highly polymorphic system, and is not helped by the fact that the nomenclature and designation of individual gene products seem to change at depressingly regular intervals.

The first observed association between HLA and IDDM was with HLA–B15. It was subsequently found that there is a stronger association with DR3 or DR4, particularly DR3/DR4 heterozygotes. Using RFLP analysis it was then established that the DQ region is more closely linked to the disease susceptibility gene than are the DR loci. Furthermore, the situation is complicated by the observation that at least two DR antigens are consistently found to be negatively associated with the disease, i.e. they appear to protect against developing IDDM. In an extensive study designed to determine which DR or DQ alleles encode class II molecules mediating susceptibility or resistance to IDDM, the sequences of the polymorphic DR and DQ loci of the haplotypes that confer susceptibility or resistance to IDDM were determined. Remarkably, only one residue, 57 of the DQ β-chain, correlated strongly with both susceptibility and resistance. All the DQ β-chains found with increased frequency in diabetics have alanine, valine, or serine at position 57. On the other hand DQ β-chains found with decreased frequency in diabetic patients have aspartic acid at this position. Even more unexpectedly this correlation crosses species; the same substitution is observed in the equivalent genes of the MHC system of the non-obese diabetic mouse. More recent studies suggest that a particular DQ α polymorphism may also be strongly related to susceptibility to IDDM.

How could these single amino acid differences in the α and β chains of the class II molecules be related to susceptibility to type 1 diabetes? It turns out that these particular residues form part of the helix that makes up one side of the putative antigen-presenting site, that is the region in which peptide antigens are 'shown' to the T cell receptor (see Chapter 3). One possibility, therefore, is that the aspartic acid-positive DQ molecules in some way mediate T cell suppression for putative islet cell antigens. Another and even more intriguing scenario is that in some way the aspartic acid-containing DQ molecules cause the elimination of potentially autoreactive T cells during T cell ontogeny in the thymus. Regardless of the underlying mechanism these remarkable observations have already taken us closer to understanding the pathogenesis of type 1 diabetes.

Despite the fact that the genetic component is stronger, less progress has been made in understanding the cause of type 2 diabetes. It is not HLA-DR related and there is no clinical or pathological evidence to suggest that it is an autoimmune disease. RFLP linkage analyses using a variety of candidate gene probes have not yet provided any clues as to the chromosomal location of the genes involved. However, there are some intriguing observations about the pathophysiology of this condition which offer possibilities for future work at the molecular level.

For example, it has been known for many years that an amorphous amyloid-like material accumulates in the pancreatic islet cells of patients with type 2 diabetes. Recently this material, variously called amylin, islet amyloid polypeptide or diabetes-associated peptide, has been isolated and its amino acid sequence determined. It turns out to have strong homology with human calcitonin gene-related peptide, a neuropeptide that may be involved in motor activity in skeletal muscle. The pancreatic peptide, amylin, and rat CGRP are both potent inhibitors of basal and insulin stimulated rates of glycogen synthesis in rat muscle. It is possible that amylin, which also occurs in very low levels in non-diabetic islet cells, is a hormone that is synthesized in these cells and may have a role in opposing insulin action in carbohydrate metabolism. Its apparent increased rate of production in diabetes, and its relationship to the pathogenesis of this condition remains to be determined. Quite recently the gene for amylin has been isolated and assigned to chromosome 12. It turns out that amylin is the product of a precursor of 89 amino acids. It should therefore be possible to investigate its genetic relationship to the pathogenesis of type 2 diabetes by RFLP analysis of affected families or sib pairs.

There are many other candidate genes for type 2 diabetes which can be explored, and because there is such a high level of heritability it should be an ideal condition for more general linkage analysis using extended pedigrees or sib pairs.

● Other autoimmune diseases

The success in defining specific residues of the products of the class II genes as being responsible for resistance or susceptibility to type 1 diabetes has led to considerable activity in applying the same analytical approaches to other disorders that are HLA-DR associated. For example, it has been found that a specific HLA–DQ β-chain polymorphism underlies the association between DR3 and myasthenia gravis. Quite recently even more spectacular results have been obtained in the case of rheumatoid arthritis (RA) and pemphigus vulgaris, a chronic skin disease.

Haplotype sharing in affected siblings has demonstrated linkage to the HLA region of a gene conferring susceptibility to rheumatoid arthritis (RA). There is also an increased concordance of rheumatoid arthritis among monozygotic twins as compared to HLA identical siblings. The condition is DR- associated in several ethnic groups. It turns out that certain DR β1 alleles occur more frequently in RA patients and that these apparent susceptibility alleles have very similar amino acid sequences at residues 65–75 of the particular DR β-chain. These observations, together with several serological studies that implicate the class II genes in the pathogenesis of this common condition, suggest that class II susceptibility alleles may create a DR or DQ site that is effective in presenting a self-peptide from the synovium to peptide-specific DR or DQ-restricted T cell clones.

The chronic skin disease, pemphigus vulgaris, has many features suggesting that it may have an autoimmune basis. In Ashkenazi Jews the frequency of the DR4 antigen is 95 per cent in patients with this condition compared with 40 per cent in non-affected controls. Similar though less striking associations are observed in other racial groups. Nucleotide sequence analyses have identified a DQ β variant in a patient with this condition which differs by only one amino acid from two other DQ alleles. Oligonucleotide dot blot analysis has shown that this variant is present in 100 per cent of DR6-positive Israeli patients with pemphigus vulgaris but in fewer than 7 per cent of controls. These findings suggest that the particular allele that carries this substitution, or a very closely linked gene, plays a major role in the pathogenesis of the condition. Coeliac disease is another autoimmune disease in which strong class II gene associations have been found, in this case both DQ and DP.

In seeking to find a pathogenetic mechanism that might relate the products of the HLD–DR genes to environmental agents their sequences have been compared with a variety of infective organisms. For example, it turns out the genomes of the rubella and Epstein–Barr viruses have short sequences with marked similarity to particular alleles of the DQ β locus. The significance of these tantalizing observations remains to be determined.

More recently attention has been directed towards the possibility that polymorphisms of the T cell receptor, which plays such a central role in immune recognition, might be associated with autoimmune diseases. Using the polymerase chain reaction, RFLPs have been identified in both the variable and constant regions of the α chain gene of the T cell receptor. Significant differences in the frequency of these polymorphisms have been identified between healthy persons and those with multiple sclerosis, myasthenia gravis, and thyrotoxicosis, conditions that are all thought to have an autoimmune basis.

These studies are particularly interesting because if it is possible to identify with certainty a T cell receptor gene that contributes to susceptibility to autoimmune disease, then it might be possible to design monoclonal antibodies which could specifically block the autoimmune T cell response. Indeed, there is some experimental evidence to suggest that this might be feasible. It is possible to produce a form of allergic encephalomyelitis in animals by injecting myelin basic protein in adjuvant. It turns out that in these animals there is a predominant expression of certain α and β chain products of the T cell receptor genes. Treatment of the affected animals with a monoclonal antibody specific for the predominant product of the T cell receptor variable region prevents the development of the disease. Whether such approaches would be feasible in the case of human autoimmune disease remains to be determined.

It appears, therefore, that many autoimmune diseases are strongly related to particular products of the HLA–DR or T cell receptor gene systems. At least in some cases it is clear that other genes must be involved in the pathogenesis of these conditions. Whether autoimmune disease will turn out to be due to the interaction of external agents acting on individuals with particular genetic susceptibility consequent on variation in the structure of their immune system, or whether the latter in some ways interferes with the identification of self antigens without the interaction of external agents, remains to be determined. However, these are the first real clues that we have to the pathogenesis of these common and important disorders and they are a valuable guide to the direction of future studies in this field.

● Cardiovascular disease

Although there are many disorders of the cardiovascular system the two most important in western societies are coronary artery disease and stroke. The major factor in the genesis of coronary artery disease is atheroma of the coronary vessels. Strokes and other cerebrovascular disorders are also related to atheroma, in this case involving the cerebral circulation, but hypertension also plays a major role. Twin studies and population surveys have shown that both coronary artery disease and hypertension have an important genetic component; first degree relatives of patients with either of these conditions are at increased risk of having the same disorder. Since heart attacks and hypertension are so important in producing premature mortality and morbidity, and since so little is known about their pathogenesis, there is considerable interest in the possibility of trying to define the important genes in the polygenic system that underlies susceptibility to these conditions.

● Vascular disease

Ischaemic heart disease and cerebrovascular disease are associated with atheromatous changes in the coronary or cerebral vessels. The pathophysiology of this condition is poorly understood. A reasonable working model suggests that atheromatous lesions result from a sequence of events starting with endothelial injury, platelet aggregation, and release of platelet growth factors which are mitogenic for arterial smooth muscle cells, a local increase in vessel wall permeability to plasma lipropropteins, and smooth muscle hyperplasia, all of which lead eventually to the formation of an atheromatous plaque, fibrosis, and ulceration. There is little doubt that the final event that occludes these diseased arteries is a thrombus formation on an ulcerated plaque. There is good epidemiological evidence that environmental factors such as obesity, stress, smoking, and lack of exercise play an important role in the pathogenesis of coronary artery disease. From the genetic vewpoint the most promising lead is the strong correlation between plasma cholesterol level and coronary artery disease, particularly in individuals under the age of 50.

Lipid metabolism

As pointed out by Goldstein and Brown, whose work on the low density lipoprotein receptor won them the Nobel Prize in 1985, cholesterol is a Janus-faced molecule. The very property that makes it useful in cell membranes, that is its complete insolubility in water, also makes it lethal. When it gets into the wrong place, the artery wall for example, it cannot be mobilized. Thus it has to be transported in a safe state in blood, its concentration must be kept low, and its tendency to escape from the blood stream must be controlled by esterification with long-chain fatty acids and packing the resultant esters in the hydrophobic (water repellant) cores of plasma lipoproteins. The main classes of lipoproteins are characterized by their behaviour in the ultracentrifuge into low density lipoprotein (LDL), very low density lipoprotein (VLDL), intermediate density lipoprotein (IDL), and high density lipoprotein (HDL). The lipoprotein family consists of at least eight different apo proteins; their nomenclature and main properties are summarized in Table 23. Some of them take part in the formation of lipoprotein particles, while others have a functional role in regulating enzymes and interacting with receptors.

   The essential features of lipid transport and metabolism are outlined in Fig. 70. It is convenient to describe these metabolic pathways as either exogenous or endogenous.

   The *exogenous pathway* of lipid metabolism describes the fate of lipids and fat-soluble vitamins derived from the diet. Initially these substances are packaged into triglyceride-rich lipoprotein particles called chylomicrons. The main structural component of chylomicrons is apolipoprotein-B48 (apo B48), with smaller quantities of the C-peptides, apo CI, apo CII, and apo CIII. Chylo-microns are secreted into the intestinal lymphatics, and enter the blood stream through the thoracic duct, and are then transported to the peripheral tissues where the core triglycerides are hydrolysed by lipoprotein lipase and the fatty acids that are released are taken up by fat cells and muscle. In this process the chylomicron is converted to a remant particle which is enriched in cholesterol esters and contains apo B48, apo CIII, and apo E. These remnants are transported to the liver where they are taken up by the LDL receptor and by hepatic receptors specific for apo E.

Table 23. *The properties of some human apolipoproteins (LDL=low density lipoprotein; LCAT=lecithin cholesteryl acyl transferase; LPL=lipoprotein lipase)*

Apoproteins	Molecular weight	Site of synthesis	Function
A-I	28 300	Intestine/liver	Activates LCAT
A-II	17 000	Intestine/liver	—
B-100	549 000	Liver	Binds to LDL receptor + Triglyceride transport
B-48	246 000	Intestine	
C-I	6331	Liver	Activates LCAT
C-II	8837	Liver	Activates LPL
C-III	8764	Liver	?inhibits LPL
E	33 000	Liver/intestine macrophage	?binds to liver receptor

Modified from Galton (1985).

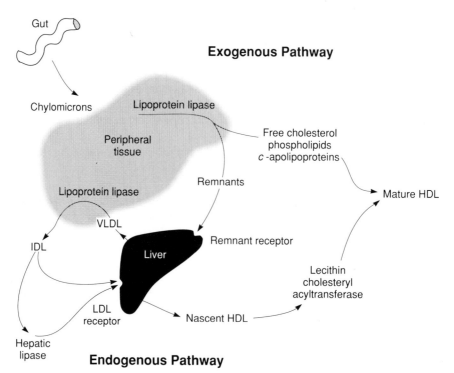

Figure 70. **The lipid transport pathways.** VLDL=very low density lipoprotein; IDL=intermediate density lipoprotein; LDL=low density lipoprotein; HDL=high density lipoprotein.

In the endogenous pathway of lipid transport triglycerides and cholesterol are synthesized in the liver and are incorporated into very low density lipoprotein (VLDL) which is secreted into the circulation. VLDL contains apo B100 as its major apoprotein, together with C-peptides and apo E. VLDL is transported to the tissues where triglyceride is hydrolysed by lipoprotein lipase. The resulting VLDL remnant, called intermediate density lipoprotein (IDL), is further metabolized in two ways. Some of the IDL is cleared directly by the liver by interaction between apo E and the LDL receptors. The remainder is acted on by another lipase, and all the residual triglyceride is hydrolysed and replaced with cholesterol ester. In the course of this conversion all the apolipoproteins, except for apo B100, are lost as the surface of the particle shrinks. The result is the transformation of the VLDL remnant particles into cholesterol-ester-rich LDL which carry 60–70 per cent of plasma cholesterol and function in the delivery of cholesterol to the tissues, where it is required for the synthesis of membranes and steroid hormones. Apo B100 is the ligand that is responsible for the cellular uptake of LDL by the LDL receptor pathway.

The elegant studies of Goldstein and Brown showed that the generation of cholesterol from LDL within lysosomes is the stimulus responsible for suppressing the intracellular pathways of cholesterol synthesis; the enzyme involved is 3-hydroxy-3-methylglutaryl co-enzyme-A reductase (HMG Co-A reductase). It appears that cholesterol or an oxygenated derivative that is formed within the cell acts at several levels including the suppression of transcription of the gene for HMG Co-A reductase and acceleration of degradation of the enzyme protein (Fig. 71).

As shown in Figs 70 and 71, the LDL receptor plays a dual role in LDL metabolism. First, it limits LDL production by enhancing the removal of its precursor, IDL, from the circulation. Second, it enhances LDL degradation by mediating the cellular uptake of LDL. It follows that a deficiency of LDL receptors causes LDL to accumulate as a result of both over-production and delayed removal. Hence the LDL receptor plays a central role in modulating the plasma LDL levels.

High density lipoprotein (HDL) is also secreted from the liver and small intestine. The major apoproteins in HDL are apo AI and apo AII. Plasma HDL acts as a receptor of free cholesterol and functions in the transport of cholesterol from tissues to the liver. Cholesterol esters are formed from free cholesterol and from fatty acid on the surface of HDL by the action of an enzyme called lecithin cholesteryl acyl transferase (LCAT). Apo AI activates LCAT. It is thought that because of its role in acting as an acceptor for excess free cholesterol, plasma HDL is an important protective agent against the development of atherosclerosis.

Genetics disorders of lipid metabolism

There are several genetically determined forms of hyperlipidaemia, most of which are associated with premature coronary artery disease. We considered the

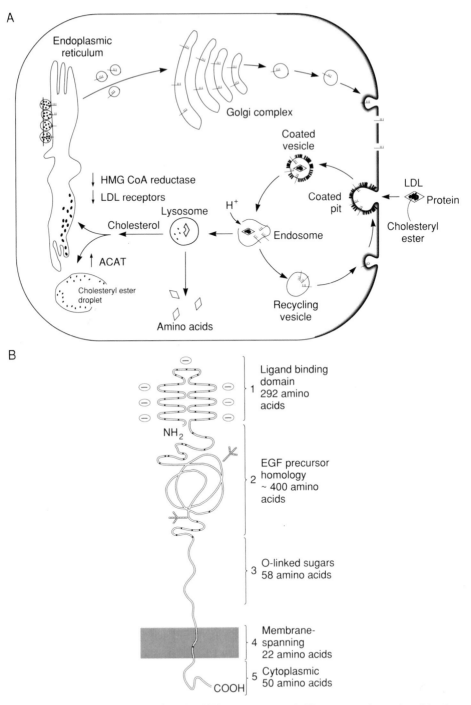

Figure 71. **The pathways for the LDL receptors.** **A** The receptor is produced in the endoplasmic reticulum from which it travels to the Golgi complex, cell surface, coated pit, endosome and back to the surface. The various metabolic interactions of cholesterol together with the abbreviations used are described in the text. **B** Structure of the receptor. Modified from Brown and Goldstein (1988).

different mutations of the LDL receptor that are responsible for monogenic hypercholesterolaemia in the previous chapter. Homozygous subjects usually die before the age of 20 years with severe atherosclerosis; heterozygotes have a greatly increased risk of early coronary artery disease. As shown in Table 24 there are several other well-defined monogenic hyperlipidaemias in which the underlying defect is established, although all of them are very rare.

Table 24. *The inherited hyperlipidaemias (modified from Galton, 1985)*

Type	Lipoprotein changes	Causes
I	Chylos increased, HDL and LDL reduced	Lipoprotein lipase deficiency, Apo-CII deficiency
IIa	LDL increased	Familial hypercholesterolaemia Polygenic hypercholesterolaemia
IIb	LDL and VLDL increased, HDL may be low	Familial combined hyperlipidaemia
III	IDL (chylo remnants) increased, LDL and HDL low	Associated with gene polymorphism of Apo E
IV	VLDL increased, HDL low	Familial hypertriglyceridaemia, Familial combined hyperlipidaemia, Polygenic hyperlipidaemia
V	VLDL, chylos increased HDL low	Familial hypertriglyceridaemia, Lipoprotein lipase deficiency

The abbreviations are as defined in the text.

Polygenic vascular disease

In dealing with complex polygenic problems of this type it is often useful to start with a well-defined genetic system. In this context the mutations of the LDL receptor that lead to monogenic hypercholesterolaemia are particularly well defined. However, as mentioned in the previous chapter, there is considerable heterogeneity in the clinical phenotype of heterozygotes for monogenic hypercholesterolaemia, particularly regarding the age of their first heart attack. Recent studies have suggested that much of this reflects polymorphisms of other plasma proteins that affect cholesterol levels. This is very encouraging, because it suggests that when we have well defined genetic systems with which to work, we will start to make some sense of phenotype/genotype relationships in premature heart disease.

   Even though the heterozygous frequency for monogenic hypercholesterol-aemia is about 1 in 500 this condition accounts for only about 5 per cent of myocardial infarctions in patients under the age of 60. It is clear, however, that inheritance plays an important role in the remainder of cases; in one large study in the US, for example, a heritability of 0.56 was observed for coronary artery disease under the age of 55 even after the exclusion of cases of monogenic hyperlipidaemia. The central question is, therefore, how might it be possible to define the important genes that underlie the polygenic system that regulates plasma lipid levels in the bulk of the population (Fig. 72).

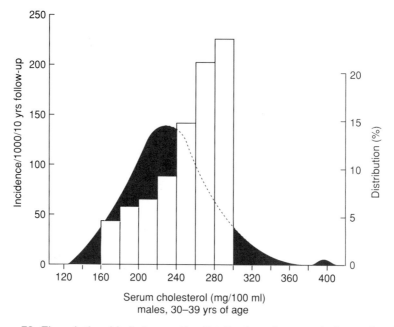

Figure 72. The relationship between the distribution of serum cholesterol and the prevalence of heart disease. (Based on data collected in Framingham, Massachusetts.)

The main difficulty in the genetics of vascular disease is the large number and diversity of possible candidate genes. Even if we restrict ourselves to those that are involved with lipid metabolism the list is daunting (Table 25). If we add to this the genes that regulate the coagulation and haemostatic systems, and the cellular elements of the arterial wall, we end up with a problem of such complexity that, at first sight, it seems unlikely that any useful answers will come from trying to break it down into its individual parts.

A start has been made however. The major effort so far has been directed at trying to define polymorphisms of the apolipoprotein genes that are related to increased plasma cholesterol concentrations or to coronary artery disease. This work has included both protein polymorphisms and RFLPs. Because of their importance in cholesterol transport much of this work has concentrated on apo E and apo B. For example, a series of alleles of the apo E locus can be demonstrated by sophisticated methods for separating proteins. It turns out that the presence of the E4 alelle, which is found in 15 per cent of individuals, increases the plasma cholesterol concentration by about 8 per cent compared with the E3

Table 25. *Some 'candidate' genes involved in lipid metabolism* (*modified from Scott, 1988*)

Class	Gene
Apolipoproteins	Apo-AI
	Apo-AII
	Apo-B
	Apo-CI
	Apo-CII
	Apo-CIII
	Apo-E
Enzymes	HMG CoA reductase
	Lecithin cholesterol acyl transferase
	Fatty acyl-CoA cholesterol acyl transferase
	Endothelial lipoprotein lipase
	Hepatic triglyceride lipase
	Fatty acid synthetase
	Phosphatidic acid phosphohydrolase
	Cholesterol ester hydrolase
	Cholesterol 7-α hydrolase
Transferase proteins	Lipid transfer proteins
Receptors	Low density lipoprotein
	Apo-E
	High density lipoprotein

'wild-type' allele, which is found in about 70 per cent of the population. On the other hand the E2 allele, which is much less common, decreases cholesterol concentration by about 13 per cent. Interestingly, these relatively small changes in plasma cholesterol concentration seem to be sufficient to produce a substantial enrichment of the E2 allele with advancing age and, incidentally, decrease the level of the E4 allele with ageing; presumably both effects reflect deaths from myocardial infarction.

It turns out that alleles at the apo B locus, as demonstrated by RFLP analysis, also have a significant effect on plasma cholesterol concentration and the risk of myocardial infarction. This is of particular relevance because apo B100 is the sole protein component of LDL and is the ligand that delivers cholesterol to the tissues by the LDL receptor pathway. Further information has been obtained by haplotype analysis of the apolipoprotein genes, that is by studying the relationship of patterns of RFLPs, as defined in Chapter 5 for the globin gene clusters, with either apolipoprotein or cholesterol levels. It has been possible, for example, to define haplotypes at the apo B locus, at the apo A1-CIII-AIV gene cluster on chromosome 11, and at the apo CI-CII and E cluster on chromosome 19. Studies relating particular haplotypes to apoprotein or cholesterol level indicate that genetic variation at the apolipoprotein loci is responsible for determining serum levels of their respective apoproteins although the effects are quite small.

How might these RFLP relationships between cholesterol levels be mediated? So far there is very little information about this critical question. However, now that many of the genes for the apolipoproteins have been isolated and sequenced it is possible to make a start to answering this question. For example, it is clear that variation at the apo B locus makes an important contribution to genetic variation in cholesterol levels. At least three of the alleles that have been defined in this context are due to charged amino acid variants, at least some of which lie near to the LDL receptor-binding domain of apo B. Whether this means that these changes are themselves responsible for altered function or whether they reflect linkage disequilibrium with other variation in the structure of the apo B gene remains to be determined.

Another interesting clue as to how genetic variability in the lipoprotein system might affect the clinical phenotype comes from studies of a variant of LDL called Lp(a). Lp(a) is an LDL that carries one or more copies of a protein called apo(a), joined to apo B by disulphide linkage. The amount of Lp(a) in plasma varies widely and it appears that high levels are strongly associated with atherosclerosis and a high risk of coronary artery disease. It turns out that apo(a) is structurally related to plasminogen, the precursor of the proteolytic enzyme plasmin which dissolves fibrin clots. Plasminogen contains five cysteine-rich sequences; these structures contain three internal disulphide bridges, producing a conformation that resembles a Danish cake called a kringle. Kringles are found in other proteases of the coagulation system including tissue plasminogen activator (tPA) and prothrombin. In plasminogen, the kringles are involved in binding to its substrate, fibrin. Plasminogen is proteolytically inactive until it has been cleaved by tPA which breaks down the chain at a single arginine residue to form active plasmin. Apo(a) is not itself a protease, because the arginine at the cleavage site for tPA is changed to serine.

These interesting structural homologies suggest a mechanism whereby apo(a) might lead to accelerated atherosclerosis. When the molecule is incorporated into an arterial wall following endothelial damage it could adhere to fibrin, forming a complex that becomes permanently fixed in the wall. There it might also block proteolysis of fibrin by inhibiting the activation of plasminogen by tPA. Quite clearly further genetic and functional analysis of apo(a) holds great promise for our understanding of premature vascular disease.

At this early stage it is difficult to see whether the intensive studies on the genetics of cholesterol metabolism over the last few years are likely to make a major impact on clinical practice in the future. Clearly, for the purposes of genetic counselling and treatment, the single gene disorders associated with grossly abnormal lipid metabolism are extremely important to identify. It is also apparent that there is a major genetic component to the remarkable variability in cholesterol levels throughout the general population and there are strong hints about some of the loci that are involved. As similar information starts to accumulate from other systems that may be involved in the pathogenesis of atheroma and thrombotic disease the relative importance of these different genetic systems will become clearer.

● Obesity

Many studies have shown a relationship between obesity and an increased likelihood of coronary artery disease. Furthermore, a variety of different analyses have shown that human obesity has a strong genetic component.

Recent work has suggested an association between certain RFLPs of the apolipoprotein B gene and obesity. Currently, the significance of this interesting association remains to be determined. Mutations of the apo B locus might cause enhanced absorption of dietary fat or secretion of VLDL from the liver. On the other hand they might enhance the association of apo B with capillary lipoprotein lipase which might favour triglyceride hydrolysis and fat deposition.

While a great deal more work needs to be done in the field of genetic predisposition to obesity these preliminary results are sufficiently encouraging to suggest that the RFLP approach may offer a valuable new method for studying this hitherto intractable problem.

● Hypertension

The distribution of blood pressure in any population is continuous. The definition of hypertension, that is a particular blood pressure above a certain level, is therefore arbitrary. In this sense hypertension is not a disease but represents the upper 15 to 25 per cent of a biological variable, a level at which there is undoubtedly an increased risk of cerebrovascular, cardiovascular, and renal disease. Twin and family studies have shown that there is a strong genetic component to hypertension. Of course, there is always the problem of a common environmental component to account for familial aggregation of cases of hypertension but careful spouse-pair and adopted child–parent-pair analyses have confirmed that genetic factors play an important role.

Like atherosclerosis there is no lack of candidate genes for hypertension. The regulation of blood pressure, intimately bound up with salt and water metabolism as it is, is extremely complex and poorly understood. The candidates range from the renin-angiotensin system through atrial natriuretic hormone to the particularly complex systems that regulate ion movement in either the smooth muscle of the vessel wall or the kidney. In fact it is the latter mechanisms that have received most attention so far. It has been argued that alterations in the calcium content of smooth muscle cells, potentially caused by changes in the intracellular content of sodium, might lead to increased smooth muscle tone resulting in augmented vascular resistance, and hence to hypertension. The altered sodium content, it has been suggested, might be due to abnormalities in intrinsic sodium transport function or to the presence of circulating factors that influence transport in the kidney or other tissues. Since it is not yet possible to study transport in renal or smooth muscle cells directly much of the work in this area has been carried out on circulating blood cells acting, optimistically perhaps, as surrogates for these tissues.

Several transport systems have been analysed in the red or white blood cells of hypertensives. For example, elevated cellular sodium content has been related to a reduced rate of the APTase-related sodium transport system, possibly reflecting the role of a serum inhibitor of the sodium pump in hypertensive persons. Differences in red cell sodium content or in sodium pump activity have not been consistent however. The sodium–potassium co-transport system, which transports sodium and potassium in concert across the cell membrane, has been shown to be less effective in hypertensive individuals than in normotensive controls. Again, these studies have been difficult to reproduce between different laboratories.

A third transport system, sodium–lithium counter transport (CT), has yielded more reproducible data, and a clear association between elevated CT and hypertension has been found in a number of studies. CT is assayed by loading red cells with lithium and measuring its rate of efflux from the cells in the presence or absence of sodium at given intervals. The physiological role of this system is unknown. Several family studies have shown that the sodium–lithium CT system is under genetic control and have provided some evidence for major locus inheritance. In an extensive study in Salt Lake City it was found that homozygotes for an allele at a major locus regulating CT activity had an increased prevalence of hypertension. It should be pointed out that the association was not complete; some homozygotes failed to develop hypertension and some non-homozygotes were hypertensive. Clearly this is a 'susceptibility gene' rather than a 'disease gene' for hypertension. These findings suggest that other susceptibility genes must exist in the population; not surprising, perhaps, considering that the inheritance of hypertension is clearly polygenic. However, the frequency of the homozygous genotype is about 5 per cent in the populations studied. These data must be viewed with caution because the families were ascertained through cases of coronary artery disease. Other studies have given broadly similar results, however.

So where is research into the genetics of hypertension moving? There is considerable activity in isolating the genes for the various transport systems, and as soon as they are available it will be necessary to find RFLPs and to repeat the family studies to see if linkage analysis turns out to be more efficient way of determining the relative importance of these genes in the genesis of hypertension. This could well be the case, because previous data are likely to have been clouded by the technical difficulties of measuring transport function in the test-tube. Currently, the sodium–lithium CT system is the prime candidate. Because of its medical importance it may well be worthwhile setting out on a 'blind hunt' for major genes involved in the genesis of hypertension, using the sib-pair approach perhaps.

Another and rather novel approach to the hypertension problem which has been developed recently re-explores the renin/angiotensin pathway, a topic which has been central to studies of hypertension for many years. Renin is normally released by the kidney and acts on its substrate angiotensin, which is secreted by the liver, to produce the decapeptide angiotension I. This in turn is split by converting enzyme to angiotensin II. The latter contracts vascular smooth muscle and promotes its growth, stimulates aldosterone secretion by the adrenal gland, and promotes sympathetic transmission at the synapse. Patients with essential hypertension have low or normal levels of plasma renin. Quite recently rats have had an additional renin gene inserted by the transgenic route. Interestingly, these animals become hypertensive despite the fact that they have low levels of plasma renin. However, it turns out that the renin gene is expressed in the adrenal glands rather than in the kidney in the transgenic animals. It is possible, therefore, that a high local concentration of angiotensin II in the adrenal gland might stimulate cell growth and lead to the overproduction of aldosterone, a situation known to occasionally cause hypertension in man. However, the experiment is not completely unphysiological because it is known that low levels of renin are present in normal human adrenal glands. Furthermore there are differences in the level of adrenal renin in salt-sensitive and salt-resistant genetically hypertensive rats.

While these observations are very preliminary, they point to further areas of research that may be of promise in sorting out these complexities of essential hypertension in Man.

● Abdominal aortic aneurysm

Aneurysms are localized dilatations of blood vessels which may rupture. They are particularly common in the abdominal aorta in middle and old age, and at this site pose an important cause of death. There is an increasing body of evidence that genetic factors play an important role in producing the pathological changes in the wall of the abdominal aorta which lead to the formation of aneurysms.

Since early surgery of aortic aneurysms is remarkably successful, and since they are so common, it would be very valuable to define a genetic marker for population screening. Recent studies have related genetic variability at the α haptoglobin and cholesterol ester transfer protein loci, both on the long arm of chromosome 16, to this disorder. Further work along these lines will be awaited with great interest.

● Neuro-psychiatric disease

● The major psychoses

The psychoses cause a major drain on health resources and virtually nothing is known about their pathogenesis. They fall into two major groups, the manic depressive illnesses and schizophrenia. There are extensive data from twin and adoption studies suggesting that the familial aggregation of these disorders is caused predominantly by genetic factors. However, the distribution of affected individuals within families does not conform to any simple Mendelian pattern of segregation, either for schizophrenia or the manic depressive illnesses. One of the major difficulties in studying the genetics of these conditions is their heterogeneity; it is far from certain whether either schizophrenia or the affective disorders are homogeneous entities or whether they represent a whole spectrum of biochemically and genetically disparate conditions.

The idea of attempting to define by genetic linkage analysis the gene or genes (as seems more likely) involved in these conditions is not new. Many studies have been carried out in an attempt to demonstrate linkage between standard protein markers or the HLA–DR system. Although some weak linkages have been obtained none of them has provided a strong and consistent clue to the chromosomal location of the genes involved. It is not surprising, therefore, that once the principle of RFLP linkage analysis was developed attempts were made to try to determine the chromosomal location of genes involved in these disorders. Both the candidate gene and 'blind hunt' approaches, as defined earlier in this chapter, have been applied to this problem. Although some early successes have been reported a great deal more work will have to be done before any conclusions can be drawn.

One of the first studies using the random linkage strategy was carried out on a large Amish family from Pennsylvania, USA, in which a manic depressive type of illness appeared to segregate as a single gene. An early hint of linkage between the disorder and the H-*ras* locus on the short arm of chromosome 11 appeared to be confirmed by a more extensive study which gave a Lod score of more than four. These promising findings were followed up by other large pedigree analyses, both in the USA and in a collaborative British/Icelandic programme; both failed to confirm this particular linkage. However, things got even more complicated when a further analysis of the Amish pedigree showed that two people in the original study had subsequently become manic depressive in the absence of the putative markers of predisposition. And, even more worrying, an additional branch of the original pedigree was now available for study and this showed no evidence of linkage. These results could mean that there are at least two genes predisposing to manic depressive in the Amish pedigree or, and this seems more likely, that the apparent linkage to a chromosome 11 locus was in fact just chance. A few families have been reported in which manic depressive illness appears to be inherited in an X-linked manner and there is a hint that linkage of this type has been confirmed using RFLPs. However, there is no suggestion that the majority of cases of manic depressive illness are inherited in this way.

Recent work on the genetics of schizophrenia has followed the same pattern. These studies were encouraged by observations of two patients, an uncle and a nephew, who had schizophrenia together with abnormal facial development and who carried an extra copy of the chromosomal region 5q11–13 on chromosome 1. Interestingly, chromosome 5q contains a gene encoding the glucocorticoid receptor, which seemed to be as good a candidate as any for a schizophrenia-susceptibility gene (every clinician who has used corticosteroids to treat patients has encountered psychotic symptoms). In fact, subsequent studies showed that the 5q11–13 region does not contain the glucocorticoid receptor but, undaunted, at least two groups set out to test the possibility of linkage of RFLPs for this region to schizophrenia.

In one study five Icelandic and two English families, with a total of 39 cases of schizophrenia, showed evidence of linkage to RFLP markers for the 5q11–13 region. Unfortunately, however, an even more detailed analysis of this region, using at least five RFLPs for 5q, in a very large Swedish family containing many schizophrenics showed no evidence whatever for linkage to this region. More recent studies have also failed to confirm this linkage.

The reader may be forgiven for thinking that psychiatric genetics is in rather a state of flux at the present time. But if further studies show that some forms of manic depressive illness or schizophrenia can be clearly localized to specific chromosomes, and if the genes involved can be isolated and their products defined, this should provide some solid evidence about the biochemical nature of these illnesses. Given the complexity of the phenotypes involved we should not be surprised that the first studies in this field suggest that there will be considerable heterogeneity in the genetics of the major psychoses. One way in which this work might be facilitated would be by better phenotypic definition. In this context we might attempt to map the genetic basis for some of the atypical biochemical or physiological responses that are characteristic of schizophrenia; pharmacological challenge studies in relatives could clarify whether such a response is a useful trait to study. For example, it is known that the amphetamine response is unusually marked in schizophrenics and shows strong concordance in twin studies.

● Dementia

Although some deterioration in intellectual capacity is acceptable or at least inevitable as one of the penalities for longevity, the serious memory deficits, gross lack of judgement, and deterioration in temperament and behaviour that form the clinical picture of dementia is one of the most tragic pictures in clinical medicine. Although dementia results from many pathological changes, one particular form, Alzheimer's disease, constitutes a specific pathological entity. This condition is characterized by neuronal loss and senile plaques together with curious structures called neurofibrillary tangles in particular parts of the brain. It accounts for at least half of all cases of dementia examined at autopsy. And it turns out to be frighteningly common. Indeed as our population ages it will become one of the most frequent causes of death, affecting at least one in twenty of those aged over 65 and as many as a quarter over 80. As well as the pathological changes found in the brains of patients with Alzheimer's disease there are widespread neuropharmacological abnormalities, including a deficit in cholinergic activity and a deficiency of other brain neuropeptides, particularly corticotrophin-releasing factor and somatostatin.

The relative roles of environmental and genetic factors in the pathogenesis of Alzheimer's disease is the subject of intense debate. A number of toxic agents have been implicated including aluminium, silicon, and free radicles. However, there is increasing evidence that genetic factors play an equal if not more important role. Although only about one in a thousand of the general population under the age of 65 has Alzheimer's disease about one in three patients with the condition have a similarly affected first degree relative. Of course this could reflect the action of an environmental toxin. However, in twin studies is was found that monozygotic twins have a concordance rate of about 45 per cent, and dizygotic twins 5 per cent. These studies, while emphasizing the role of genetic factors, also suggest that environmental agents are involved.

One of the most tantalizing observations in research into Alzheimer's disease is the pathological finding that the brains of patients with this condition are morphologically indistinguishable from those of middle-aged patients who have died with Down syndrome. Not surprisingly, this directed attention towards the possibility that a gene on chromosome 21 might be involved in the pathogenesis of Alzheimer's disease. It was also observed that the plaques that occur in the brains of patients with Alzheimer's disease have, as one of their main components, a protein consisting of amyloid filaments. Vascular amyloid is part of a much larger precursor and it turns out that its structure is also controlled by a gene on chromosome 21. Could this be the gene involved in Alzheimer's disease?

In 1987 the pedigrees of four families in which Alzheimer's disease seemed to be inherited in an autosomally dominant fashion were published. Using appropriate RFLP markers it appeared that the determinant for Alzheimer's disease in these families was linked to two chromosome 21q21 loci, one of which is linked to the amyloid β gene. However, in a further study this linkage was not confirmed in 6 out of 15 families with multiple members with Alzheimer's disease. To complicate matters further a more recent study has found evidence for linkage. In these latter families linkage between the putative disease locus and a chromosome 21 locus designated D21S1/S was demonstrated. These findings are consistent with the multiple recombinants that have been reported between the 'Alzheimer's disease locus' and the β amyloid gene, since it is now clear that the latter is telomeric to D21S1/S.

What are we to make of these apparent discrepancies? First, of course, there is the possibility that genetic susceptibility to Alzheimer's disease can be determined by more than one locus. However, the different studies are not entirely comparable because one of those that failed to show linkage made use of inbred populations or pedigrees that contained a high proportion of late-onset cases. At the time of writing the bulk of evidence suggests that there may be a susceptibility locus on chromosome 21, which is not that for β amyloid but which plays an important role in the likelihood of developing Alzheimer's disease. If this is the case it is an important step forward towards our understanding of this extremely important condition.

● Alcoholism

Disorders due to alcoholism are assuming an increasingly important burden on the health services of many advanced societies. Surprisingly many adoption, twin, and half-sibling studies have demonstrated a significant hereditary contribution to the likelihood of becoming addicted to alcohol.

At first sight it is difficult to imagine the kind of candidate genes that might be involved in susceptibility to over-indulgence in alcohol. One approach might be to attempt to define certain inherited personality traits. Another avenue, perhaps more amenable to direct measurement, is the biochemical reactions that cause individual variability in response to alcohol. For example, it is known that many individuals develop acute flushing reactions after ingestion of alcohol which have been attributed to an inherited polymorphism in the metabolism of ethanol and acetaldehyde. There may also be inherited variability in the formation of diols or in the hepatic P450 microsomal oxidising system. To take these arguments a step further it is possible that genetically determined variation in susceptibility to toxic metabolites of alcohol might influence the risk of developing cirrhosis of the liver, cardiomyopathy, or the fetal alcohol syndrome.

Recently, using DNA technology it has been possible to make a start in dissecting some of these possibilities. The two enzyme loci analysed in this way were those for alcohol dehydrogenase (ADH) and mitochondrial aldehyde dehydrogenase (ALDH). It has been known for some time about 50 per cent of orientals are deficient in activity of ALDH. This enzyme is the first line of defence in metabolizing acetylaldehyde. A standard dose of alcohol produces acute flushing symptoms and higher blood acetylaldehyde concentrations in deficient individuals. Recent studies using RFLPs related to the ALDH locus have pointed to a high frequency for this defect in the Japanese population. Furthermore, a deficiency of ALDH associated with flushing attacks was found in patients with alcoholic liver disease in Japan. This is a particularly intriguing finding because it suggests that the inheritance of the flushing reaction may lead individuals to avoid ingesting excessive alcohol and therefore protect them from developing the complications of alcoholism.

The ALDH polymorphism does not occur in Caucasians, although alcohol-induced flushing does occur in non-oriental populations. There is some evidence that variant forms of ADH may be involved. Another variant of cytosolic ALDH has been found to be associated with alcohol-induced flushing in Caucasians. Very recently a strong association has been found between an allele of the dopamine D_2 receptor and alcoholism. The work suggests that a gene that confers susceptibility to at least one form of alcoholism is located on the q22–q23 region of chromosome 11. The dopamine receptor is a good candidate for being the gene locus involved. These studies offer a further 'candidate gene' approach to the dissection of the genetic factors that underlie alcoholism.

● Hereditary variability in response to drugs

Iatrogenic diseases, that is disorders that result from the side-effects of medical treatment, play an increasingly important role in modern practice. Although few drugs are free of side-effects it has been apparent for some time that at least some of the differences between ways in which individuals respond to drugs is genetically determined. For example, it has been calculated that for the anti-rheumatic agent, phenylbutazone, at least two-thirds of variation in response is due to genetic factors.

Some unusual responses to drugs can be defined in simple Mendelian terms. For example there is clear evidence that individual variation to the anti-tuberculous agent isoniazid depends on genetic variability in the rate of acetylation of the agent; slow acetylators may show toxicity while fast acetylators often have a diminished response to the drug. Similarly, individuals are encountered occasionally who have severe and prolonged apnoea (cessation of breathing) following the administration of suxamethonium. These conditions are inherited as an autosomal recessive. On the other hand, the malignant hyperthermia that is observed occasionally following the use of anaesthetic agents such as halothane and suxamethonium is inherited as an autosomal dominant.

As knowledge of drug metabolism has increased it has been possible to apply some of the methods of molecular biology to the study of the basic mechanisms that underlie individual response to drug administration. For example, about 5 to 10 per cent of individuals suffer severe side-effects from the antihypertensive agent debrisoquine. This agent is metabolized primarily by a cytochrome P450 enzyme, P450db1. Susceptible individuals inherit a defect in debrisoquine hydroxylation due to abnormal function of this particular cytochrome. Recent molecular studies have shown that poor metabolizers have a variety of different mutations involving the P450db1 gene. Furthermore, these are quite novel lesions which occur within the introns and give rise to a series of incorrectly spliced messenger RNAs that are unable to code for a protein product. So far the nature of these mutations is unknown.

It seems likely that mutations of the genes for the products of the members of the cytochrome P450 family will have a variety of clinical manifestations. It appears, for example, that there are strong epidemiological associations between debrisoquine hydroxylation phenotypes and some chemically induced diseases including lung cancer, bladder cancer, and Balkan nephropathy.

Recently the molecular basis for other types of drug sensitivity has been unravelled. For example, the prolonged inhibition of neuromuscular transmission caused by succinylcholine has been shown to result from a point mutation Asp→Gly in serum cholinesterase, causing a reduced affinity for choline esters.

As mentioned earlier malignant hyperthermia, a condition characterized by sustained muscle contracture and an elevation in body temperature triggered by a variety of anaesthetics and muscle relaxants, is usually inherited in an autosomal dominant fashion. Because calcium is the chief regulator of muscle contraction and metabolism it has been suspected for some time that the primary defect in this condition lies in calcium regulation. Recently the gene for the human ryanodine receptor, the calcium release channel of sarcoplasmic reticulum, has been cloned and mapped to the region q13.1 of chromosome 19. Linkage studies in families with malignant hyperthermia have shown that there is a high probability that the condition results from mutations at the ryanodine receptor locus.

In Chapter 2 we saw how millions of individuals are affected with an X-linked deficiency of glucose-6-phosphate dehydrogenase (G6PD) which makes them prone to haemolytic anaemia after receiving certain antimalarial drugs or other oxidants. Recent work has shown that the G6PD variants result from different amino acid substitutions and a start has been made in relating modifications of enzyme stability and function to these structural changes.

Although the molecular basis for the human acetylation polymorphism has not yet been worked out it was found recently that the slow-acetylation phenotype in the New Zealand white rabbit is due to a deletion of genes for arylamine N-acetyltransferase.

There is no doubt that molecular pharmacogenetics will be an extremely productive field over the next few years, not only for helping us to understand individual variation in response to drugs but also for evaluating the problem of why some individuals are more prone than others to the harmful effects of a wide variety of environmental agents. The single gene mediated reactions to drugs outlined here are probably only the tip of the iceberg of genetic variability of the way in which we handle these substances.

● Infectious disease

Although it has been speculated for a long time that genetic factors may play an important role in determining the way in which individuals respond to infection, this important subject has been neglected in recent years. Although there has been much speculation that the unequal distribution of blood groups among the world population may reflect protection or susceptibility to major epidemics in the distant past, it has been very hard to provide any convincing evidence that this is the case. Indeed studies of this complex problem and of the possible relationships of other genetic polymorphisms to susceptibility to infection, have been bedevilled by problems of founder effect and gene drift within populations. Only very recently, with the availability of DNA technology, has it been possible to start to re-evaluate this difficult field.

It has been suspected for many years that the common haemoglobin disorders such as sickle cell anaemia and thalassaemia may have reached their high frequencies because heterozygotes are, or have been in the past, protected against *Plasmodium falciparum* malaria. Now that it is possible to analyse these conditions at the molecular level it is becoming clear that this is indeed the case. For example there is abundant evidence that the different forms of α and β thalassaemia have arisen in different populations by independent mutations. Furthermore, by studying large numbers of neutral DNA polymorphisms, and by comparing the distribution of the haemoglobin disorders between malarious and non-malarious populations, it has been possible to provide unequivocal evidence that malaria is a major factor in maintaining these polymorphisms.

It should now be possible to use the same type of approach to study other genes that may be involved in susceptibility or resistance to infection, the class I and II genes of the HLA-DR system for example. This should be a particularly productive area of reasearch because there is considerable serological evidence that the products of these genes are involved in determining individual response to a variety of important infections including hepatitis, AIDS, tuberculosis, and leprosy. It should also be possible to analyse some of the single gene disorders that are associated with increased susceptibility to infection, including the various immune deficiency states and inherited defects of white cell function. Indeed, as we saw in Chapter 6, elucidation of the molecular basis for chronic granulomatous disease is close to solution. In this way it should be possible to build up a number of candidates genes for broader studies of susceptibility or resistance to infections within communities.

● Allergy and atopy

In finishing this brief account of the molecular approach to common diseases we must not forget a particularly widespread condition that undoubtedly afflicts many readers of this book. About a quarter of most European populations have allergic responses to common inhaled proteins. Such atopic individuals suffer at some stage in their lives from the symptoms of rhinitis (a runny nose) or asthma. Indeed, asthma is the commonest cause of admission of young people to hospital, affecting between 4 and 8 per cent of all children. Recent studies have shown that atopy appears, at least in some families, to be inherited as an autosomal dominant. Even more remarkably it has been possible to demonstrate that the putative gene for atopy is linked to a DNA polymorphism on chromosome 11q13.

The formation of immunoglobulin E (IgE) in response to allergens is thought to be central to the generation of the atopic state. In sensitized persons the disease appears to be initiated by the interaction of inhaled allergen with specific IgE bound to mucosal mast cells. Atopic individuals have a propensity to prolonged and exaggerated IgE responses to minute amounts of antigen. The factors that promote enhanced IgE responses in this way are not known. The putative gene on chromosome 11 might produce a protein that acts at epithelial barriers, on antigen-presenting cells, on regulator T cells, or indeed on IgE-secreting B cells.

Interestingly, chromosome 11 carries a number of genes for cell surface antigens, including some on T cells.

If these intriguing findings are confirmed they offer a genuine opportunity to start to dissect the molecular and cellular basis for some extremely common and incapacitating disorders that afflict all racial groups.

● Postscript

In this chapter we have touched briefly on an intriguing new field which is young and still unformed. It is impossible to say where it will take us, but we probably know enough already to suggest that it has the potential for providing a completely new level of understanding of some of the common disorders that afflict western societies. We must not expect it to produce clean answers to these difficult problems overnight, but its long-term possibilities are enormous.

● Further reading

Bell, J. and Todd, J.A. (1989). HLA class II sequences infer mechanisms for major histocompatibility complex-associated disease susceptibility. *Mol. Biol. Med*, **6**, 43–53.

Blum, M., Grant, D.M., Demierre, A., and Meyer, U.A. (1989). *N*-acetylation pharmacogenetics: a gene deletion causes absence of arylamine *N*-acetyltransferase in liver of slow acetylator rabbits. *Proc. Natl. Acad. Sci. USA*, **86**, 9554–7.

Bock, G. and Collins, M.M. (eds) (1987). *Molecular approaches to human polygenic disease. Ciba Foundation Symposium*, **130**, Wiley, Chichester.

Bodmer, W.F. (1987). HLA, immune response, and disease. In *Human genetics*, (eds. F. Vogel and K. Sperling), pp. 107–13. Springer-Verlag, Berlin.

Brown, M.S. and Goldstein, J.L. (1988). Receptor mediated pathway for cholesterol synthesis. *Science*, **232**, 34–47.

Deary, I.J. and Whalley, L.J. (1988). Recent research on the causes of Alzheimer's disease. *B. Med. J.*, **297**, 807–9.

Demaine, A.G. (1989). The molecular biology of autoimmune disease. *Immunology Today*, **10**, 357–61.

Field, L.L. (1988). Insulin-dependent diabetes mellitus: a model for the study of multifactorial disorders. *Am. J. Hum. Genet.*, **43**, 793–8.

Galton, D.J. (1985). *Molecular genetics of common metabolic diseases*. Edward Arnold, London.

Goate, A.M., Haynes, A.R., Owen, M.J., Farrall, M., James, L.A., Lai, L.Y.C., Mullan, M.J., Roques, P., Rossor, M.N., Williamson, R., and Hardy J.A. (1989). Predisposing locus for Alzheimer's disease on chromosome 21. *Lancet*, **ii**, 352–5.

Gordis, E., *et al.* (1990). Finding the gene(s) for alcoholism. *J. Am. Med. Assoc.*, **263**, 2094–5.

Hasstedt, S.J., Wu, L.L., Ash, K.O., Kuida, H., and Williams, R.R. (1988). Hypertension and sodium-lithium countertransport in Utah pedigrees: evidence for major-locus inheritance. *Am. J. Hum. Genet.*, **43**, 14–22.

Kahn, C.R. and Goldstein, B.J. (1989). Molecular defects of insulin action. *Science*, **245**, 13.

MacLennan, D.H., Duff, C., Zorzato, F., *et al.* (1990). Ryanodine receptor gene is a candidate for predisposition to malignant hyperthermia. *Nature*, **343**, 559–61.

Mullins, J.J., Peters, J., and Ganten, D. (1990). Fulminent hypertension in transgenic rats harbouring the mouse *Ren*-2 gene. *Nature*, **344**, 541–3.

Omenn, G.S. (1988). Genetic investigations of alcohol metabolism and of alcholism. *Am. J. Hum. Genet.*, **43**, 579–81.

Rajput-Williams, Knott, T.J., Wallis, S.C., Sweetnam, P., Yarnell J., Cox, N., Bell, G.I., Miller, N.E., and Scott, J. (1988). Variation of apolipoprotein-B gene is associated with obesity, high blood cholesterol levels, and increased risk of coronary heart disease. *Lancet*, **ii**, 1442–6.

Scott, J. (1987). The molecular genetics of lipid metabolism. *Molecular Medicine*, **2**, 27–40.

Scott, J. (1989). The molecular and cell biology of apolipoprotein-B. *Mol. Biol. Med.*, **6**, 65–80.

Sherrington, R., Brynjolfsson, J., Pertusson, H., Potter, J., Dudleston, K., Barraclough, B., Washmuth, J., Dobbs, M., and Gurling, H. (1988). Localization of a susceptibility locus for schizophrenia on chromosome 5. *Nature*, **336**, 164–7.

Todd, J.A. (1990). Genetic control of autoimmunity in Type 1 diabetes. *Immunology Today*. (In press).

Todd, J.A., Bell, J.I., and McDevitt, H.O. (1987). HLA-DQ$_\beta$ gene contributes to susceptibility and resistance to insulin-dependent diabetes mellitus. *Nature*, **329**, 599–604.

Cancer

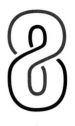

In the last few years there have been some remarkable discoveries about the molecular basis for the disordered proliferation, growth, and differentiation of cells which is the hallmark of all the common cancers. It is likely that many aspects of this work will have important practical implications for clinical medicine in the near future. These advances have stemmed from an amalgamation of information from studies of tumour viruses, cytogenetics, pedigree analysis of families with familial cancers, and epidemiology. Here we will review briefly each of these areas of research and attempt to synthesize current ideas about the general nature of cancer.

It is worth prefacing this brief description of current thinking about the pathogenesis of cancer by pointing out that we are moving into an area of human genetics that has not been touched on so far in this book. Up to now we have considered single gene disorders or polygenic conditions resulting from inherited variability of information which is transmitted through parental germ cells. In the cancer field, however, we are extending the definition of genetic disease to include acquired changes in the genome of somatic cells. Every time a cell divides there is the opportunity for genetic errors to occur. It is becoming apparent that many forms of cancer result from somatic mutations in cells, the progeny of which lose their facility for regulated division and proliferation. Even more interestingly, it turns out that some cancers result from the interaction of both germ cell and somatic mutations; i.e. we may inherit genes that by themselves are incapable of producing malignant transformation, but which will do so if there is a second (somatic) mutation that somehow allows them to express their malignant phenotype.

● Tumour viruses and oncogenes

The first oncogenic virus to be fully characterized was the Rous sarcoma virus, which produces tumours in chickens. This is an RNA virus, or retrovirus, which, when it enters cells, has its RNA genome transcribed into DNA which subsequently becomes inserted into the host chromosomal DNA. Many retroviruses have been identified, as well as several classes of DNA tumour viruses. Viruses seem to cause neoplastic proliferation of cells in two ways. First, the integration of viral DNA into the host genome may cause changes in the level of expression of adjacent host cell genes, a process called insertional mutagenesis.

Second, many tumour viruses carry one or more specific genes called oncogenes that appear to be responsible for their neoplastic transforming properties. Hence these genes are called viral oncogenes (v-onc genes).

One of the most remarkable findings of recent years, and the discovery for which Michael Bishop and Harold Varmus won the 1989 Nobel Prize, is that sequences that are homologous to v-onc genes are found in the genomes of all vertebrate species; these homologues of the viral oncogenes are called cellular oncogenes (c-onc genes), or protooncogenes. The c-onc genes, which seem to have been highly conserved throughout evolution, have been found in every species examined so far, from yeast to man. It turns out that they are part of a cell's normal genetic machinery, responsible for the control of proliferation, differentiation, and development. It appears, therefore, that viruses have 'picked up' normal cellular genes which, in their new home, have undergone changes that render them capable of inducing neoplastic transformation under appropriate conditions. This extraordinary discovery led to the notion that tumours might be caused by mutations involving cellular oncogenes.

During the last few years many oncogenes have been identified. A representative list, together with an explanation of the nomenclature used to describe viral and cellular oncogenes, is shown in Table 26.

● Transforming properties of human oncogenes

The story of the discovery of the transforming properties of human oncogenes is one of the most interesting in modern biology. The introduction (transfection) of DNA isolated from normal or neoplastic human and other mammalian cells into certain cell lines has turned out to be a valuable analytical tool for studying the action of oncogenes. The cell line that has been used most extensively was derived from murine fibroblasts (NIH 3T3). DNA sequences from human tumour cells were found to be capable of inducing transformation, that is disordered growth, in NIH 3T3 cells. As we shall see in Chapter 10 it is possible to insert calcium microprecipitates of DNA into cells. In experiments of this type a precipitate of calcium phosphate and the tumour DNA was added to NIH 3T3 cells, which were then grown for about 2 weeks. Those that were transformed continued to divide and formed visible foci. DNA from these cells was then used to transform further NIH 3T3 cells. After several rounds of transfection the murine cells contained only the minimal amount of human DNA required for transformation. The transforming human DNA sequences were then isolated from libraries prepared from the DNA of the transformed murine cells or analysed directly by Southern blotting of DNA prepared from these cells.

Molecular hybridization of v-onc genes to restriction-endonuclease-cleaved DNAs isolated from transformed NIH 3T3 cells established the presence of homologies between certain v-onc genes and activated c-onc genes in the DNA of several human tumours; human bladder and lung carcinoma onc genes were found to be homologous to the Harvey (Ha-*ras*) and Kirsten (Ki-*ras*) sarcoma

Table 26. *Examples of retrovirus oncogenes (v-onc) and the chromosomal location of their human cellular oncogene (c-onc) counterparts (PK = protein kinase, EGF = epidermal growth factor, PDGF = platelet derived growth factor)*

onc	v-onc origin	Virus disease	Product or activity	Human chromosome
abl	Mouse	pre B cell leukaemia	PK (tyr)	9q34
erb B	Chicken	Erythroblastosis	Truncated EGF receptor	7p13-q11.2
fms	Cat	Sarcoma	M-CSF receptor	5q34
fos	Mouse	Osteosarcoma	DNA binding	14q21-31
Ha-ras1	Rat	Sarcoma	GTP binding	11p15
Ha-ras2	Rat	Sarcoma	GTP binding	X
Ki-ras1	Rat	Sarcoma	GTP binding	6p23-q12
Ki-ras2	Rat	Sarcoma	GTP binding	12p12
Mos	Mouse	Sarcoma	PK (ser. thr)	8q22
Myc	Chicken	Myelocytomatosis	DNA binding	8q24
sis	Monkey	Sarcoma	Truncated PDGF (β chain)	22q12-q13
src	Chicken	Sarcoma	PK (tyr)	20q12-q13

virus oncogenes, respectively. It was also found that an Ha-*ras* gene cloned from a bladder carcinoma cell line was capable of transforming NIH 3T3 cells after transfection, while alleles of this gene from normal placenta did not have this property. Even more remarkably, the difference between the two genes was only a single nucleotide within the protein coding sequence; non-transforming alleles coded for glycine (GGC) at the 12th residue from the N-terminal end, while the bladder-carcinoma-transforming allele coded for valine (GTC) at this position.

Using this type of approach many human cellular oncogenes have been discovered and their chromosomal location defined (Table 26). Although tumours of the same cell types may show the same active oncogene, it is now apparent that the situation is more complex than this. It has been found that the same oncogenes can be activated in many different tumours, Ki-*ras* in ovary, lung, pancreas, and bowel for example. Furthermore, different oncogenes may be activated in the same tumour, *neu* or *myc* in breast cancer for example, and while some tumours show point mutations in particular oncogenes, colon and lung cancer in the case of *ras* for example, not all tumours of these tissues show altered oncogenes of this type. Thus, although the role of oncogene expression seems to have been established as being an important part of neoplastic transformation, these apparent inconsistencies obviously raise questions about the primary role of altered oncogenes in producing a neoplastic phenotype.

Another question posed by these tantalizing observations is how far the experimental systems used to study oncogenes mirror cancer in the real world. For example, although a single mutant gene may be sufficient to transform cultured mouse cells, epidemiological analysis of human and animal cancers suggests that several independent mutations are required to transform a normal human cell. One answer to this paradox may lie in the properties of the NIH 3T3 cell, which by no stretch of the imagination can be considered to be normal. Indeed it may well have already undergone some of the steps required for neoplastic transformation; the mutant *ras* gene extracted from bladder carcinoma cells will not transform normal human cells. However, further experiments have provided a link between oncogenes and the epidemiologists 'multiple hit' model of malignant transformation.

Certain DNA tumour viruses require two separate genes to produce neoplastic transformation of normal cells. One of the genes enables the cells to go on growing indefinitely; the other produces changes in the shape and behaviour of the cells that are associated with loss of constraints on growth. These two classes of genes are called immortalizing and transforming, respectively. It was guessed, therefore, that the NIH 3T3 cell line might already be 'immortal' and that the mutant *ras* oncogene described earlier might be the equivalent of a virus transforming gene. This idea was tested by introducing an immortalizing gene from adenovirus together with a *ras* gene into normal rat kidney cells; the two genes together produced a full transformation. Several other combinations of oncogenes are capable of similar transformation of normal cells in culture; neither work on their own and the effect is only produced when both genes are inserted into the cells.

● The nature of cellular oncogenes

It is apparent, therefore, that cancer-producing genes in animal retroviruses are related to normal cellular genes. So far about 25 different cellular oncogenes have been defined, some of which are listed in Table 26. It has been estimated that of our 50 000 different genes perhaps fewer than 100 are potential oncogenes. It is unfortunate that cellular oncogenes are so named because it is now quite clear that they are normal regulatory genes and are only oncogenic in the sense that if they are abnormally activated, or if their function is changed in other ways, they may be involved in transforming the properties of normal cells to those of cancer cells.

The ways in which cells respond to external regulatory factors involved in their growth and differentiation were outlined in Chapter 3. It was pointed out that normal cells produce growth factors, proteins that regulate cell division, differentiation, and maturation. Many of these molecules act on their target cells by binding to specific surface receptors, after which their activity may be mediated by enzymes (kinases) that are part of the cytoplasmic domain of the receptor, through intracellular second messenger systems, or by interacting with proteins that bind directly to DNA. Growth factors have several properties that may be involved with carcinogenesis. Some of them transform normal cells *in vitro*. Conversely, the induction of cell transformation can result in increased production of a growth factor. These observations suggest that, since growth factors can both initiate and be the end product of transformation, they may be involved in self-perpetuating, positive-feedback loops which, if inappropriately controlled, could result in unregulated cell division and growth. This phenomenon, called autocrine secretion, has been implicated in a variety of situations in which there is rapid growth of cells such as wound repair and embryogenesis, as well as in malignant transformation.

It turns out, in fact, that oncogene products may be involved in many different aspects of cellular regulation (Fig. 73). They may be growth factors or their receptors, enzymes associated with these receptors, tyrosine kinases involved in the intracellular activation of enzymes, or DNA binding proteins. For example, the c-*erb*-B oncogene product is a truncated form of the epidermal growth factor receptor; it does not bind epidermal growth factor but appears to fire signals into cells as if they were permanently activated by the growth factor. The c-*cis* gene encodes a protein with strong sequence homology with one of the polypeptide chains of platelet-derived growth factor. Oncogenes such as c-*src* or c-*myc* encode protein kinases or nuclear proteins that bind to DNA. Altered tyrosine kinase activity is exemplified by the c-*fms* oncogene, which codes for the receptor for the colony-stimulating factor, CSF-1, involved in macrophage differentiation. In fact, the c-*fms* oncogene has a point mutation in the region coding for the external domain of the receptor. The transforming viral gene v-*fms* has an enhanced kinase activity compared with its cellular counterpart.

One of the best studied examples of oncogene involvement at the level of

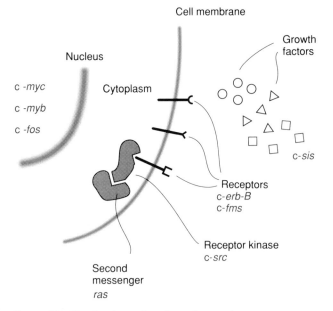

Figure 73. **Mechanism of action of some human oncogenes.**

intracellular messengers is the *ras* family. Its gene products have structural homology with proteins called G and N which control adenylate cyclase activity. Some *ras*-encoded products have also been shown to have GTPase activity. These proteins are thought to be important in the regulation of the 'second messenger' system (see Chapter 3). Several oncogenes including *myc*, *myb*, and *fos* code for nuclear-associated proteins. Their precise localization and function is not yet fully worked out. It is likely that they are involved in the control of gene expression, acting to modulate the production of growth factors for example.

● Mechanisms of abnormal oncogene function

One of the most important activities in the cancer field is to try to understand the genetic changes that cause normal cellular regulatory genes to alter their function, so leading to a neoplastic phenotype. A number of mechanisms have already been worked out, at least in outline. As already mentioned, point mutations may be sufficient. We have seen how c-*ras* may become oncogenic by a single base change resulting in an amino acid substitution in its gene product. Apparently even such a minor alteration at a critical point in a protein may alter the phenotype of a cell, at least if it is already primed in some way. Although it is not yet clear how these point mutations alter the function of their products some progress has been made.

The molecular mechanism for abnormal *ras* activation has been studied intensively over the last few years. The *ras* genes encode proteins with a molecular weight of 21 kd and called p21 which are 188 or 189 amino acids long and which are found at the inner surface of cell membranes. There is extensive evidence that p21 is essential for the proliferation of mammalian cells *in vitro* and that it is required for the viability of certain strains of yeast. Interestingly, human p21 *ras* can restore viability to yeast mutants in which the endogenous yeast genes have been inactivated. All transforming *ras* genes detected by gene transfer have been found to contain point mutations that lead to an amino acid substitution at codons 12, 13, or 61. Like other members of the family of guanine nucleotide-binding regulatory proteins, or G proteins, p21 binds guanosine diphosphate and guanosine triphosphate. It is thought that they function as regulators of the signal transduction pathway from plasma membrane into cells. It is therefore of particular interest that the codons at positions around 12, 13, and 61, which have been found to contain mutations in neoplastic cells, are either critical sites for GTP or GDP binding or, in the case of codon 61, seem to be physically linked to these sites. Furthermore, p21 which is altered at these codons has been shown to have a reduced intrinsic GTPase activity and it is thought that the inability to hydrolyse GTP blocks the p21 molecule in a biologically active, GTP-bound state.

Quite recently, a cytoplasmic protein called GAP (<u>G</u>TPase <u>a</u>ctivating <u>p</u>rotein) has been identified which interacts with p21 *ras* to stimulate its GTP hydrolytic activity by as much as 50-fold. The *ras* proteins that have mutated at codons 12, 13, and 61 do not show elevation of GTPase activity in the presence of GAP. It appears that GAP interacts with *ras* at the p21 effector site. Mutations in this domain destroy the ability of *ras* proteins to transform cells without affecting guanine nucleotide binding. These and related studies seem to identify GAP as a putative target molecule for regulation of p21 within the cell. To complicate matters it appears that another signal generated by p21 is activation of protein kinase C. Furthermore, it turns out that *ras* activation can affect other pathways including TGFα (see Chapter 11). Transforming *ras* proteins will only initiate DNA synthesis in cells with intact protein kinase C, and down regulation of protein kinase C tends to abolish the mitogenic response to *ras* proteins though not to other growth factors. Thus although we are starting to have some insights into the way in which an altered *ras* protein functions, the story is becoming more complicated with each new research finding and there is still a long way to go before we understand the precise role of these point mutations in the genesis of the neoplastic phenotype.

Another example of the way in which point mutations can alter oncogene function comes from work on *Neu*, which is frequently activated in tumours of the nervous system in rats and which directs the synthesis of a protein called p185. This is glycosylated and can be identified by antisera made against intact cells, suggesting that at least part of it is localized to the cell surface. In fact its gene sequence is similar to that for the epidermal growth factor receptor. Recent studies suggest that it is a trans-membrane protein consisting of an extracellular region of about 650 amino acids, a trans-membrane domain, and an intracellular portion of about 580 amino acids, part of which consists of a tyrosine kinase domain. It turns out that a single point mutation, valine to glutamic acid, is enough to endow transforming properties on this oncogene. It has been suggested, therefore, that this substitution causes the receptor to be active in the absence of ligand and hence to deliver a continuous proliferative signal to an affected cell. The effects of the amino acid substitution could be mediated by clustering of the receptor, stabilization of interactions between it and its substrate or other effectors in the membrane, or simply by exerting a physical constraint that shifts the receptor slightly inward or outward in the membrane.

Another well-defined mechanism for the abnormal activation of cellular oncogenes is amplification. This simply means the repeating of DNA sequences, sometimes by as many as 100 times. This in turn may lead to over-production of the gene product; amplification of the c-*myc* oncogene has been found in the white cells of patients with acute leukaemia, in the late stages of metastasizing neuroblastoma, and in tumours of breast, ovary, and lung. Although only a few leukaemias show c-*myc* amplification, N-*myc* amplification associated with neuroblastoma is common enough to provide an extremely useful prognostic marker. Similarly, there is increasing evidence that c-*erb B*-2 amplification may be a useful marker for the prognosis of breast cancer.

Finally, cellular oncogenes may become abnormally activated by chromosome translocation. This is one of the most interesting areas of cancer research because it is starting to provide a molecular basis for some long-standing observations about specific cytogenetic abnormalities in malignant cells.

● Oncogenes and chromosomal translocations

The chromosomal location of many human cellular oncogenes is now known (Table 26). This information, together with the observation that there are specific chromosomal alterations associated with certain cancers (Table 27), has resulted in the unfolding of a fascinating if incomplete story about some of the events that may occur as a prelude to neoplastic transformation.

Burkitt's lymphoma (BL)

This tumour has been studied in great detail in this context. This is a common cancer in parts of tropical Africa, is found predominantly in young children, and is remarkably amenable to chemotherapy. It is known that BL cells have specific chromosomal changes; 90 per cent of patients have an 8/14 translocation (Fig. 74), while others have 8/2 or 8/22 translocations. As mentioned in Chapter 4, chromosomes 14, 2, and 22 carry the genes coding for the immunoglobulin heavy chain, and κ and λ light chains, respectively. The cellular equivalent of the viral oncogene, c-*myc*, is located on chromosome 8. It turns out that the breakpoint of all three translocations is at the site of the c-*myc* gene. In the case of the 8/14 translocation the heavy chain gene is actually split by the

Table 27. *Some cytogenetic changes associated with cancer*

Chromosomal rearrangement	Disease
del(1)(p32-36)	Neuroblastoma
t(1;3)(p36;q21)	Acute non-lymphocytic leukaemia (ANLL)
del(1)(p12-p22)	Malignant melanoma
t(1;19)(q23;p13.3)	Acute lymphatic leukaemia (ALL)
t(2;8)(p12;q24)	Burkitt lymphoma (BL)*
t(2;11)(p21;q23)	ANLL, myelodysplasia (MD)
del(3)(p14-p23)	Bronchial carcinoma
t(6;14)(q21;q24)	Ovarian carcinoma
t(9;22)(q34;q11)	Chronic myeloid leukaemia (CML), ALL, ANLL
del(11)(p13)	Wilms tumour
t(11;17)(q23;q25)	ANLL-M4, ANLL-M5
t(11;19)(q23;p13)	ANLL
t(11;22)(q24;q12)	Ewing sarcoma
del(12)(p11-p13)	ANLL
del(13)(q14.1)	Retinoblastoma
inv(14)(q11;q32)	T-cell chronic lymphocytic leukaemia (CLL)
del(14)(q22-q24)	B-cell CLL
del(22)(q11)	Meningioma, glioma

*Other translocations described in text.

translocation. The coding sequences for the constant region remain on chromosome 14 while the more distally placed coding sequences for the variable region are usually translocated to chromosome 8; the c-*myc* gene is moved from chromosome 8 to the rearranged chromosome 14. In the less common translocations involving the genes for the immunoglobulin light chains on chromosomes 2 and 22, the c-*myc* gene remains on chromosome 8 while a variable portion of the unrearranged light chain loci is translocated to that chromosome.

The c-*myc* gene is composed of three exons, the first of which encodes for the 5' untranslated region. The initiation codon for the c-*myc* protein is close to the 5' end of exon 2. The gene has two promotors, p1 and p2, which initiate transcription of two distinct messenger RNAs. The c-*myc* gene product is found exclusively in the nuclei of cells, where it appears to have DNA binding properties that are due to its highly conserved C-terminal segment. Although many details remain to be worked out it appears that the *myc* protein may in some way be involved in the modulation of cell replication.

The central question, therefore, is the role of the translocated oncogene in the pathogenesis of BL. The breakpoints of several translocations have been analysed by gene mapping and cloning and have been found to be very heterogeneous. The only consistent feature is that the c-*myc* coding sequences, that is exons 2 and 3, are preserved. The breakpoints are distributed both

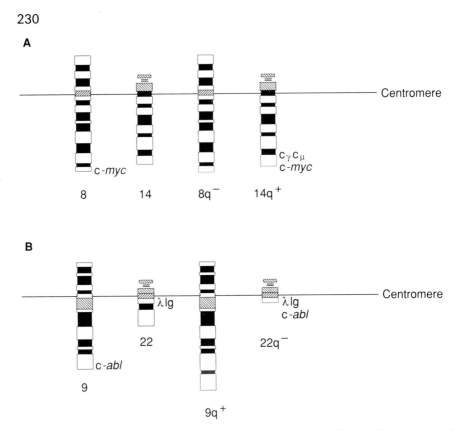

Figure 74. Chromosomal translocations and oncogenes **A** One of the chromosomal translocations found in Burkitt's lymphoma. The c-*myc* oncogene translocates to the region of the heavy-chain locus on chromosome 14. **B** Reciprocal translocation responsible for the Philadelphia chromosome (9;22) (q34;q11). The translocation involves the movement of the c-*abl* oncogene from chromosome 9 to 22.

upstream and downstream of c-*myc*, in the immediate 5′ flanking region, and within the gene itself. When both breaks are located within the first intron or first exon of c-*myc*, that is downstream from the normally used promotors of the gene, transcription is initiated from cryptic promotors in the first intron. In these cases, because the concensus splice sequence at the 5′ end of the first intron is lost, intron sequences downstream from the cryptic promotor are not spliced out from the nascent mRNA transcript. The processed mRNA from tumours of this type contains 5′ intron sequences not present in those with breakpoints upstream or downstream of the c-*myc* promotors. The functional significance of these abnormal molecules is not clear, although, as mentioned later in this chapter, they may be of interest as abnormal products of a cancer cell and hence targets for antitumour agents.

Of course, the fact that all these translocations are into the immunoglobulin loci suggests that the particular environment in which the c-*myc* gene finds itself may also be of considerable importance. As we saw in Chapter 4 the immunoglobulin genes in B cells undergo a remarkable series of rearrangements during the generation of antibody-producing cells. In this context, many rearranged c-*myc* alleles are subject to potential damage by point mutations in the promotor control regions and/or exon 1; somatic point mutations are common within the Ig loci as one of the mechanisms for generating antibody diversity. It is possible that translocation of the c-*myc* gene to an Ig locus may interfere with the normal regulatory processes that link c-*myc* gene expression to stimuli that control proliferation and differentiation. Regardless of the mechanisms, however, cell fusion experiments have provided good evidence that the rearranged c-*myc* gene escapes normal regulatory mechanisms and it is now believed that this is an essential feature of BL cells. Although this may be reflected in the generation of abnormal quantities of c-*myc* protein it seems likely that these changes are less important than the inability of the altered c-*myc* gene to be modulated by normal regulatory influences.

A great deal is known about the epidemiology of BL and it is clear that the chromosomal translocation leading to the rehousing of an oncogene cannot be the only factor responsible for this tumour. It has been realised for a long time that BL occurs in two distinct settings. First, it is found quite frequently in localized areas of Africa and there is good epidemiological evidence that a factor that may be involved in its pathogenesis in this part of the world is chronic antigenic stimulation due to *P. falciparum* malaria infection. Second, BL may occur sporadically in any part of the world. In addition, there is strong evidence that infection with Epstein–Barr (EB) virus plays a major role in causing BL. Thus, there are at least three threads to the story of the pathogenesis of BL, a particular geographical distribution, an identified infective agent, and a well-defined chromosome translocation.

Can we fit all this together into a coherent story? Unfortunately, this is not yet possible, though a few facts are clear. EB virus infection leads to polyclonal expansion of B cells, either by antigenic stimulation or integration into the genome. Chronic malaria may also provide a source of antigenic stimulation. The translocation event might be more likely to occur in cells in this state, with subsequent deregulation of the c-*myc*. Of course, there are numerous other combinations and permutations of these different events which are equally likely.

Chronic myeloid leukaemia (CML)

Chronic myeloid leukaemia is another condition in which it is sometimes possible to trace the evolution of events leading up to the emergence of an aggressive neoplastic cell line. This disorder is characterized by a long chronic phase in which there is disordered white blood cell production but in which the predominant cell in the peripheral blood is a mature granulocyte, or one of its immediate precursors. This can be regarded as the pre-neoplastic (or pre-leukaemic) phase of the illness. At any time the condition may dramatically change into acute myeloblastic leukaemia; this is heralded by the appearance of extremely immature myeloid precursors in the blood. Patients with CML have a specific chromosomal abnormality in their blood cells, even in the chronic phase of the illness, called the Philadelphia (Ph^1) chromosome, which usually results from a translocation between chromosomes 9 and 22, with breakpoints at 9q34 and 22q11 (Fig. 74). It turns out that this translocation involves the movement of another oncogene, c-*abl*, which is normally situated on chromosome 9, to chromosome 22.

A great deal of work has been directed towards the molecular analysis of the new home of the c-*abl* gene following the generation of the Philadelphia chromosome. Although the breakpoints in chromosome 9 are variable, those in chromosome 22 all occur within a region of about 5.8 kb. For this reason this part of chromosome 22 has been designated a breakpoint cluster region (*bcr*). From studies of an abnormal messenger RNA containing c-*abl* sequences found in the cells of patients with chronic myeloid leukaemia it appears that a new transcription unit must be created by the *bcr*/c-*abl* fusion event. This type of messenger RNA, which seems to be specific to chronic myeloid leukaemia cells, is about 8500 nucleotides long in contrast to the normal c-*abl* messenger RNAs which are approximately 6800 and 7400 nucleotides long. Even more interestingly, complementary DNAs derived from the mRNA of 8500 nucleotides contain coding sequences derived from the *bcr* region of chromosome 22. Thus it appears that at least two genes, c-*abl* and *bcr*, and perhaps more, are involved in this fusion event.

The c-*abl* gene, which is normally found on the long arm of chromosome 9 has a 7 kb coding sequence spread over more than 100 kb of DNA. Part of the c-*abl* protein has homology to members of the tyrosine kinase family. Human and mouse c-*abl* genes have a similar structural organization with remarkable conservation of much of their coding sequence. Four different c-*abl* cDNAs have been cloned using messenger RNA from mouse cells. Each encodes a different protein with identical C-terminal ends but with different N-terminal sequences. These different messenger RNAs are produced by differential splicing of the c-*abl* RNA. The c-*abl* messenger RNAs encode 145 or 150 kD phosphoproteins in both mouse and human cells. It seems likely that these products function as the tyrosine kinase portion of a receptor complex. So far little is known about the products of the *bcr* gene except that they include 130 and 160 kD proteins.

It turns out that cells of patients with chronic myeloid leukaemia contain a protein called p210 which is precipitated by antibodies directed against determinants of both the c-*abl* and *bcr* encoded proteins. This abnormal protein undergoes autophosphorylation of its tyrosine residues and functions as a tyrosine kinase. It appears that it is the abnormal product of the fused *bcr* and *abl* genes, as shown in Fig. 75. Because of the variable breakpoints on chromosome 22, two different messenger RNAs may be produced depending on whether one of the small exons of the *bcr* genes is included in the Philadelphia chromosome. Recent studies in which the *bcr*/*abl* fusion gene was inserted into mice via the transgenic route have shown marked changes in white cell production in the offspring, though no consistent pattern has emerged. One of

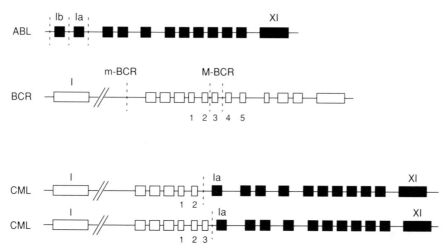

Figure 75. The *Abl* and *Bcr* genes and the *Abl/Bcr* fusion genes. The boxes represent exons and the introns are shown as lines. The numbers below the *Bcr* gene identify the exons in the classical breakpoint cluster region. The breakpoints in CML and Ph positive ALL are shown as vertical dashed lines. The breakpoint region involved in CML is called the major *Bcr* (M-*Bcr)* and that in ALL is called the minor region (m-*Bcr*). Two different fusions genes that have been found in patients with chronic myeloid leukaemia are shown below.

the most remarkable outcomes of these studies is that, even in patients with chronic myeloid leukaemia who appear not to have a typical Philadelphia chromosome, there are rearrangements of *bcr* that are undetected even by high resolution cytogenetic analysis; the c-*abl* gene is not involved in such cases.

How are these intriguing observations related to the clinical phenotype of chronic myeloid leukaemia? Analysis of B lymphocytes from patients with this disorder suggests that they are the product of a single stem cell population that lacks the Philadelphia chromosome. This suggests that the latter may develop in a pre-existing clone of already abnormal cells. The major characteristic of the disease that appears to be most directly associated with the *bcr/abl* fusion gene product is marked hyperplasia of the white cell line with a variable increase in megakaryocytic and even erythroid lineages. On the other hand the maturation of these lines is relatively normal. Thus to generate the chronic phase of myeloid leukaemia it appears that at least two steps are required. Many patients enter a more acute phase of their illness, in which white cell maturation is defective and primitive progenitor cells accumulate in the marrow; these appear to be myeloid in origin although in at least one-quarter of patients the cells have the morphological and surface-marker characteristics of lymphoblasts. At this stage additional cytogenetic changes become apparent including multiple Philadelphia chromosomes, various trisomies, and a variety of translocations and other chromosomal changes. Thus it appears that the disease goes through the type of multi-step generation that is becoming the rule for many types of cancer. Currently, it is very difficult to establish a causal relationship between molecular events and changes in the phenotype although it seems very likely that the *bcr/abl* gene product is in some way responsible for the abnormal proliferation of white cell progenitors in the chronic form of the illness; but even this is uncertain.

A variety of other cytogenetic abnormalities with the potential for involving oncogenes have been observed in different forms of leukaemia and related conditions. Some of these are summarized in Table 27. At the moment all they offer is a tantalizing clue to at least one of the changes that may form a series of somatic mutations that, collectively, give rise to the neoplastic phenotype.

In this short account of cancer cytogenetics we have only touched on a few aspects of a rapidly expanding field. We shall return to this theme at the end of the chapter.

● The overall relevance of abnormal oncogene function in human cancer

In the previous sections we have seen how cellular oncogenes may be abnormally activated by point mutation, amplification or, presumably, by chromosomal translocation. Although we have considered in some detail the possible mechanisms of oncogene activation associated with the well-defined chromosomal abnormalities of Burkitt's lymphoma and chronic myeloid leukaemia, the question remains as to how often altered oncogene function occurs in other human tumours. Over the last few years a vast amount of work has been carried out in this field and a few examples will have to suffice.

One of the most extensively studied disorders with regard to oncogene function is acute myeloid leukaemia (AML). This condition is of particular interest because it may present in a pre-malignant phase called the myelodysplastic syndrome, it can be followed through remission and relapse and, in particular, it is possible to obtain relatively pure cell populations from patients at all stages of the illness. At presentation between 25 and 50 per cent of patients with AML have activated *ras* genes. In most cases it is the Ki-*ras* that is affected although occasionally activation of Ha-*ras* occurs. The use of the polymerase chain reaction has allowed the study of the mutations which occur in the *ras* genes of patients with AML. The most frequent finding is a G-A transition at codons 12 or 13 leading to an aspartate substitution. However, a number of other base substitutions have been found. Interestingly, these mutations do not appear to be in all myeloblasts in the acute phase of AML, an observation which suggests that the *ras* gene mutations may not be the initiating event in leukaemogenesis. On the other hand, after successful treatment leading to haematological remission the mutant *ras* genes cannot be identified in the peripheral blood white cells. This suggests that the treatment has either suppressed or eradicated the mutant *ras*-containing clones. Even more interestingly, although other evidence suggests that the neoplastic white cells are derived from the same clone as the initial presenting clone in AML, recent studies have shown that in four patients in which a mutant *ras* gene was detected at presentation the same mutations were not present at relapse. Although these studies require confirmation, as they stand they suggest that the *ras* mutations may arise early during leukaemogenesis but that they are not the initial event that fires off the leukaemic transformation. Rather, it appears that *ras* mutations occur commonly during the progression of leukaemia, a finding consistent with their presence in only a fraction of the malignant cell population.

Studies of the myelodysplastic syndrome, a pre-leukaemic condition for AML, have also turned up a number of mutant *ras* genes. The significance of their presence at this stage in the evolution of myeloid leukaemia is unclear.

Mutations of the *ras* gene family have been found in many other human cancers. As mentioned earlier, point mutations in the c-Ha-*ras* gene have been found in human bladder cancers and point mutations in the c-Ki-*ras* have been found in colonic and lung cancers and many others. Amplified oncogenes have been found in a wide variety of tumours. One of the best examples of gene amplification is n-*myc* in neuroblastomas. The oncogene c-*myc* is a normal cellular gene. A variant form, n-*myc*, was originally found in a human neuroblastoma cell line. Subsequent studies showed that n-*myc* could transform other cell lines under certain conditions. It turns out that multiple copies, sometimes up to 300, of n-*myc* are found in fresh specimens in many cases of neuroblastoma. Interestingly, amplification of n-*myc* seems to be associated with a poor prognosis, that is with a shorter tumour-free survival and a greater tendency to metastasize. Amplification of both c-*myc* and n-*myc* is also found in small-cell lung cancers and other human tumours although the correlation with prognosis is not so clear-cut. Amplification of many other oncogenes has been observed in a wide variety of human tumours, both in cell lines and in fresh pathological specimens.

One of the major characteristics of malignant tumours is their ability to spread by invasion and metastasis. There is some experimental evidence that introduction of altered oncogenes, *ras* for example, into fibroblasts can confer the capacity for metastasis to develop. Again, the significance of these studies remains to be clarified further.

We shall return to the theme of the spectrum of altered oncogenes in human cancers later in this chapter.

● Cancer suppression and 'anti-oncogenes'

One of the most remarkable developments in the cancer field of recent years is the discovery that certain tumours may result from the recessive inheritance of single mutant genes. It appears that the cancer-producing properties of these genes may become unmasked by a variety of mechanisms, all of which have in common the inactivation of the normal allele which somehow is able to repress the action of its abnormal partner. Although at first this phenomenon seemed to be restricted to rare childhood cancers, more recent evidence suggests that it may occur in many common adult neoplasms.

● Anti-oncogenes

The ideas that led to the elucidation of the molecular basis of cancers of this type pre-dated the development of methods for their verification. They stem largely from the work of Knudson on the inheritance of the childhood cancer, retinoblastoma. Knudson proposed a 'two-hit' hypothesis for the generation of these neoplasms. In essence this suggests that in familial cases the first mutation is inherited in the germ-line and that tumour development requires only one further specific event in any single cell of the appropriate tissue. Indeed, in the case of retinoblastoma, because this second event is so frequent, the pattern of inheritance of the tumour appears to be dominant. In sporadic cases two separate mutations are required to produce a malignant phenotype. Furthermore, Knudson invented the term 'anti-oncogene' to describe the normal alleles of these mutant genes which seem to behave as dominant repressors of malignancy. When it later turned out that chromosomal deletions are a common cause of loss of anti-oncogenes, and since by definition both alleles must be involved before a tumour will develop, it is not surprising that there have been major efforts in recent years to define regions of the genome that are consistently deleted in tumour tissue, as a rational approach to the identification of new anti-oncogenes.

● Retinoblastoma and Wilms' tumour

There is compelling evidence that chromosomal rearrangements involving specific gene loci may cause retinoblastomas, malignant tumours of the eye, and certain other rare childhood cancers. It appears that these tumours, which probably arise in embryonal cells, may be the result of as few as two events, one of which can be inherited. Solid tumours in childhood occur in two types of patients. One group carry a germinal mutation, have multiple tumours (in the case of retinoblastoma the tumours occur in both eyes), and are at risk of developing a second primary cancer. The other is comprised of children who do not carry a germinal mutation, have unilateral disease, and do not seem at risk for carrying a second malignancy. The time of appearance of the tumours in the second group is significantly later than that in the first. These two patterns of childhood cancer are particularly common in children with retinoblastoma but are also seen in other malignancies of early life such as Wilms' tumour (a kidney tumour of childhood) and neuroblastoma.

The locus that is involved in retinoblastoma (Rb) has been assigned to chromosome 13 (13q14). It is closely linked to the locus for esterase D which therefore acts as a useful genetic marker for the region of chromosome 13 that carries the Rb locus. It is now believed that a retinoblastoma involves two mutational events at the *rb* loci. Hereditary cases are thought to result from a germ-line mutation which is present in all the somatic and germ cell lines and can be transmitted from one generation to another. Tumour formation only results when a second, and in this case somatic, mutation occurs in a retinal cell at the *rb* locus on the other homologous chromosome. In sporadic cases it is assumed that both mutations occur as chance events in the same retinal cell.

There are several ways in which the normal allele, the presumed anti-oncogene, of the *rb* gene carrying an oncogenic mutation might be inactivated in somatic cells (Fig. 76). One involves mitotic non-dysjunction, whereby the chromosome carrying the normal gene is lost because of an error during cell division in a retinal cell. It could also result from mitotic non-dysjunction with subsequent reduplication of the chromosome carrying the *rb* locus or from meiotic recombination between the *rb* locus and the centromere resulting in homozygosity of the *rb* locus as well as the distal part of the chromosome. A similar effect would be produced by a point mutation of the normal allele. Many of these predictions have now been confirmed by RFLP analysis using markers flanking the *rb* locus (Fig. 76). For example, in cases that proved to be heterozygous for DNA markers in normal somatic tissues it was found that only one of them was present in the tumour, indicating loss of the normal allele. Similar findings have been observed in Wilms' tumour in childhood; in this case the locus is at 11p13.

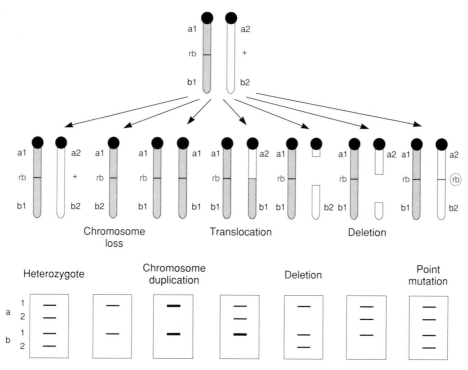

Figure 76. **Various ways in which a recessive mutation at the retinoblastoma (rb) locus might be activated.** The alleles a1 and 2, and b1 and 2 are closely linked RFLPs which can be used to identify some of these mechanisms. The RFLP patterns for each different molecular mechanism are indicated.

These remarkable results emphasize the great strength of recombinant DNA technology. By demonstrating loss of heterozygosity for RFLPs flanking potential anti-oncogenes it is possible to begin to study how abnormal alleles may be involved in the production of a neoplastic phenotype. Not surprisingly, therefore, this approach has been extended to the study of a variety of other malignancies.

● Familial adenomatous polyposis

One of the most interesting and potentially important advances arising from this field of cancer research is the chromosomal assignment of the gene for familial adenomatous polyposis (FAP). This is a dominantly inherited condition characterized by the development of multiple polyps throughout the large bowel which are very prone to change from benign tumours into adenocarcinomas, an event that is so common that prophylactic removal of the colon is carried out routinely. The assignment of the FAP locus to chromosome 5 followed the discovery of an interstitial deletion of this chromosome in a mentally retarded patient with multiple developmental abnormalities and FAP. Using five polymorphic DNA probes which had been previously assigned to chromosome 5, and by studying their segregation in 13 large families with FAP, it was found that one showed evidence for close linkage to the disease locus. In order to relate this finding to the previously reported interstitial deletion, *in situ* hybridization was carried out. This clearly localized the FAP locus to 5q21/q22, quite consistent with the site of the deletion observed in the mentally retarded patient with FAP. It was then found that, using flanking RFLP markers and comparing tumour tissue with normal tissue, about 20 per cent of sporadic colorectal cancers had become homozygous or hemizygous for chromosome 5 alleles. These observations suggest that becoming recessive for a gene in the region of 5q21/q22 is a key step in the progression of at least some forms of colorectal cancer, both sporadic and familial.

● 'Loss of heterozygosity' in other tumours

Considering the potential importance of these findings it is not surprising that searching for loss of heterozygosity in tumour DNA compared to constitutional DNA has become a major industry in the cancer field. Similar results have been reported in acoustic neuromas and meningiomas (chromosome 22), breast cancer (chromosome 13), and lung cancer (chromosome 3, p21). Furthermore, more extensive studies of colon cancers, in addition to confirming loss of heterozygosity on the long arm of chromosome 5, have demonstrated a high frequency of a similar phenomenon on the short arm of chromosome 17. The list grows longer by the week.

Some even more remarkable observations are appearing. For example, there has been considerable interest in the behaviour of the *rb* gene in cancers other than retinoblastoma. This stemmed from the observation that patients who are successfully treated for these tumours have an increased likelihood of developing other forms of cancer, particularly osteosarcoma and, even more surprisingly, cancer of the breast. Furthermore, it appears that the mothers of children with osteosarcoma have an increased risk of developing breast cancer. Could the *rb* defect increase susceptibility to other forms of cancer? It now appears that the same kind of abnormalities of the *rb* gene that are found in retinoblastomas occur in at least some breast cancers, osteosarcomas, synovial sarcomas, and small-cell lung carcinomas. It should be pointed out that much of this work has utilized breast-tumour cell lines, although more recently similar findings have been observed in a small proportion of primary tumours. These changes have also been observed in cell lines from cancers of the lung. Obviously, all this work needs repeating and extending using fresh tumour material.

Of course, it is still very difficult to understand how loss of a particular allele can give rise to localized abnormalities of growth such as colonic polyps. One possibility is that these changes reflect a threshold effect involving, for example, negative control over the production of growth factors. In the case of the FAP locus on chromosome 5, it is suggested that a normal homozygote produces enough of the FAP gene product so that random fluctuations of its concentration cannot go below a threshold that permits localized excessive growth. On the other hand a deficient heterozygote, that is an individual with a defect in one 'FAP locus', might synthesize a reduced level of the FAP product so that abnormal cell proliferation may occur; in the case of the colonic epithelium this might give rise to polyps. Presumably a second mutation involving the normal allele is required in this setting for malignant change to occur. We shall return to this theme in a later section.

● The molecular basis of anti-oncogene activity

The term 'cancer suppression' was used originally to describe the loss of malignant phenotype observed in fusions between cancer cells and normal cells including fibroblasts and lymphocytes. The effect was thought to be mediated in some way by dominant suppressive factors derived from normal cells. These classical cell fusion experiments suggested that at least some of the suppressive factors were genetic since the phenomenon of suppression seemed to be more common when particular chromosomes were present in the fused cells. For example, if a normal chromosome 11 was introduced into Wilms' tumour cells the neoplastic phenotype was suppressed, whereas the X chromosome or chromosome 13 did not have this effect.

The experiments outlined in the previous sections provide another body of evidence for the existence of cancer suppressor genes or, as they are sometimes called, anti-oncogenes. There is no doubt, therefore, that if we understood the action of these genes we might have a much better idea of the general mechanisms underlying neoplastic transformation.

Over the last year or two there has been intense activity in the cancer field directed towards trying to isolate the gene products of the retinoblastoma (*rb*) locus and similar loci that seem to be involved with the generation of tumours. A gene from the *rb* locus, chromosome band 13q14, has been cloned and appears to have properties that are at least consistent with it being the *rb* gene. A 4.7 kb mRNA transcript of this gene was present in all normal tissues examined but was absent or altered in retinoblastomas cells, and deletions within the gene have been detected in many retinoblastomas. The next step was to identify the protein product of the *rb* gene. It turned out to be a nuclear phosphoprotein of about 110 kD that has DNA binding activity. DNA sequences homologous to *rb* cDNA, and proteins antigenically related to *rb* protein, have been found in all vertebrate species examined to date. Quite recently the *rb* protein has been shown to associate with large T antigen and E1A, the transforming proteins of the DNA tumour virus SV40 and adenovirus, respectively. These intriguing results suggest, at least indirectly, that the *rb* protein has a role in regulating the expression of other cellular genes, and may therefore mediate the oncogenic effects of some viral transforming proteins.

And even more direct proof of the involvement of the *rb* gene in neoplastic transformation has been obtained. Experiments have been carried out in which a cloned *rb* gene was introduced, attached to a retroviral vector, into retinoblastoma or osteosarcoma cells that had inactivated endogenous *rb* genes. Expression of the exogeneous *rb* gene affected morphology, growth rate, colony formation, and the ability to form tumours in nude mice. These experiments appear to provide clear evidence of suppression of a neoplastic phenotype by a single gene and hence demonstrate directly the central role of the *rb* gene in cancer formation.

Evidence is already amassing about the extraordinary diversity of mutations that may involve the *rb* gene. Using the polymerase chain reaction it has been possible to sequence the gene from tumour tissue. Several different lesions have been found, including deletions, mis-sense and nonsense mutations, splice–donor mutations, and frameshifts. In some cases these are restricted to the tumour; in others they are also found in normal somatic cells although less often in the parents, suggesting that in many cases they are new germ-line mutations. These observations have important implications for genetic counselling.

Quite recently a candidate gene for the Wilms' tumour locus in 11p13 has been isolated. The predicted amino acid sequence contains four tandem zinc-finger motifs which, as described in Chapter 3, are known to be associated with transcription factors. The putative gene shows very little similarity to other known genes. It spreads over approximately 60 kb of genomic DNA and maps to a region between 60 and 170 kb in size that is homozygously deleted in two independent Wilms' tumour cell lines. However, the situation with regard to Wilms' tumour will undoubtedly turn out to be much more complex than for retinoblastoma. Studies of the Beckwith–Wiedemann syndrome, a disorder characterized by hyperplasia of the kidneys and other organs, macroglossia and other congenital abnormalities, which is also associated with a high likelihood of Wilms' tumour as well as other neoplasms, have pinpointed the lesion to 11p15. Furthermore, some families have been studied in which the genetic predisposition to Wilms' tumour is not linked to either 11p13 or 11p15. These observations suggest that at least three gene loci may be involved in the generation of Wilms' tumour. A great deal more work will be required to define the products of the other Wilms' tumour genes and to determine whether the evolution of this particular neoplasm follows a similar pattern in most cases, or, as seems more likely, there are many different pathways towards the development of this tumour.

Another interesting thread in the story of tumour suppressor genes has also come from the colon carcinoma field. As mentioned earlier, allelic deletions of the short arm of chromosome 17 occur frequently in colorectal cancer. Extensive mapping and sequencing studies have provided strong evidence that the gene that is lost in these deletions codes for p53, a transformation-associated protein implicated in the genesis of neoplasia. Two tumours were studied in particular detail. In both cases there were allelic deletions of chromosome 17p, but considerable amounts of p53 mRNA were expressed from the allele that remained. It turned out that this particular allele contained a mutation in both tumours, in one case an alanine was substituted for valine at codon 143, and in the other a histidine was substituted for arginine at codon 175. These remarkable findings suggest that p53 mutations may be involved in colorectal cancer, perhaps through inactivation of a putative tumour suppressor function of the normal p53 gene.

What are we to make of these intriguing observations? It is reasonable to speculate that the normal p53 gene product interacts with other molecules to suppress neoplastic growth of colorectal cells. It follows that this suppression is relieved by loss of the p53 gene or if mutations prevent the normal interaction of p53 with other cell constituents. Again there are major possibilities for a 'two-hit' generation of neoplasia. For example, the first mutation in a p53 gene might not be manifest provided there were normal p53 products present in the cell; if a second mutation removed the normal allele the effect of the mutated p53 gene might be expressed. Another intriguing scenario follows the observation that, at least *in vitro*, mutated p53 genes can cooperate with mutant *ras* to transform primary rodent embryo cells. As mentioned earlier, colorectal tumours often have *ras* mutations. It is possible, therefore, that the occurrence together of p53 and *ras* mutations could produce a neoplastic phenotype.

More recent studies suggest that mutations in the p53 gene occur in many other human tumours. It has been found that many tumours with allelic deletions contain p53 point mutations resulting in amino acid substitutions. Furthermore, such mutations are not confined to tumours with allelic deletion, but also occur in at least some tumours that have retained both parental alleles. Finally, it appears that p53 gene mutations are clustered in four hot-spots which coincide exactly with the four most highly conserved regions of the gene. These observations, together with the widespread occurrence of p53 mutations in tumours including those of the brain, breast, lung, and colon indicate the central importance of the p53 gene in the generation of cancer.

Recently yet another extraordinary facet of the anti-oncogene story has emerged. Studies of sporadic Wilms' tumours, retinoblastomas, and osteosarcomas have shown that loss of maternal alleles and retention of paternal alleles is a recurrent pattern. Based on these findings it has been suggested that parental imprinting (see Chapter 3) may play a role in the genesis of these tumours. The argument goes along the following lines. Cells in the target tissue have both paternal and maternal alleles of, say, the Rb gene. On some maternal chromosomes these genes may be repressed by methylation imprinting. If the first hit (mutation) occurs on the paternal allele of such a repressed locus this population of cells will expand. The expanded population offers an increased target for a second event, loss of the maternal allele by somatic recombination for example. If the second event does not occur there will be no tumour. Whether this idea is correct remains to be determined. But whatever the mechanism, it is beginning to look as if parental imprinting may play a role in the development of these tumours.

From this brief outline of this intriguing field of cancer research, another excellent example of the meeting place between cytogenetics and molecular genetics, it is clear that dominant repressors of malignancy exist and that there are a variety of ways in which their activity can be rendered defective. It seems reasonable to suppose, therefore, that further analysis of the products of these loci, and the multi-step changes involved in the generation of tumours of this type, will provide genuine insights into the basic mechanisms of neoplasia.

● How many mutations are required to produce a cancer cell?

Given all this new information about the molecular pathology of cancer can we start to understand the complexities of malignant transformation? In particular, how many different mutations or related changes in the genome of a cell are required?

In the previous section we saw how it now seems likely that two events are probably all that is necessary to produce a retinoblastoma in a child who has inherited a mutation at the *rb* locus. But it seems likely that many human cancers will be much more complicated than this. Some indication of the type of complexity involved has come from recent studies on the generation of colon cancer.

We have already met some of the genes involved in cancer of the large bowel. These include the FAP locus on chromosome 5, the p53 locus on chromosome 17, and the K-*ras* locus. Quite recently another gene, in this case on chromosome 18q, has been identified as a major player in the development of colon cancer. It was found that there is a very high frequency of allele loss in this region in these tumours. By using a conventional chromosomal walking technique a 2–3 megabase gene with a 12 kb mRNA was identified in this area. It has been called DCC (deletion in colon cancer) and is expressed in normal colonic mucosa but usually not in tumours. It turns out to be a hot-spot for somatic mutation. In many tumours specific mutations of this gene have been found and there is a high frequency of allele loss in this region. It is particularly interesting to note that the gene product of the DCC locus is homologous to several cell surface adhesion molecules, such as the neural cell adhesion molecule. Further studies of colon cancer have also revealed frequent allele loss on chromosomes 18, 22, 6, 1, 8, and 9.

From detailed analysis of colon cancers at different stages, it is now believed that the progression to adenocarcinoma involves at least eight mutational events involving K-*ras*, FAP, p53, and DCC. Such events need not be the same in all cases, nor need they occur in the same order. One possible scenario would involve either a somatic or germline mutation in the FAP gene on chromosome 5, which might lead to the formation of an adenoma. Similarly, allele loss on chromosomes 17 and 18 is also found in large adenomas. On the other hand, K-*ras* mutations are not seen in early adenomas but only in larger adenomas or after malignant transformation. Similarly, allele loss from chromosomes 17 and 18 increases dramatically in carcinomas.

Thus although many of these concepts may require some revision, a pattern of a complex multistep process, leading first to the production of a benign adenoma and followed by malignant transformation, is starting to emerge.

● Rare genetic disorders that predispose towards cancer

Since it is now well established that somatic mutations play an important role in the genesis of cancer it is reasonable to ask whether there are any inherited conditions associated with instability of the genome that may make such events more likely to occur. There are in fact a number of rare chromosome fragility syndromes including Fanconi's syndrome, Bloom syndrome, and ataxia telangiectasia, in which there appears to be a genuine increase in the likelihood of developing cancer. It is beyond the scope of this book to describe these conditions in detail but, since they are interesting models for understanding the genesis of cancer, it is worth outlining the main features of one of them.

Ataxia telangiectasia (AT) is a rare autosomal recessive condition character-ized by disordered movement due to defective cerebellar function, small vascular tumours of the skin and eyes called telangiectases, immune deficiency, a high incidence of cancer, increased chromosomal breakage, an unusual sensitivity to DNA damaging agents, and failure of DNA repair following ionizing radiation. The disease is also characterized by the high frequency of non-random chromosomal translocations. Approximately 10 per cent of patients with AT develop cancers during their lifetime, over 80 per cent of which involve the lymphatic system and include lymphatic leukaemia, lymphoma, and Hodgkin's disease. Surprisingly, most of these tumours seem to be of T cell origin.

It has been found that the majority of AT-associated translocations in T cell leukaemia and lymphoma involve band 14q32. Indeed, clonal expansion of cells carrying abnormalities of this region has been documented in some patients before the development of overt malignancy. The fact that this region seems to be involved in many human T cell tumours suggests that there is a locus near the chromosomal breakpoint which plays an important role in oncogenesis.

It is not yet possible to put together a fully satisfactory hypothesis that links AT, the development of T cell neoplasms, and these interesting cytogenetic changes. Although the cause of chromosomal instability in AT is not yet fully elucidated there is recent evidence that it may be due to faulty activity of the enzyme recombinase. This might account for the defective DNA repair and also for the associated immunodeficiency since this enzyme is required for appropriate rearrangements of the genes of the immunoglobulin superfamily. It has been suggested that, because many of the chromosomal translocations in AT involve T cells, this might reflect faulty recombinational machinery in a cell lineage in which recombination is particularly active.

It turns out that the common 7/14 translocations that are found in AT are close to the heavy chain locus of the immunoglobulin gene on chromsome 14 and to the T cell receptor β chain locus on chromosome 7. It has been suggested, therefore, that the development of lymphoid malignancies in patients with AT follows several steps. A fundamental defect in recombinase activity may promote translocations involving band 14q32 leading to the juxtaposition of a T cell receptor locus with a cellular oncogene. The deregulation of the cellular oncogene involved in the translocation would then cause clonal expansion of the cells carrying the translocation. In other words, we have a similar scenario to that described earlier for Burkitt's lymphoma and chronic myeloid leukaemia; only in this case there is an underlying genetic defect which makes the chromosomal translocations more likely.

There are other rare familial cancers which may offer us clues about the general nature of neoplasia. For example, the dominant disorder multiple endocrine neoplasia 2a has recently been assigned to chromosome 10 by RFLP linkage. It should soon be possible to define the mutations that underlie this condition.

Studies of rare genetic diseases of this kind promise to offer us considerable insights into the ways in which mutational events may be generated and lead to malignant transformation.

● Viruses and human cancer

As mentioned earlier in this chapter, following the pioneering experiments of Peyton Rous over 70 years ago animal retroviruses have served as the main models of viral carcinogenesis and, of course, as the basis for the discovery of oncogenes. Retroviruses are so-called because there is a 'backwards step' in the movement of genetic information during their replication cycle. Retrovirus particles contain genes in their single-stranded RNA which is converted to a double-stranded DNA provirus by the viral enzyme reverse transcriptase soon after infection. The DNA provirus is then inserted into the chromosomal DNA of the host and this establishes a persistent infection. The latter may remain latent or be expressed and produce progeny virus. We shall consider the genetic makeup of retroviruses in more detail in Chapter 10 when we discuss their potential as vectors for gene transfer.

Until a few years ago no infectious human retroviruses had been identified. Currently, at least four human pathogens of this type are recognized: human T cell leukaemia virus type 1 (HTLV-1), human T cell leukaemia virus type 2 (HTLV-2), human immunodeficiency virus type 1 (HIV-1), and human immunodeficiency virus type 2 (HIV-2). There is now compelling evidence that HTLV-1 is the causal agent responsible for adult T cell leukaemia (ATL), a condition that is most prevalent in Japan and the Carribbean. HTLV-1 was first isolated from a cell line derived from an American patient with ATL, but epidemiological studies together with further isolates provided clear evidence that HTLV-1 infection is the cause of leukaemia in Japanese and Carribean populations. Infection with this agent also causes a chronic degenerative disease of the nervous system called tropical spastic paraparesis.

Less is known about the distribution of HTLV-2. It appears to be associated with the pathogenesis of a rare blood disease called hairy cell leukaemia, a condition associated with massive enlargement of the spleen and the presence of morphologically distinct lymphocytes in the peripheral blood. Although this tumour usually involves B cells it appears that there are rare T cell variants which may well be due to HTLV-2 infection.

The oncogenic capacity of HTLV-1 and 2 is reflected in the capacity to transform lymphocytes of the T4 class into immortal cell lines. HTLV transformed cell lines, and ATL tumour cells, show over-expression of surface receptors for the growth factor interleukin-2 (IL-2). IL-2 is a protein that has various immunological functions, the most important of which is the ability to initiate proliferation of activated T cells (see Chapter 12). High affinity receptors for IL-2 are absent on resting T cells but appear within hours of activation. The binding of IL-2 to these receptors gives rise to the clonal expansion of T cells activated by specific antigen. Recent evidence suggests that a *trans*-activating gene product, called P40X, of HTLV acts directly or indirectly on enhancer sequences of both the IL-2 and IL-2 receptor genes thus producing an autocrine loop, as defined earlier in this chapter, for the establishment of uncontrolled T cell proliferation.

The activation of genes by retroviruses in this way provides a model of viral oncogenesis which is different from earlier models in that the retrovirus genome either incorporates an oncogene or integrates into the host chromosome next to a cellular oncogene. Interestingly in this respect, examination of ATL cells from different patients has shown that there are no common sites of viral integration, an observation that is compatible with this more novel mechanism for viral oncogenesis.

There is now overwhelming evidence that HIV-1 is the aetiological agent responsible for the acquired immune deficiency syndrome (AIDS). Unlike HTLV, HIV does not immortalize cells *in vitro*, but in active replication is usually lytic and causes cell death. HIV shows a specific predilection for cells that express the T4 antigen including lymphocytes and cells of the intestine and brain.

One of the well-recognized features of AIDS is the high prevalence of malignant disease of an unusual pattern. For example, a proportion of young homosexual males in the United States with AIDS develop Kaposi's sarcoma, an otherwise rare tumour. Other tumours with a high relative risk in AIDS are non-Hodgkins lymphoma, anogenital warts, and squamous cell carcinoma. It seems likely that these tumours arise because of the immunosuppressive action of HIV-1; they also have a relatively high incidence in patients who are immunosuppressed by drugs, particularly those who have had an organ transplant. It has been suggested that Kaposi's sarcoma may result from the action of another virus in this background of immune suppression. This idea is based mainly on epidemiological observations. For example, although Kaposi's sarcoma is particularly common in male homosexuals it is rare in haemophiliacs and recipients of blood transfusions with AIDS. Kaposi's sarcoma has always been relatively common in Africa and only a new atypical and aggressive form is associated with HIV infection. If this is so, and there is a veterinary parallel in the case of canine venereal sarcoma, then there may well be other viruses to be discovered that are able to produce malignant transformation.

It remains to be determined whether other human cancers will turn out to be related to retrovirus infection. Clearly HIV is transmissible only by blood or sexual contact. In contrast to HIV, cell-free plasma and blood products do not seem to present a risk for HTLV-1 infection which requires the transfer of latently infected cells. Mother to infant transmission is also well documented for both HTLV-1 and HIV, although it is not known what proportion of infants become infected transplacently, perinatally, or postnatally through milk. Given the rather limited ways for transmission of retroviruses it seems unlikely that the great bulk of human malignancies will turn out to have a retroviral origin.

We shall return to this topic in Chapter 11.

● Tumour immunology

The increasing occurrence of cancer with ageing, the relatively high frequency of certain tumours in immunosuppressed individuals, and the association of certain lymphomas to particular HLA-DR types suggests that the immune system must be related in some way to the development or progression of the neoplastic process. Although many putative 'cancer antigens' have been described over the years, they have all fallen by the wayside as it has become apparent that they are normal developmental antigens that are inappropriately expressed by cancer cells. Furthermore, attempts at non-specific immunotherapy of cancer have, in general, led to disappointing results.

Recently, however, there has been a major resurgence of interest in this field. For example the availability of powerful cytokines has made it possible to expand lymphocyte populations and to use them, with some success, to stimulate immune responses to tumours. Similarly, the ability to 'humanize' mice monoclonal antibodies has enabled potential anti-cancer agents to be produced; we shall return to this topic in Chapter 11. The recent developments in the oncogene field described earlier in this chapter may, ultimately, provide some of the most valuable leads in cancer immunology.

We have seen how oncogenes like K-*ras* and p53 may develop mutations that lead to structural changes in their products. As described in Chapter 3, T cells recognize degraded fragments of molecules expressed on cell surfaces in association with HLA products. It is possible that these altered oncogene proteins might present a target for immune destruction by cytotoxic T cells. Interestingly it is becoming clear that some tumours seem to lose specific HLA alleles on their surface, a phenomenon that might provide them with a major proliferative advantage by protecting them from such immune attack. These concepts are all open to experimentation, particularly now that it is possible to establish T cell lines and clones to see whether they react with synthetic peptides containing sequences representing altered oncogene products.

● Metastatic disease

Another important area of the cancer field that is just starting to open up is an understanding of the changes in the genetic makeup of cancer cells that allow them to metastasize and change their behaviour during the evolution of the malignancy. Already progress has been made in this area by comparing the function of a variety of oncogenes in primary tumours with their metastases; a number of studies have suggested that allelic deletions are commoner in metastases than in primary tumours and that c-*myc* shows a higher degree of amplification in metastases. Obviously further studies of this type, together with an analysis of expressed surface molecules that may modify the relative degree of anchoring and adhesion of cells, offer a valuable approach to understanding the phenomenon of tumour metastasis.

● Molecular aspects of cancer chemotherapy

● Drug resistance genes

Recent studies have started to throw some light on the problems of multi-drug resistance that develops in many human tumours. A multi-drug resistance gene has been discovered, of which the deduced amino acid sequence suggests that it is a membrane glycoprotein which includes six pairs of trans-membrane domains and a cluster of potentially N-linked glycosylation sites near its amino-terminus. The particular interesting feature of the amino acid sequence of the product of this gene is that it has strong homology with a series of bacterial transport genes. These observations suggest that an energy-dependent transport mechanism is responsible for the multi-drug resistant phenotype.

The multi-drug resistant gene is expressed at a very high level in the adrenal gland and at lower levels in lung, liver, bowel, and other tissues. Of particular interest is the observation that this gene is expressed at unusually high levels in some tumours at the time of relapse following initial chemotherapy. Clearly this recent and important aspect of the molecular pathology of cancer has considerable practical implications.

● Topoisomerases

Another area of study that holds promise for practical application is the DNA topoisomerase enzymes. In Chapter 2 we described how DNA in mammalian chromosomes is packaged into chromatin fibres which are themselves organized into loop domains that project from the backbone of the chromosome. It was pointed out that DNA replication, chromatin separation, and gene transcription all necessitate unravelling of the double helix. Hence mechanisms must exist that somehow overcome the remarkable torsional stresses of DNA. DNA topoisomerases are nuclear enzymes that help to deal with some of these problems by catalysing the interconversion of topological isomers of DNA. There are two classes; type I introduces single strand DNA breaks, and type II cleaves both strands of a DNA helix. It turns out that topoisomerases are the molecular targets for a variety of agents including antibiotics and antibodies, and, of particular relevance to the cancer field, many of the drugs that are used for the treatment of tumours.

Topoisomerase II is an enzyme that catalyses the passage of one double-stranded DNA segment through a reversible break in another DNA segment, a mechanism that entails the formation of a transient covalent DNA enzyme linkage called a cleavable complex. It turns out that a number of important cytotoxic drugs all stabilize the cleavable complex and thus induce protein-linked DNA strand breaks. There is now compelling evidence that interaction with topoisomerase II plays a major role in the cytotoxic effect of these agents. This observation may have important implications for designing cancer chemo-therapy in the future. For example, it turns out that oestrogen enhances DNA cleavage induced by the drug etoposide in human breast cancer cells. This suggests that there may be a rational basis for using both oestrogen and topoisomerase II interactive drugs for treating breast cancer. Furthermore, there is increasing evidence that both qualitative and quantitative changes in topoisomerase II may be involved in drug resistance; both qualitative abnor-malities of the enzyme and reduced levels have been found to be associated with resistance to etoposide. Similarly, it has been suggested that low levels of topoisomerase II may explain resistance to the anti-leukaemic agent, doxorubicin. Interestingly, and in contrast to the type II enzyme, the topoisomerase I content of tumour cells is independent of their proliferative status. Thus it might be possible to develop analogues of the cytotoxic agent camptothecin which is known to act on topoisomerase I.

These recent studies, showing as they do two totally different mechanisms for drug resistance in tumours, suggest that the generation of resistance may be almost as complex as the induction of the malignant process itself! More importantly, they are also starting to suggest more logical approaches to *in vitro* testing of drug resistance and for designing better approaches to cancer chemotherapy.

● Therapy targeted against unique products of cancer cells

As the biology of cancer cells becomes better understood, it may be possible to tailor-make chemotherapy directed at products of these cells that are unique to the malignant phenotype. A number of efforts of this type have been made already. For example, as mentioned earlier in this chapter, some cases of Burkitt's lymphoma are associated with the production of an abnormal messenger RNA which contains part of the first intron of c-*myc*, a sequence which is not found in normal cells. It turns out that antisense oligonucleotides inhibit not only c-*myc* protein synthesis but also proliferation of cell lines derived from lymphomas bearing this particular breakpoint product. Normal lymphocytes or lymphoma cells without the product are not affected. Antisense technology is also being used to switch off genes involved in growth control including c-*myc* and fibroblast growth factor. It appears, therefore, that there is the possibility of developing specific antitumour agents if particular cancer cells produce novel messenger RNAs or proteins. Since, as we have seen, many cancers are associated with mutations, gene rearrangements, amplification, or enhanced transcription, this approach may have more general applicability although the problems of introducing antisense oligonucleotides into tumour cells will be formidable.

Because many tumours show mutations involving specific oncogenes or related genes, the p53 mutations in colonic cancers and many others for example, it may be possible to produce antibodies against the mutant products of these genes for diagnosis or therapy. Here again, the effect of the antibody should be highly specific and should not be exhibited by normal cell populations. We shall return to this theme in Chapter 11.

● What is cancer? Practical applications

It is clear from this brief consideration of the molecular and cell biology of cancer that we know a great deal more about the mysteries of neoplastic transformation than we did 10 years ago. It is apparent that most cancers reflect the clonal proliferation of a cell population that is derived from a progenitor, the genome of which has developed somatic mutations that fundamentally alter its capacity for ordered growth and differentiation. It is also clear that more than one molecular event must be involved in the generation of most cancers. There is equally compelling evidence that at least some cancers result from the action of recessive 'cancer' genes, the expression of which requires inactivation of their dominant allele; the mutations at these loci may be inherited or acquired. Enough is known about the ways in which oncogenes can be activated, and about their abnormal function, to suggest that it is unlikely that the oncogene story is just an epiphenomenon of malignant transformation. The growing evidence for abnormal activation of oncogenes by mutations or chromosomal changes provides a direct link between somatic cell genetics and environmental carcinogens.

What is not yet clear is how all these threads hang together. A few years ago Michael Bishop proposed a tentative interpretation. The proliferation of cells is, he points out, controlled by an elaborate circuitry which stretches from the surface of the cell to the nucleus. The products of cellular oncogenes may represent some of the junction boxes in this circuitry: polypeptide hormones that act on the surface of the cell, receptors for these hormones, proteins that carry signals from the receptors, and nuclear functions, which may all interact to orchestrate the genetic response to afferent commands. Altered oncogene function may therefore act to short circuit these junction boxes. Although all this conjecture is highly speculative, it provides a conceptual framework on which to try to understand further the multi-step process that must be the basis of many common cancers. In particular, it underlines the notion that there is no single cause of cancer. Most of the common cancers must reflect the action of many different environmental carcinogens, inherited or acquired mutations of several oncogenes, a failure of immune destruction of cells expressing their abnormal products and, in particular, a complex series of chance events that combine to allow these different changes the opportunity to lead to uncontrolled cell proliferation and defective maturation.

The recent studies outlined earlier on the evolution of the different mutations that appear to underline colon cancer provide us with some insights into the many routes that may lead to a malignant phenotype and to the hierarchy of molecular events that are required for neoplastic transformation. Vogelstein, who with his colleagues at Johns Hopkins University has done much to develop these new concepts, uses the analogy of a motor car to describe these different mutational events. He describes the oncogene mutations as the accelerator pedal being permanently on the floor! On the other hand, the various suppressor genes can be likened to the brake. Various permutations of excessive use of the accelerator together with defective braking may lead to the accident which is the neoplastic transformation. In addition to providing an outline of the interactions of the multiple-hit events that lead to the production of cancer, these new concepts also underline their complexity and, in a sense, how difficult it is to produce a malignant phenotype! The idea of multiple mutations occurring in a variety of patterns is compatible with the genesis of malignancy by factors that increase mutational rates, such as exposure to environmental carcinogens and increasing age.

From the medical viewpoint the major question that arises from the work outlined in this chapter is whether we shall have to wait for a detailed understanding of how all these threads hang together before we can make use of our new knowledge in clinical practice. Probably not. In the situations in which there are consistent changes in the cytogenetic makeup of tumour cells, or where there are similarly consistent alterations in the structure or function of oncogenes, it should be possible, as is indeed already the case for some tumours, to use these characteristics for diagnostic and prognostic purposes. And as we understand more about the mechanisms of defective oncogene function we should be able to devise more rational forms of treatment for different cancers based on attempts to interfere with the effects of their abnormal action, or by enhancing immune responses to their altered products. Similarly, as the functions of recessive cancer genes are determined we will be able to develop more definitive screening programmes for those at particular risk for developing cancers due to changes in their normal alleles. Thus, although it seems likely that the clinical fall-out from these remarkable scientific advances will not occur overnight, in the long-term these new approaches to the cancer field should provide us with invaluable tools with which to prevent, diagnose, and treat many of the common cancers.

● Further reading

Baker, S.J., Fearon, E.R., Nigro, J.M., Hamilton, S.R., Preisinger, A.C., Jessup, J.M., van Tuinen, P., Ledbetter, D.H., Barker, D.F., Nakamura, Y., White, R., and Vogelstein, B. (1989). Chromosome 17 deletions and p53 gene mutations in colorectal carcinomas. *Science*, **244**, 217–21.

Bargmann, C.I., Hung, M.-C., and Weinberg, R.A. (1986). Multiple independent activations of the *neu* oncogene by a point mutation altering the transmembrane domain of p185. *Cell*, **45**, 649–57.

Barnes, D.M. (1989). Breast cancer and a proto-oncogene. *Br. Med. J.*, **299**, 1061.

Bishop, J.M. (1983). Cancer genes come of age. *Cell*, **32**, 1018–20.

Bodmer, W.F., Bailey, C.J., Bodmer, J., Bussey, H.J.R., Ellis, A., Gorman, P., Lucibello, F.C., Murday, V.A., Rider, S.H., Scambler, P., Sheer, D., Solomon, E., and Spurr, N.K. (1987). Localization of the gene for familial adenomatous polyposis on chromosome 5. *Nature*, **328**, 614–16.

Bodmer, W.F., Cottrell, S., Frischauf, A.-M., Kerr, I.B., Murday, V.A., Rowan, A.J., Smith, M.F., Solomon, E., Thomas, H., and Varesco, L. (1990). Genetic analysis of colorectal cancer. (In press.)

Bock, G. and Marsh, J. (eds.)(1989). *Genetic analysis of tumour suppression*. Ciba International Symposium, **142**. Wiley, Chichester.

Cavanee, W.K., Dryja, T.P., Phillips, R.A., Bendict, W.F., Godbout, R., Gallie, B.L.,

Murphree, A.L., Strong, L.C., and White, R.L. (1983). Expression of recessive alleles by chromosomal mechanisms in retinoblastoma. *Nature*, **305**, 779–84.

Cleaver, J.E. and Karentz, D. (1987). DNA repair in main: regulation by a multigene family and association with human disease. *BioEssays*, **6**, 122–7.

Downes, C.S. and Johnson, R.T. (1988). DNA topoisomerases and DNA repair. *BioEssays*, **8**, 179–84.

Editorial. Molecular mechanisms in familial and sporadic cancers. (1988). *Lancet*, **i**, 92–4.

Epstein, R.J. (1988). Topoisomerases in human disease. *Lancet*, **i**, 521–4.

Ferrari, S. and Baserya, R. (1987). Oncogenes and cell cycle genes. *BioEssays*, **7**, 9–12.

Franks, L.M. and Teiah, N. (eds.) (1986). *Introduction to the cellular and molecular biology of cancer*. Oxford University Press.

Glover, D.M. and Hames, B.D. (1989). *Oncogenes*. Oxford University Press.

Gros, P., Croop, J., and Housman, D. (1986). Mammalian multidrug resistance gene: complete cDNA sequence indicates strong homology to bacterial transport proteins. *Cell*, **47**, 371–80.

Harris, H. (1988). The analysis of malignancy by cell fusion. *Cancer Res.* **48**, 3302–6.

Holt, J.T., Morton, C.C., Neinhuis, A.W., and Leder, P. (1989). Molecular mechanisms of hematological neoplasms. In *The molecular basis of blood diseases*, (ed. G. Stamatoyannopoulos, A.W. Neinhuis, P. Leder., and P.W. Majerus), pp. 347–6. W.B. Saunders, Philadelphia, P.A.

Huang, H.-J., Yee, J.-K., Shew, J.-Y., Chen, P.-L., Bookstein, R., Friedmann, T., Lee, E.Y.-P., and Lee, W.-H. (1988). Suppression of the neoplastic phenotype by replacement of the RB gene in human cancer cells. *Science*, **242**, 1563–6.

Kerr, I.B.C. (1989). Molecular genetics of colorectal cancer. *Br. Med. J.*, **299**, 637–8.

Lehmann, A.R. (1989). Trichothiodystrophy and the relationship between DNA repair and cancer. *BioEssays*, **11**, 168–71.

McManaway, M.E., Neckers, L.M., Loke, S.L., *et al.* (1990). Tumour-specific inhibition of lymphoma growth by antisense oligodeoxynucleotide. *Lancet*, **335**, 808–10.

Murphree, A.L. and Benedict, W.F. (1984). Retinoblastoma: clues to human oncogenesis. *Science*, **223**, 1028–33.

Nowell, P.C. (1988). Molecular events in tumor development. *New Engl. J. Med.*, **319**, 575–77.

Nyhan, W.J. (1987). Retinoblastoma—genetic insights into neoplasia. *BioEssays*, **6**, 5–8.

Reik, W. and Surani, M.A. (1989). Genomic imprinting and embryonic tumours. *Nature*, **338**, 112–13.

Russo, G., Isobe, M., Pegoraro, L., Finan, J., Nowell, P.C., and Croce, C.M. (1988). Molecular analysis of a t(7; 14) (q35; q32) chromosome translocation in a T cell leukaemia of a patients with ataxia telangiectasia. *Cell*, **53**, 137–144.

Slamon, D.J. (1987). Proto-oncogenes and human cancers. *New Engl. J. Med.* **317**, 955–7.

Smith, P.A. (1990). DNA topoisomerase dysfunction: A new goal for antitumour chemotherapy. *BioEssays*, **12**, 167–72.

Sobol, H., Narod, S.A., Yakamura, Y., *et al.* (1989). Screening for multiple endocrine neoplasia type 2a with DNA-polymorphism analysis. *New Engl. J. Med.*, **321**, 996–1001.

Steel, C.M. (1989). Peptide regulatory factors and malignancy. *Lancet*, **ii**, 30–4.

Toguchida, J., Ishizaki, K., Sasaki, M., Nakamura, Y., Ikenaga, M., Kato, M., Sugimot, M., Kotoura, Y., and Yamamuro, T. (1989). Preferential mutation of paternally derived RB gene as the initial event in sporadic osteosarcoma. *Nature*, **338**, 156–8.

Toksoz, D., Farr, C.J., and Marshall, C.J. (1989). *Ras* genes and acute myeloid leukaemia. *Br. J. Haematol.* **71**, 1–6.

Varmus, H. (1987). Cellular and viral oncogenes. In *The molecular basis of blood diseases*, (ed. G. Stamatoyannopoulos, A.W. Leder, and P.W. Majerus), pp. 271–346. W.B. Saunders, Philadelphia, PA.

Weinberg, R.A. (1989). The Rb gene and the negative regulation of growth. *Blood*, **74**, 529–32.

Weiss, R.A. (1987). Retroviruses and human disease. *J. Clin. Pathol.* **40**, 1064–2069.

Yandell, D.W., Campbell, T.A., Dayton, S.H., *et al.* (1989). Oncogene point mutations in the human retinoblastoma gene: their application to genetic counselling. *New Engl. J. Med.*, **321**, 1689–95.

Carrier detection and prenatal diagnosis of genetic disease

9

Until gene replacement becomes a reality the only approaches to the control of genetic disease are prevention and avoidance. Except for trying to ensure that we are not exposed to excessive ionizing radiation or other mutagens in our environment, there is little we can do to control the mutation rate in man. After all, mutation is the mechanism whereby natural selection improves the species. Most of the common genetic diseases must have been maintained by an advantageous effect on survival or transmission, and the rare diseases are merely the inevitable scars of the random events that have made us what we are.

It follows that when we talk about trying to 'prevent' the viable birth of an infant with a serious genetic disability we really mean avoidance rather than prevention. Most clinical geneticists agree that our first priority for controlling serious genetic disease is to develop programmes for screening and avoidance. Medical intervention of this type raises many ethical and economic problems which we will touch on in a later chapter. Here, I shall outline the role of the 'new genetics' in the avoidance of common genetic diseases.

● The avoidance of genetic disease

There are several approaches to the avoidance of genetic diseases (Table 28). In populations in which a particular genetic disorder is common, and for which

Table 28. *Control of genetic disease*

Primary prevention
  Mutagen control
Population screening
  Prospective counselling
Retrospective counselling
Antenatal screening
  Prenatal diagnosis
  Selective termination
Neonatal screening

there is a simple diagnostic test for carriers, schoolchildren or young adults can be screened and given appropriate advice about the choice of marriage partners. Prospective genetic counselling of this kind requires an intensive education programme in the community and has only been carried out extensively in countries or in racial groups within countries in which genetic disorders like thalassaemia or Tay–Sach's disease affect a large proportion of the population. Having observed the mating habits of my fellows I am not optimistic about the beneficial effect of screening on the choice of partners; the only study of which I am aware where it was evaluated thoroughly it was a complete failure. However, screening for common diseases does provide the basis for efficient prenatal detection programmes.

More commonly, prospective screening for genetic diseases or congenital malformation is restricted to pregnant women or newborn babies. Programmes are designed to identify conditions that occur frequently in all populations or are restricted to particular racial groups. For example, screening of pregnant women is carried out in many countries to identify neural tube defects by analysing serum alphafetoprotein levels. Screening programmes for common chromosome defects are also applied widely, particularly in high-risk age groups. Screening for Down syndrome in women over the age of 35 is a good example. In appropriate populations maternal screening for haemoglobin disorders or Tay–Sachs disease has been carried out with varying success. This is usually with a view to prenatal detection of the particular disease. Neonatal screening programmes are confined to conditions that are amenable to treatment and for which a reliable test exists. They are most cost-effective if several tests can be included. For example, large-scale programmes have been set up to screen newborn infants for phenylketonuria and congenital hypothyroidism; occasionally, tests for other inborn errors of metabolism have been included.

Genetic counselling is often retrospective, that is there has already been one affected child, or a relative has a child with a genetic disorder, and parents wish to know the risk for a future pregnancy and whether anything can be done to avoid having another affected infant. In appropriate cases chromosome analysis can be carried out on the parents or other family members or, if a metabolic disorder is suspected, it is sometimes possible to obtain an accurate diagnosis on the affected family member, after which potential parents can be studied for 'heterozygous' levels of an enzyme or protein. If a particular disorder can be identified in a fetus, either by amniocentesis or fetal blood sampling, a couple at risk for having a child with a serious genetic disease can be offered the possibility of prenatal diagnosis followed, where appropriate, by termination of the pregnancy. Alternatively, the parents may opt not to have any children, to adopt, or if the circumstances are right, to use artificial insemination with the sperm from a donor.

Space does not permit a wider discussion of the problems of the avoidance of genetic disease. We shall concentrate on prenatal diagnosis, since it is here that the recent advances in molecular genetics have such an important role to play, both in carrier detection and for facilitating the identification of genetic disease in fetal life.

● Current methods for prenatal diagnosis

Some of the current methods for prenatal diagnosis are summarized in Table 29. Until recently it was carried out either by amniocentesis or by direct examination or biopsy of the fetus. Analysis of amniotic fluid cells has been one of the major tools of prenatal diagnosis. Cytogenetic studies after short-term culture enable many different chromosome disorders to be identified. By analysing cultured amniotic fluid cells it is also possible to diagnose many metabolic disorders; a partial list is shown in Table 30. Examination of amniotic fluid is used mainly for the confirmation of neural tube defects by measurement of alphafetoprotein or acetyl cholinesterase levels.

Table 29. *Prenatal diagnosis*

Second trimester
    Direct inspection of fetus. Ultrasound
    Amniocentesis
        Fluid
        Cells
    Fetal blood sampling
    Biopsy of fetal skin or liver
First trimester
    Chorion villus sampling
    ?Preimplantation

The development of better techniques for fetal blood sampling led to the diagnosis of several genetic disorders which had hitherto been impossible to identify in the fetus. One of the main applications has been for the prenatal diagnosis of haemoglobin disorders such as sickle cell anaemia and thalassaemia. In these conditions, fetal blood samples are incubated with radioactive amino acids and the relative rates of synthesis of the fetal globin chains are determined or, if a sickling disorder is suspected, traces of newly synthesized sickle cell haemoglobin are sought (Fig. 77). Despite its relative sophistication this technique has been used widely in the United States, Europe, and the Mediterranean for the prenatal diagnosis of thalassaemia. It has the great advantage that it measures directly the product of the mutant gene locus.

Fetal blood sampling has also been used successfully for the prenatal diagnosis of haemophilia, Von Willebrand's disease, and various red cell enzyme defects. Rare genetic disorders of white cell function such as chronic granulomatous disease have also been identified in this way. The major problem is the small amount of fetal blood that can be obtained, which makes it necessary to develop microtechniques for the various measurements that are required. Furthermore, its use is limited to genetic blood diseases or to conditions in which there are

Table 30. *Some examples of inborn errors of metabolism which have been successfully diagnosed* in utero *(modified from Miles and Kaback 1978). The enzymes that are assayed are indicated for each condition*

Lipid metabolism
    Fabry's disease   α-Galactosidase A
    Gaucher's disease   β-Glucosidase
    Gangliosidoses   β-Galactosidases A, B, or C
                                          Hexosaminidases A, or A and B
    Krabbe's disease   Galactocerebroside β galactosidase
    Metachromic leukodystrophy   Arylsulphatase A
    Mucolipidosis   Multiple lysosomal hydrolases
    Neimann–Pick disease   Sphingomyelinase

Mucopolysaccharidoses
    Hurler syndrome   α-L-iduronidase
    Hunter syndrome   Iduronic acid sulphatase
    Sanfillipo A   Heparin sulphamidase
    Maroteaux–Lamy   Arylsulphatase B

Carbohydrate metabolism
    Galactosaemia   Galactose-1-phosphate uridyl transferase
    Glycogen storage II   α-1,4-glucosidase

Amino acid metabolism
    Arginosuccinic aciduria   Arginosuccinase
    Homocystinuria   Cystathione synthetase
    Maple syrup urine disease   Branched chain ketoacid decarboxylase
    Methylmalonic acidaemia I   Methylmalonic-CoA mutase

Others
    Adenosine deaminase deficiency   Adenosine deaminase
    Congenital erythropoietic porphyria   Uroporphyrinogen III co-synthetase
    Lesch–Nyhan syndrome   Hypoxanthine-guanine-phosphoribosyl
                                          transferase
    Xeroderma pigmentosa   Defective DNA repair
    Hypophosphatasia   Alkaline phosphatases

altered levels of metabolites in the blood. Fetal blood sampling is associated with a fetal mortality of between 2 and 5 per cent and an increased maternal morbidity due to infection and haemorrhage.

Direct examination of the fetus can be carried out non-invasively by x-ray or ultrasound analysis. These approaches are of particular value for demonstrating major congenital malformations, though recent technical advances in ultrasound have expanded the scope for detecting more subtle developmental lesions. The fetus can also be examined directly by fetoscopy, and techniques have been developed for biopsying fetal skin or liver for the diagnosis of rare genetic diseases.

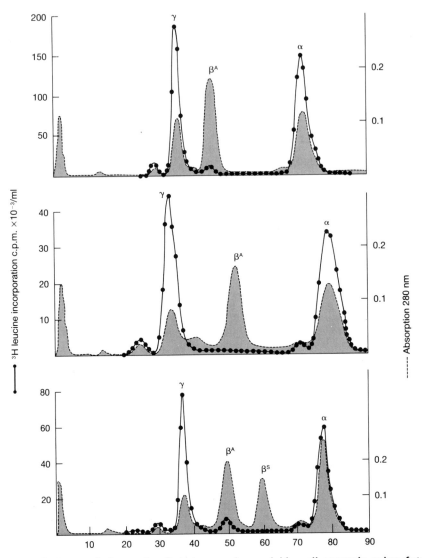

Figure 77. **Prenatal diagnosis of thalassaemia or sickle cell anaemia using fetal blood sampling**. Fetal blood samples were incubated with radioactive amino acids and the labelled globin chains separated by chromatography. The continuous line represents radioactivity eluted from the column; the shaded area shows the position of the fetal globin chains as indicated by non-labelled globin from appropriate haemoglobin markers or fetal blood. The profile shown at the top is from a normal fetus; note the small radioactive β globin chain peak which makes up about 10 per cent of the total non-α globin. The second profile is from a fetus homozygous for β^0 thalassaemia; there is no radioactivity under the β globin peak. The third profile is from a fetus at risk for sickle cell anaemia. Note the absence of radioactivity in the β^S region; this fetus was normal and the pregnancy was allowed to continue.

The major problem with fetoscopy, amniocentesis, and fetal blood sampling is that they cannot be done until the second trimester. Many of the conditions for which prenatal diagnosis is required necessitate the growth of amniotic cells in culture for several weeks and hence a diagnosis cannot be made until late in the second trimester. As mentioned earlier, fetal blood sampling is not feasible until about 18 weeks gestation, and since the analytical methods take at least a week, a decision to terminate the pregnancy cannot be made until nearly 20 weeks gestation. These late second-trimester prenatal diagnoses mean that the mother has a long wait, and by the time they are made she is already feeling fetal movements and the pregnancy is obvious to her friends and relatives. Thus, although second trimester prenatal diagnosis has been a major advance in preventive genetics, it causes a considerable degree of maternal emotional trauma and often ends in a difficult termination of pregnancy.

Over the last few years methods for obtaining fetal tissue much earlier in pregnancy have become available. This important advance, coming at the same time as the new technology of DNA analysis, has revolutionized the whole field of prenatal detection of genetic disease. It is now possible to examine fetal DNA directly and to identify genetic disease very precisely during early development. Furthermore, these new approaches make it feasible to diagnose genetic disorders in the fetus for which the cause is not known and even before the precise location of the disease locus is worked out.

● Sources of fetal DNA

The first prenatal diagnoses of genetic disorders by analysis of DNA utilized amniotic fluid cells. Sometimes this can be done directly on the cells obtained from 20–30 ml of amniotic fluid. However, the yield is variable and often it is necessary to grow the cells in culture for up to several weeks to obtain sufficient DNA to carry out a prenatal diagnosis.

More recently, a technique called chorion villus sampling (CVS) has been developed which has already greatly expanded the prenatal diagnosis of genetic disorders by DNA analysis. After implantation of the embryo, the chorionic plate derived from the trophoblast layer of the blastocyst spreads over the uterine wall; by about the 8th week of gestation it is much larger than the fetus. The cells of the trophoblast are diploid and of fetal origin. The chorion is composed of an outer layer, the trophoblast, an inner mesodermal layer, and fetal blood vessels supplying the villi that extend over the gestation sac until the end of the second month. As the fetus develops, continuing growth of the sac causes thinning of the decidua capsularis and a reduction in its circulation leading to atrophy of the villi. From about 9 to 12 weeks gestation it is possible to biopsy the chorion by the cervical route using either an aspiration needle, cannula, or forceps, under ultrasound guide (Fig. 78). It is also possible to carry out CVS transabdominally, which seems less prone to cause infection and can be done safely up to 14 weeks gestation. It is usual to obtain about 20–40 micrograms of DNA, though as much

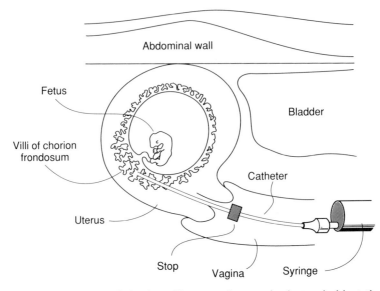

Figure 78. **The principle of chorion villus sampling to obtain trophoblast tissue for fetal DNA analysis.**

as 100 micrograms can be obtained with larger biopsies. Because of the physical properties of chorionic tissue it is usually quite easy to separate it from any contaminating maternal tissue.

Information about the safety of CVS is gradually being amassed. One of the best ways of obtaining this kind of data is by carrying out large multi-centre clinical trials comparing the results of CVS with amniocentesis. Quite recently the first report of the Canadian Collaborative CVS/Amniocentesis Clinical Trial Group has been published. The results are very encouraging, particularly as each group consisted of over 1000 pregnancies. The total fetal losses, made up of spontaneous and induced abortion and late losses, were 7.6 per cent in the CVS group and 7.0 per cent in the amniocentesis group. Mean birthweights for each week of gestation were similar in both groups. Perimortality was slightly greater in the CVS group. There was no evidence of any excess of intrauterine growth-retarded babes in the CVS group. Maternal morbidity was similar in both groups. Similar results were obtained in a comparable trial in the US. Although in both trials there were no obvious deleterious effects on the infants from the pregnancies that had undergone CVS it must be emphasized that some years of careful follow-up will be required before it is absolutely certain that CVS has no side-effects on development. However, as judged by the limited data that are available it appears that CVS is likely to be a safe and acceptable procedure for prenatal diagnosis. The fetal loss rate directly related to the procedure is falling with increasing experience; most recent series quote figures in the region of 2 per cent.

There is little doubt that if CVS turns out to be safe it will revolutionize prenatal diagnosis. This is because it provides an opportunity to diagnose genetic diseases within the first trimester of pregnancy, a time that is much more acceptable to many women. Chorionic tissue can be used for cytogenetic and biochemical analysis, or as a source of DNA. Here, we shall restrict our discussion to the study of fetal DNA for the diagnosis of genetic disorders.

● How is fetal DNA analysed for single gene disorders?

Currently, there are several ways to analyse fetal DNA for single gene disorders (Table 31). First, the mutation can be identified directly by restriction endonuclease mapping. Second, there is linkage analysis using restriction fragment length polymorphisms (RFLPs). The latter approach has wide application to intrauterine diagnosis; its major limitations are complexity and expense, and the necessity of first being able to establish a linkage by studying appropriate family members. Finally, and in the long term the most promising, is the use of oligonucleotide probes designed to detect individual mutations.

Table 31. *Fetal DNA analysis for the prenatal detection*

Direct
    Deletions. Rearrangements
    Mutations that change restriction enzyme sites
    Oligonucleotide probes
        Genomic DNA
        PCR
        Direct sequencing

Indirect
    RFLP linkage analysis (genomic DNA or PCR)
        RFLPs in linkage disequilibrium with mutation
        RFLP analysis in individual family to determine affected chromosome

---

● The diagnosis of single gene disorders directly by restriction endonuclease mapping

In an earlier chapter we considered how human genes can be analysed by restriction endonuclease mapping. It is sometimes possible to use this approach for fetal DNA samples. To be successful the particular mutation that we are looking for must produce a new restriction enzyme site or remove a previously existing one, or there must be a major gene rearrangement or a deletion of sufficient size to be identified by gene mapping.

The first disorder that was shown to be amenable to direct detection by

Southern blotting analysis was sickle cell anaemia. This condition results from an A→T substitution in the sixth codon of the β globin gene which, when it changes from GAG to GTG, leads to the substitution of valine for glutamic acid. The alteration in sequence CTGAG→CTGTG eliminates the recognition site for the restriction enzyme *Dde*I. After digestion with this enzyme, DNA from a chromosome with a β^S gene yields a different sized fragment to one carrying a β^A gene. It turned out that this analysis is technically difficult, but there is another enzyme which also identifies the sickle mutation and is more convenient to use in practice. The sequence CCTGAGG in the region coding for amino acids 5 to 7 in the normal β globin gene sequence is recognized by the enzyme *Mst*II. Cleavage of normal DNA with this enzyme generates several fragments which 'light up' with a β gene probe; the main one is of 1.1 kb. A β globin gene containing the sickle mutation has the sequence CCTGTGG which is not recognized by *Mst*II; cleavage generates a 1.3 kb fragment (Fig. 79).

While this is a very useful method for identifying the sickle cell mutation, certain technical snags must be borne in mind. Incomplete digestion by the enzyme or the possible, if unlikely, occurrence of normal variation in the structure of DNA in this region could obscure the diagnosis. For example, a normal β gene might contain the sequence GAA instead of the usual GAG sequence, both coding for glutamic acid at position 6. Although this unusual sequence would code for normal β globin it would not be recognized by *Mst*II. In addition, there is a form of β thalassaemia caused by a single base mutation in the same codon as that involved in sickle cell anaemia. This also removes the *Mst*II site. With these reservations, however, the diagnosis of sickling disorders with

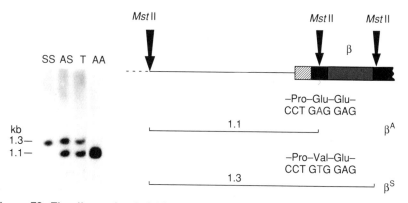

Figure 79. The diagnosis of sickle cell anaemia by restriction enzyme analysis of fetal DNA. The base substitution which causes sickle cell anaemia removes an *Mst* II site. In normal DNA a *Mst* II fragment of 1.1 kb is generated, as shown. The absence of the *Mst* II site in DNA from individuals with the sickle cell mutation generates a longer *Mst* II fragment of 1.3 kb. Heterozygotes show both 1.1 and 1.3 kb bands while homozygotes show only a 1.3 band. The inset shows the results of this type of analysis on a pregnancy at risk for a fetus with sickle cell anaemia. The trophoblast DNA (T) is compared with normal (AA), sickle cell trait (A), and sickle cell anaemia (SS) DNA. Clearly, the fetus (T) is heterozygous for the sickle cell gene.

this restriction enzyme is very reliable. Some of the mutations that cause β thalassaemia and that can be identified directly with restriction enzymes are summarized in Table 32; they constitute about a quarter of those known to be responsible for this condition. No doubt more mutations that can be identified directly will be discovered.

Table 32. β *Thalassaemia mutations directly detectable by restriction enzyme analysis*

Mutation	Restriction enzyme
β° Thalassaemia	
1. Indian deletion	Various enzymes, −619 bp*
2. American Black deletion	Various enzymes, −1.35 kb*
3. Dutch deletion	Various enzymes, −10 kb*
4. Czech deletion	Various enzymes, −4.2 kb*
5. Turkish deletion	Various enzymes, −300 bp*
6. −1 codon 6	*Mst* II
7. IVS 2 splice junction	*Hph* I
8. IVS 1 (−25 bp)	*Fnu* 4H, *Mst* II
9. IVS 1 (−17 bp)	*Fnu* 4H, *Mst* II
10. IVS 1-position 116	*Mae* I
11. IVS 1 position 6	*Sfa* N1
12. IVS 2 3′ end AG→GG	*Alu* I
13. β°39	*Mae* I
14. β°17	*Mae* I
15. β°37	*Ava* II
16. β°121	*Eco* RI
β⁺ Thalassaemia	
17. IVS 2 position 745	*Rsa* I
18. −87 C→G	*Avr* II
19. Hb E	*Mnl* I

*Indicates size of deletion.

Recently the development of the polymerase chain reaction (PCR) has greatly facilitated the identification of mutations that alter restriction enzyme sites. For example, in the case of the sickle cell mutation an appropriate fragment of the β globin gene is amplified approximately 30 times, after which the DNA fragments are digested with the restriction enzyme *Dde*I which, as we have just seen, has a recognition site which is abolished by the A→T mutation at codon 6. Normal DNA is cleaved into two fragments, of about 150 and 201 bp, while DNA from patients with sickle cell anaemia yields a 351 bp fragment; in heterozygotes all three fragments are generated. Because PCR produces so much DNA, these fragments can be detected by either ethidium bromide or silver staining of DNA bands on gels; no radioactive probes are required (Fig. 80).

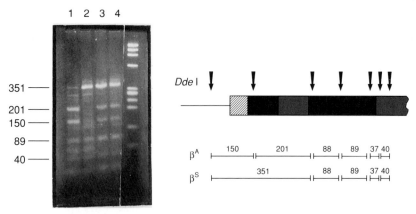

1 2 3 4

351 —
201 —
150 —
89 —
40 —

AA SS AS CVS

Dde I

β^A   150   201   88   89   37 40

β^S   351   88   89   37 40

Figure 80. **The diagnosis of sickle cell anaemia using the polymerase chain reaction.**
The region of DNA shown is generated by PCR and then treated with the enzyme *Dde* I. The absence of *Dde* I site due to the sickle cell mutation generates a larger fragment as shown. In this case a fetus was at risk for having sickle cell anaemia but the fetal DNA showed the pattern of the sickle cell trait.

The major advantage of this new approach is its simplicity; PCR can be carried out on lysed chorionic villus samples without prior extraction of DNA. The electrophoretic separation of the samples is no more complicated than ordinary haemoglobin electrophoresis. And, most importantly, the entire procedure can be completed in 3 to 4 hours.

As mentioned in Chapter 6, gene deletions underlie a number of single gene disorders and can be diagnosed by Southern blotting. For example it is easy to identify the different forms of α^+ thalassaemia and α° thalassaemia and the one common form of β thalassaemia that occurs in some Indian populations, all of which are due to major deletions of the α or β globin genes (Figs 81 and 82). The δβ thalassaemias, which result from major gene deletions, can also be detected in this way. Similarly, some of the haemoglobin disorders that result from major gene rearrangements with the production of fusion genes, the δβ gene of haemoglobin Lepore for example, are easily identified by gene mapping.

So far, prenatal diagnosis by direct demonstration of point mutations, deletions, or gene rearrangements has been restricted mainly to the haemoglobin disorders. However, as we saw in Chapter 6, several other single gene disorders result from deletions. These include hypoxanthine phosphoribosyl transferase deficiency (Lesch–Nyhan syndrome), growth hormone deficiency, ornithine transcarbamylase deficiency, haemophilia and Christmas disease, Duchenne muscular dystrophy, and cystic fibrosis. One of the difficulties in developing prenatal diagnosis programmes for single gene disorders is that many X-linked conditions are due to heterogeneous new mutations. For example, partial gene deletions account for about 50 per cent of cases of Duchenne muscular dystrophy (DMD), and approximately one-third of all cases of this condition result from a

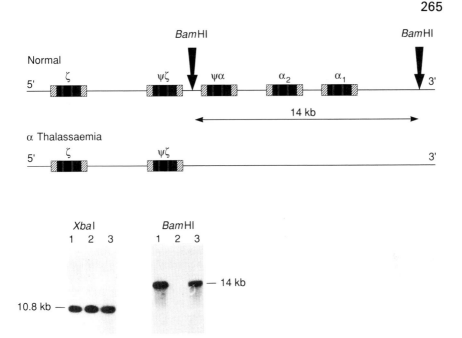

Figure 81. Gene mapping to demonstrate the loss of both α globin genes on chromosome 16. The diagram shows the normal arrangement of the α and ζ globin genes on chromosome 16 (described in detail on page 170). When normal DNA is digested with the enzyme *Bam* HI the α genes are found on a 14 kb fragment. Below is shown a chromosome 16 from an infant homozygous for a form of α thalassaemia in which both α genes are deleted. The gels show DNA digested with *Bam* HI and analysed with an α gene probe or digested with *Xba* I and analysed with a β probe. The right-hand gel shows normal DNA (i.e. normal α gene fragments) in lanes 1 and 3, and the absence of α fragments in the DNA from the infant in lane 2. (To ensure that the infant's DNA was otherwise normal, the filter was rehybridized with a β gene probe. The β genes are normally found on a 10.8 kb *Xba* I fragment. It is clear that the β gene pattern in the infant is normal, indicating that the absence of the α gene fragment is not an artefact due to unsatisfactory DNA preparation.)

new mutation. The gene for dystrophin, the site of the lesions that cause DMD, is very large and difficult to analyse by standard Southern blotting techniques. Although deletions can be demonstrated by pulsed field gel electrophoresis this approach has limited applicability to routine prenatal detection.

Quite recently an ingenious method has been developed for the rapid prenatal identification of deletions at the DMD locus which could easily be used for defining deletions at other loci (Fig. 83). Essentially, the idea is to use PCR to amplify multiple widely separated sequences and hence to permit deletion scanning of a hemizygous locus. For the identification of deletions in the DMD gene six oligonucleotide probes are prepared and tested against appropriately amplified regions of the DMD locus. This procedure, which takes about 5 hours, precludes the need for further analysis in about 40 per cent of samples. Cases in which deletions are not detected can be examined subsequently by standard

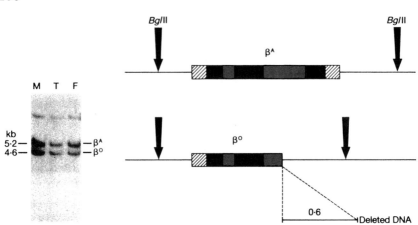

Figure 82. The intrauterine diagnosis of β⁰ thalassaemia resulting from a small deletion of the β globin gene. The 0.6 kb deletion shortens the distance between two *Bgl* II sites. Thus heterozygotes have two bands when their DNA is digested with this enzyme and analysed with a β gene probe, the longer from the normal chromosome and the shorter from the thalassaemia chromosome. In this case both parents (M, F) showed this pattern, as did DNA obtained by villus sampling (T). Thus the fetus must also be a heterozygote.

Southern blotting analysis using full-length DMD cDNAs subdivided into 7 to 9 separate probes, a process that takes 1 to 2 weeks. As further sequence data for the DMD locus are obtained it should be possible to extend the PCR screening procedure to cover an even higher proportion of deletions.

This new and ingenious application of PCR is applicable to any hemizygous locus susceptible to deletion. It will also be useful for detecting homozygous deletions of autosomal genes although, as currently applied, it will not detect all heterozygous deletions because of amplification from the non-deleted allele.

● Prenatal diagnosis using restriction fragment length polymorphisms (RFLPs)

In Chapter 5 we saw how the use of RFLP linkage analysis has been used to determine the chromosomal location of loci involved in single gene disorders. One of the beauties of this approach is that it is not necessary to know anything about the gene or its product and hence it is possible to define the chromosomal site of genes for conditions of completely unknown cause.

RFLP linkage has been used very successfully for prenatal diagnosis. Currently its main application is for single gene disorders of known cause in which there is considerable molecular heterogeneity, or for the detection of conditions of unknown cause in which the locus has been pin-pointed by linkage analysis. Although this method may be replaced once individual mutations have been defined and can be identified by oligonucleotide probes, as described in the

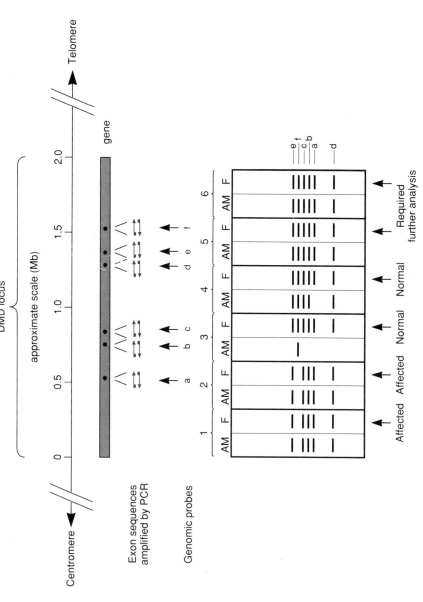

Figure 83. Scanning of the Duchenne muscular dystrophy (dystrophin) gene using different oligonucleotide probes for exons a–f. The gel shows the results from six families in which DNA from an affected male (AM) is compared with that of a potentially affected fetus (F). In families 1 and 2 there is a deletion involving region f. In family 3 the affected male is deleted for all regions except f while the fetus is normal. In family 4 the affected male is deleted for region a and the fetus is normal. In families 5 and 6 no deletion was detectable. Based on Chamberlain *et al.* (1988).

next section, it is likely to be a mainstay of many prenatal diagnosis programmes for the foreseeable future.

The principle of RFLP analysis for carrier or prenatal detection of genetic disease is very simple, and entails three steps. First an appropriate RFLP marker is chosen which is either within or closely linked to the disease locus and for which an individual at risk of transmitting the disease is heterozygous. Second, it is necessary to determine which of the marker alleles is on the chromosome carrying the disease allele; this involves the study of family members, ideally a previously affected or normal child. It is sometimes possible to solve this problem by examining the DNA of grandparents or other relatives. Finally, using the markers fetal DNA is examined to see whether the fetus has inherited the chromosome(s) carrying the gene(s) for a particular disease, or its normal allele. In dominant disorders the inheritance of one allele is all that is necessary to produce the abnormal phenotype; in the case of recessive conditions the fetus must have inherited markers from both parental chromosomes that carry the abnormal allele.

The various approaches to disease tracking using linked RFLPs are summarized in Table 33 and some of the diseases for which appropriate RFLP markers exist, and which can be identified prenatally using this approach, are summarized in Table 34. It is possible to use single linked markers, bridging markers, intragenic RFLPs or, because in some cases loci carrying mutations for a particular disorder are in strong linkage disequilibrium with a particular marker or markers, to identify disease-associated haplotypes.

Table 33. *Prenatal detection disease by RFLP linkage analysis*

Detection of linkage by individual family members
    Intragenic RFLP
    Linked RFLP
    Bridging markers
RFLP in strong linkage disequilibrium with mutation

Single linked RFLPs

The first prenatal diagnoses using single linked RFLP markers were carried out for the detection of the haemoglobin disorders. Figure 38 (page 109) shows the pattern of RFLPs in the β globin gene cluster. An example of the use of an RFLP for prenatal diagnosis of β thalassaemia utilizing one of these markers is shown in Fig. 84. By establishing that both parents are heterozygous for the RFLP, and by analysing the RFLP pattern of the marker in a previously affected sibling, it is possible to determine which of the parental chromosomes carries the β thalassaemia mutation and hence whether the fetus has inherited these chromosomes. Figure 39 (page 113) shows a similar approach to the prenatal

Table 34. *Some genetic diseases for which genomic probes or linked RFLPs are available for prenatal diagnosis**

Genomic probes and RFLPs
  α and β thalassaemia. Haemoglobinopathies
  Cystic fibrosis
  Growth hormone deficiency
  Antithrombin III deficiency
  Haemophilia A and B. von Willebrand's disease
  α_1 anti-antitrypsin deficiency
  Duchenne muscular dystrophy
  Phenylketonuria
  Lesch–Nyhan syndrome
  Retinoblastoma
  Monogenic hypercholesterolaemia
  Gaucher disease
  Chronic granulomatous disease

RFLPs†
  Huntington's disease
  Adult polycystic disease of the kidney
  Osteogenesis imperfecta (dominant form)
  Ornithine transcarbamylase deficiency
  Adrenoleucodystrophy
  Retinitis pigmentosa
  Neurofibromatosis. Types 1 and 2

---

*A more extensive list will be found in Antonarakis (1989).
†In some cases the genomic probes are available but reports on prenatal diagnosis to date have used RFLP linkage.

diagnosis of cystic fibrosis. Linked markers for which each parent is heterozygous were established; a sibling was used to find out which allele in each parent marked the chromosome carrying the cystic fibrosis mutation; and, finally, the fetus was examined to determine which parental chromosomes it had inherited.

It is possible to carry out exclusion testing for Huntington's disease, which has a dominant form of inheritance, using RFLPs. The offspring of an affected individual has a 1 in 2 chance of carrying the disease gene. Although symptoms do not usually appear until middle age some younger people wish to know whether they are affected because of the risk of passing the gene on to their own children. The exclusion of Huntington's disease using this approach is illustrated in Fig. 85.

Recently PCR has been applied to prenatal diagnosis using RFLPs. The principle is exactly the same as outlined in the previous paragraphs. In this case,

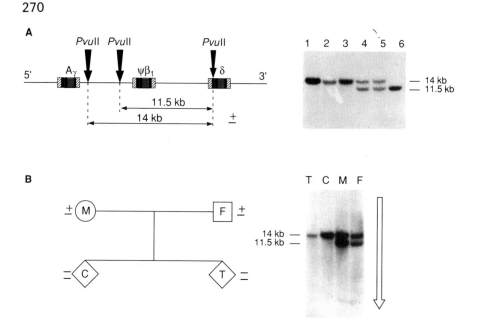

Figure 84. Prenatal diagnosis of β thalassaemia using an RFLP in the β globin gene cluster. A The site of a *Pvu* II polymorphism in the β globin gene cluster. Using a pseudo β1 gene probe either 14 kb or 11.5 kb *Pvu* II fragments are generated depending on the presence or absence of this polymorphic site. The bands which are generated on gene mapping are shown above. If the site is absent (−) only 14 kb bands are generated as shown in tracks 1, 2, and 3. Maps for heterozygous individuals, with both bands, are shown in tracks 4 and 5, and the map of an individual homozygous for this polymorphism, which shows only the 11.5 kb band, is shown in track 6. **B** Use of this polymorphism for prenatal diagnosis. The parents (M and F) were both heterozygous for this polymorphism, and a previousy born child (C) homozygous for β thalassaemia was found to have only the 14 kb band. Thus the β thalassaemia mutation must be on the chromosome which does not carry the polymorphism (− chromosome). In the next pregnancy trophoblast sampling was carried out and the fetal DNA analysed (T). Clearly this fetus was also homozygous for the β thalassaemia mutation.

however, the regions containing appropriate polymorphisms are amplified and it is possible to analyse the DNA directly by ethidium bromide staining of gels without the necessity of using radioactively labelled probes. An example of this approach for the prenatal detection of cystic fibrosis is shown in Fig. 86.

The major snag with prenatal detection of genetic disease using RFLP linkage is that it is always necessary to establish which chromosome carries the particular mutation by analysis of affected or normal siblings or other relatives. The other disadvantage, in cases in which the RFLPs are not within the particular gene, is recombination. Thus it is absolutely essential to determine recombination values for any linked RFLP which it is proposed to use for this purpose. We shall return to the practical aspects of crossovers as a source of error in prenatal diagnosis by DNA analysis later in this chapter.

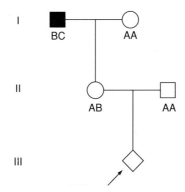

Figure 85. Prenatal detection of Huntington's disease. The fetus in the third generation is at risk. Because the disease is present in her father (I1) the mother has a 50 per cent risk of being affected. Different RFLP haplotypes designated A, B, C, and D have been identified for RFLPs close to the Huntington's locus (see text). The mother has inherited haplotype A from her unaffected parent and therefore haplotype B is associated with a 50 per cent risk. If the fetus types AB, then its risk of developing Huntington's will increase from 25 per cent to nearly 50 per cent. On the other hand if the fetus types AA its risk of inheriting Huntington's will decrease from 25 per cent to 2.5 per cent, allowing for the possibility of crossover. In carrying out this test the risk to the parent in generation 2 has not been altered. From Harper *et al.* (1988).

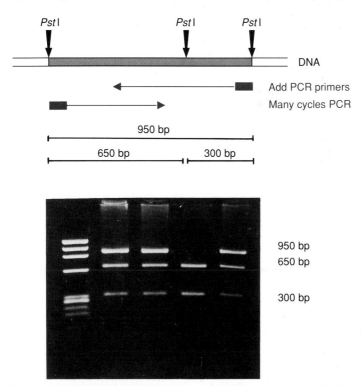

Figure 86. The use of the polymerase chain reaction for detection of RFLPs close to the cystic fibrosis gene. This polymorphism is detected by the enzyme *Pst* I; the different sized fragments are indicated.

Bridging markers

Another way of using RFLP markers is to find RFLPs that lie on either side of a particular disease locus. This has the advantage that only double recombinants will produce diagnostic errors. Hence it is particularly valuable in situations in which single RFLPs show appreciable recombination. It has been very useful for detecting Duchenne muscular dystrophy (DMD) (Fig. 87). The two particular markers used each show about 10 per cent recombination with the disease gene, so that the risk of double recombination is 1 per cent and hence it is possible to provide a 99 per cent probability of a correct diagnosis.

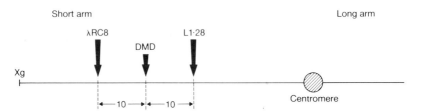

Figure 87. A representation of part of the X chromosome which contains the locus for Duchenne muscular dystrophy (DMD). Two RFLPs have been defined: each has a 10 per cent recombination frequency with DMD. However, when used in combination they can provide valuable information for carrier detection or prenatal diagnosis of DMD in appropriate cases.

Intragenic RFLPs

Because of the problems of recombination an ideal approach to RFLP linkage analysis is to use polymorphisms within the gene itself rather than close to it. Furthermore, the polymorphisms may be within introns and hence unrelated to the mutations that are responsible for the particular disease. Obviously if enough is known about the structure of a particular gene to reach this stage it may be better to construct specific oligonucleotide probes with which to detect the disease in carriers or in fetal life. However, where a genetic disorder is particularly heterogeneous, like β thalassaemia for example, the intragenic RFLP approach is still useful.

Linkage disequilibrium

The first description of the use of fetal DNA for a prenatal diagnosis followed the discovery that when normal DNA is digested with the enzyme *HpaI*, the β globin gene is located on a fragment approximately 7.6 kb long. However, if the same enzyme is used to cut the DNA of many American Blacks with sickle cell disease, the β globin gene is found on a longer fragment of approximately 13 kb. Thus it appears that the sickle mutation is on a chromosome which also carries an RFLP outside the coding area for the β globin gene (Fig. 88). The most likely

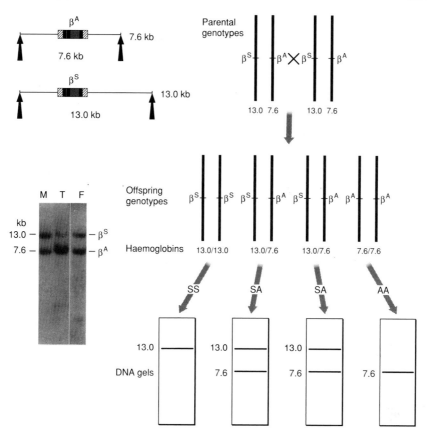

Figure 88. The prenatal diagnosis of sickle cell anaemia using an allele-linked restriction fragment length polymorphism. The gel shows a prenatal diagnosis using this approach with fetal DNA obtained by chorion villus sampling. The parents (M and F) and the fetus (T) are sickle-cell heterozygotes.

explanation is that, before the introduction of the sickle gene into west Africa, most individuals had the 7.6 kb type of β chromosome. There were probably a few 13 kb types in the population, however. Presumably the haemoglobin S mutation occurred on one of the latter chromosomes, which then achieved a high frequency by 'hitch-hiking' with the sickle cell gene as it came under strong selection. This type of RFLP linkage can be used for prenatal diagnosis as shown in Fig. 88. If fetal DNA has both 7.6 and 13 kb fragments, and if the sickle mutation is linked to the 13 kb RFLP in the particular family, the fetus must have the sickle cell trait; if it has only the 13 kb fragment it must be homozygous for the sickle cell mutation. This approach has been superseded by the development of more direct methods for identifying the sickle cell mutation. Furthermore it is now clear that the sickle cell mutation is not always linked to this particular RFLP, particularly in individuals of non-African origin.

Other examples of RFLPs in strong linkage disequilibrium with particular mutations have been found. For example the β thalassaemia determinant which is common in Sardinia is associated with a 9.3 kb *Bam*HI fragment, whereas the normal β globin gene in this population is contained within a 22 kb fragment. Furthermore, the β thalassaemia chromosome in Sardinia is nearly always linked to an *Ava*II polymorphism which is 16 bp 3′ to the 5′ splice junction of the second intervening sequence of the β globin gene, i.e. an intragenic RFLP.

The value of finding RFLPs in strong linkage disequilibrium to particular mutations was highlighted by the discovery of an *Ava*II polymorphism in the β globin gene cluster in Mediterranean populations. This site is absent in over 50 per cent of β thalassaemia chromosomes but in less than 4 per cent of normal chromosomes. This finding greatly increases the feasibility of prenatal diagnosis of β thalassaemia by RFLP analysis in these populations. For example, in Cypriots it increases the likelihood of being able to detect β thalassaemia in fetal life from about 30 to 70 per cent, and in Italian populations from 70 to nearly 100 per cent.

More recently, RFLP haplotypes associated with cystic fibrosis and phenyl-ketonuria have been found in North European populations although a different haplotype has been found in association with cystic fibrosis in Spain. It seems unlikely, however, that this phenomenon will be very common. It probably requires a particular set of circumstances; the original mutation must occur on a chromosome with the particular RFLP or group of RFLPs that forms a haplotype, it must then come under selection or be distributed among a population by a founder effect, and different mutations giving rise to the disease must not occur commonly in the particular population.

● Detection of mutations using oligonucleotide probes

The principles underlying the use of oligonucleotide probes for detecting single base changes in DNA were described in Chapter 4. Once the particular mutation that causes a disease has been defined it is usually possible to synthesize an appropriate oligonucleotide probe. This is the most direct approach to carrier detection and prenatal diagnosis (see Fig. 21, page 76). Oligonucleotide probes have been used successfully for the prenatal detection of sickle cell disease, several forms of β thalassaemia, α_1 antitrypsin deficiency, Lesch–Nyhan syndrome, and other conditions.

The development of PCR, combined with the use of oligonucleotide probes, offers a variety of new approaches for facilitating the speed and accuracy of carrier detection and prenatal diagnosis. As mentioned earlier, it is possible to amplify DNA from blood, amniotic fluid cells, or chorion villus material without previous purification, and to analyse some genetic disorders without the need for gene probes; if a particular mutation can be recognized directly with a restriction enzyme the fragments can be identified simply by ethidium bromide or silver staining of the gel. Point mutations can be identified directly using labelled oligonucleotide probes and amplified DNA. But perhaps the most important application of PCR in the long term is to enable us to do away with any form of electrophoresis or radioactively labelled gene probes.

As described in Chapter 4, considerable progress has been made towards the development of non-radioactive probes by the use of biotinylated nucleotides. The biotin incorporated into the probe can be coupled to avidin, and antibodies that identify the biotin/avidin complex can be raised and labelled in a variety of ways. Currently, these avidin-activated probes give a good though short-lived colorimetric signal. Thus it is becoming possible to identify single base changes by simple dot blot analysis. The amplified DNA is simply plated out into wells and probed with appropriate oligonucleotides labelled by a non-radioactive method. This method has been used to identfy the sickle cell mutation and several forms of β thalassaemia (see Fig. 34, page 97) and, particularly as it can be automated, may well be the way in which the prenatal diagnosis of single gene disorders will move in the future.

Another variation on this theme has been reported recently. Oligonucleotide homologues to normal or mutant DNA are labelled with fluorescein or rhodamine, respectively. After PCR, products with the normal sequence fluoresce green whereas those with the mutant sequence fluoresce red; heterozygous DNA is yellow! The results can be read by eye. Again the method could be automated.

● Current progress

It will be apparent from the previous sections that there have been remarkable technical advances in our ability to identify single gene disorders in fetal life by DNA analysis over the last few years. But results obtained in a research laboratory are one thing; how much progress has been made in the clinic? Because new methods are coming along so quickly there has been little opportunity to test them thoroughly in practice. Many centres that are running prenatal diagnosis programmes are finding that by the time they have mastered one technique it is already out of date! However, despite the rapidly changing technology enough information has been amassed to suggest that the first trimester prenatal diagnosis of single gene disorders is feasible and is here to stay.

● The genetic disorders of haemoglobin

The genetic disorders of haemoglobin, particularly sickle cell anaemia and the α and β thalassaemias, were the first conditions to which fetal DNA analysis was applied for carrier or prenatal detection. The first diagnoses relied on RFLP linkage analysis, and DNA obtained from amniotic fluid cells. The first successful prenatal diagnoses using DNA derived from CVS, and thus late in the first trimester, were reported in 1982. In 1986 we published our experience of over 200 first trimester prenatal diagnoses of haemoglobin disorders, including 133 cases at risk for β thalassaemia and 55 for sickle cell anaemia. Most of these analyses were carried out using RFLP linkage and a successful diagnosis was made in all but one case, an error due to plasmid contamination. This study included two sets of twins; a successful diagnosis was made on each of the pair.

With the introduction of synthetic oligonucleotide probes, and the elucidation of the mutations that underlie many forms of β thalassaemia, direct determination of the mutations in fetal DNA started to be applied in community programmes, notably in Sardinia. Quite recently the group in Sardinia have described their experience on 1000 prenatal diagnoses using oligonucleotide probes. Remarkably, there was only one failure, and no mis-diagnoses. Although these results are extremely encouraging it should be pointed out that the majority of patients in Sardinia have the same β thalassaemia mutation and therefore one pair of oligonucleotide probes is sufficient to run the programme.

In a country like Great Britain, where patients with β thalassaemia come from many different racial backgrounds, the provision of a comprehensive prenatal diagnosis programme poses rather more problems. Recently, we have analysed our experience of over 700 first trimester diagnoses. There were six failures and five mis-diagnoses. In this series a variety of techniques were used; sickle cell anaemia was usually identified using *Mst*II digestion, whereas the bulk of the β thalassaemias were diagnosed by RFLP linkage analysis. Preliminary studies in the United Kingdom had suggested that it would be possible to carry out prenatal diagnosis by RFLP linkage in approximately 80 per cent of the immigrant families. More recently both PCR and oligonucleotide probe technology have been introduced.

As mentioned in the previous section, it should soon be possible to identify the sickle cell mutation and the various β thalassaemia mutations by dot blot analysis using specific oligonucleotide probes. But because there are over 60 different β thalassaemia mutations, and since many potentially affected persons are compound heterozygotes for two different mutations, just how many oligonucleotide probes will be required and what will be the most efficient approach to setting up community programmes? Fortunately it turns out that the many different β thalassaemia mutations are not distributed at random across all populations. Rather, each population has a few very common mutations and a variable number of rare ones. It follows that for any particular population it should be possible to identify the bulk of the mutations with a few oligonucleotide probes, perhaps half a dozen. Once PCR becomes applied more widely it should be possible to determine the variety of β thalassaemia in each parent and then to use the appropriate oligonucleotide probes for prenatal diagnosis.

Another important factor in determining the strategy for developing prenatal diagnosis programmes using these new techniques, particularly PCR and specific oligonucleotide probes, is the marital practices of the population. For example, in Great Britain it has been found that in the Afro-Asian immigrants, in whom cousin marriages are the rule, homozygosity is particularly common. A pilot study has shown that, using about six oligonucleotide probes, it should be possible to provide a prenatal diagnosis service for over 90 per cent of this population. On the other hand, in populations in which consanguinity is less common, there will be a much higher proportion of compound heterozygotes in the seriously affected β thalassaemia population. In this case, although a few probes may cover a reasonable proportion of the population, it may be necessary to screen heterozygous parents with a large number of probes to identify fetuses that are at risk of inheriting one common and one rare β thalassaemia allele, or two rare alleles. It seems likely that RFLP linkage analysis will have to be kept as a back-up for prenatal diagnosis in these populations, at least for the forseeable future. The recent improvements in methods for the rapid detection of point mutations may make it feasible to define rare forms of β thalassaemia in parental DNA as part of the prenatal diagnosis screening programme. For the immediate future a comprehensive programme will require a diversity of techniques, including fetal blood sampling, if it is to be applicable to entire 'at risk' populations.

● Duchenne muscular dystrophy and other X-linked disorders

Duchenne muscular dystrophy is a common X-linked disorder, and because at least 30 per cent of cases represent new mutations, poses a challenging problem for prenatal diagnosis. Like every single gene disorder the techniques for the prenatal detection of DMD are changing rapidly with the acquisition of new knowledge about the molecular basis of the condition. Initially, RFLPs closely linked to the DMD locus were sought. Although these 'early' markers showed 10 per cent recombination with the disease gene, bridging markers, that is one mapping on either side of the disease locus, were discovered which when used in combination greatly improved the detection rate. Thus although the individual markers have a 10 per cent recombination frequency with the disease locus, risk of double-recombination, that is a crossover involving both markers, is only 1 per cent. As soon as the DMD locus was defined it became possible to find RFLPs within the gene itself; and the development of cDNA clones made it possible to start to identify deletions of the gene. As mentioned earlier, it has now been possible to prepare batteries of oligonucleotide probes against different regions of the DMD gene that are capable of detecting the majority of the deletions that affect it.

    Given these advances what is the current approach to carrier detection and prenatal diagnosis of DMD? Since about a third of all cases result from new mutations it would only be possible to develop a completely comprehensive programme by screening every birth. Although, as we shall see in a later chapter, this may become feasible, for the forseeable future we are likely to be dealing with families in which there has already been an affected child. Probably the most effective approach using current technology is to analyse DNA from the mother and affected child for the presence of a deletion, which will be found in approximately 50 per cent of cases. Initially, the most efficient approach is to use

PCR as outlined in a previous section. If this fails to show a deletion the DNA can be examined further by Southern analysis using full-length DMD cDNAs divided into about eight separate probes. If this does not demonstrate a deletion the DNA should be analysed for RFLPs with appropriate restriction enzymes to attempt to determine which of the maternal chromosomes carries the DMD mutation; prenatal diagnosis is then carried out by linkage analysis using either intragenic or closely linked markers.

It has been found recently that intron sequences in the DMD gene contain a high frequency of polymorphisms, many of which do not occur at restriction enzyme recognition sites. It is possible, therefore, that these polymorphisms can be detected by amplification of intron-containing sequences followed by hybridization with specific oligonucleotide probes. Indeed, PCR technology is advancing so rapidly that it may be possible to identify polymorphisms directly by the PCR amplification procedure. Thus future technological developments along these lines should permit the diagnosis of most cases of DMD, provided that appropriate family members are available. Even where facilities for this type of work do not exist at present, it is vitally important to store tissue from affected children for future diagnostic use.

Similar approaches can be used for other X-linked disorders. For example, considerable experience has been gained in the prenatal detection of haemophilia. As described in Chapter 4 this condition is also very heterogeneous at the molecular level and a proportion of cases result from new mutations, both deletions and point mutations. Carrier detection and prenatal diagnosis follow the same principles as outlined for DMD. Deletions or mutations that are detectable directly by restriction enzyme analysis can sometimes be defined in patients, and then identified in the mother and other family members. If a molecular lesion of this type is found in the mother it may be identified by fetal DNA analysis in future pregnancies. Both intragenic and flanking RFLPs have been identified for the factor VIII gene which, if appropriate family members are available, can be used to determine which of the maternal X chromosomes carries the mutation; this approach can be used in appropriate families for carrier detection or prenatal diagnosis.

● Cystic fibrosis

The first linkage between a polymorphic marker and the cystic fibrosis (CF) locus was with the serum protein, paraoxonase. This was followed by the demonstration of linkage to several DNA markers located on the long arm of chromosome 7. Further studies showed that the two closest markers, *Met* and D7S8, flank the CF locus and are each located from it a distance of approximately 1 centimorgan. It turned out that there is strong linkage disequilibrium between three RFLPs and CF, at least in North European populations. The findings suggested that the majority of cases of CF in these populations result from the same mutation.

Further markers in the region of the CF locus have been defined and used extensively for carrier testing and prenatal diagnosis. Currently it appears that the closest probes have a recombination fraction in the order of 0.1 cM. Like other parts of the genome there appears to be a clear-cut sex difference in recombination frequencies in this region of chromosome 7. This has to be considered when calculating genetic risks for families seeking prenatal diagnosis or carrier detection. As is the case for other single gene disorders, errors due to recombination can be reduced if it is possible to track the CF gene using flanking markers.

Now that the molecular pathology of cystic fibrosis is known (see Chapter 6) it should be possible to replace these linkage methods by direct detection of the mutation. Initial studies in the UK have shown that about 75 per cent of mutations in patients with CF are the same: the loss of phenylalanine at position 508 of the putative gene product. Earlier RFLP haplotype studies had suggested that a number of different mutations will be found in other populations. Preliminary screening has suggested that in Spain and Italy the position 508 mutation occurs in only 40–50 per cent of cases. Using an appropriate oligonucleotide probe it should be possible to screen parents for the position 508 mutation and to identify homozygotes in fetal DNA as a means of prenatal detection. Thereafter the field will develop in the same way as that described for thalassaemia. In some families we shall continue to use RFLP analysis, but as more mutations are identified it will be possible to carry out direct detection with specific oligonucleotide probes.

● Huntington's disease

Huntington's disease was one of the first conditions in which the genetic location of the determinant for a disorder of completely unknown aetiology was located using RFLPs. Huntington's disease is a severe neurodegenerative disorder that follows a typical autosomal dominant pattern of inheritance with a penetrance close to 100 per cent by old age but very low during the years of reproductive life. This is the reason why the condition presents so many distressing problems for affected families; individual members often do not know whether they have inherited the gene until they are approaching middle age, and hence whether they are likely to pass it on to their children.

Linkage studies using a variety of RFLPs have localized the HD gene to a site on the short arm of chromosome 4. The probe used to determine this linkage, G8, detects two invariant and several variable HindIII fragments. In fact it turns out that there are several polymorphic sites for this enzyme in relative close proximity to the HD locus so that the frequency of recombination between them is negligible, that is they are inherited together as a unit or haplotype. The particular haplotypes can be designated A, B, C, and D. In the first large family studies the A haplotype was associated with Huntington's disease while in the second family the association was with the C haplotype. More recently other RFLPs linked to the Huntington's locus have been defined.

The availability of tests for the likelihood of developing Huntington's disease raise many ethical difficulties. The problem arises in any family in which there is an affected individual. Have their offspring inherited the Huntington's gene and could their grandchildren be affected? Surveys of large numbers of patients with this condition suggest that about half of 'at risk' individuals wish for predictive testing for themselves. There are many different motives. In particular, they may wish to know whether they could transmit the disease to their children and, if this is the case, whether prenatal diagnosis could be attempted. Of course, for prenatal diagnosis to be carried out a family study must be done and therefore the likelihood of the particular 'at risk' parent being affected will be disclosed. Living with the knowledge that they are very likely to develop this crippling disease is a burden that many at-risk individuals, and their families, find intolerable.

An example of pregnancy exclusion testing for Huntington's disease is shown in Fig. 85 (page 271). In this family the mother in the second generation has a 50/50 chance of having Huntington's disease. It is clear that the HD locus must be linked to marker B if she is indeed affected. Thus if the fetus types AB the risk of it being affected would increase from 25 per cent to nearly 50 per cent. On the other hand, if the fetus types AA its risk of being affected will decrease from 25 per cent to 2.5 per cent, the latter figure allowing for the possibility of a crossover. This type of study does not 'alter' the parental risk.

Although RFLPs closer to the HD locus have now been found, the problem of recombination still exists and the unequivocal determination of whether an individual or a fetus is affected will await the determination of the molecular lesion(s).

● Other single gene disorders

Some of the other single gene disorders in which the carrier state can be identified and for which prenatal diagnosis can be carried out are summarized in Table 34. In some cases the mutation can be identified directly whereas in others RFLP linkage analysis is required. The feasibility of different approaches to prenatal diagnosis will rest ultimately on the heterogeneity of these conditions. For example, it turns out that the point mutation associated with phenylketonuria is associated with an RFLP haplotype that seems to be constant throughout many North European populations. This suggests that the condition is genetically homogeneous, at least in these populations. Thus carrier detection or prenatal diagnosis can be carried out simply by using an appropriate oligonucleotide probe or RFLP marker. On the other hand there is increasing evidence that other monogenic disorders such as growth hormone and anti-thrombin III deficiency are very heterogeneous at the molecular level. This will certainly be the case for all the important X-linked disorders.

There is another important problem relating to the heterogeneity of disease to consider when developing prenatal diagnosis programmes. As well as the fact that some monogenic disorders are due to different mutations at the *same* locus there is increasing evidence that in others the same clinical phenotype may result from mutations at completely *different* loci. Adult polycystic kidney disease is a good example. The genetic determinant for this condition was originally found to be close to the α globin gene cluster at the tip of the short arm of chromosome 16. Extensive studies of families with this condition from a variety of racial backgrounds suggested that the condition always mapped to this location. Subsequently, several probes were developed for which recombination was considerably less than the original 5 per cent figure obtained with a probe for the hypervariable region close to the α globin genes. Thus it appeared that we were dealing with a homogeneous genetic disease which always mapped to the short arm of chromosome 16. However, exceptions started to appear, and there have been well-documented reports of families in which it is clear that the genetic determinant for this condition is not on the short arm of chromosome 16.

These observations have important implications for developing prenatal diagnosis programmes. First, once a linkage has been established for a monogenic disorder it is very important to study many families from different racial backgrounds in order to establish homogeneity. Second, if heterogeneity is demonstrated it means that RFLP linkage analysis can only be used for prenatal diagnosis in families where it has been possible to establish quite unequivocally that the particular RFLP is linked to the disease locus. In the case of adult polycystic kidney disease it appears that lack of linkage to the α globin genes is rare, but even so it is not possible to use linkage analysis for carrier detection or prenatal diagnosis in this condition unless the appropriate linkage can be demonstrated in the individual family. More examples of this problem are likely to be uncovered.

● Sources of error

Prenatal diagnosis using fetal DNA analysis is open to a number of errors. Contamination of tissue obtained by chorion villus sampling (CVS) with maternal tissue may occur, particularly in the hands of inexperienced operators. This can usually be assessed during the initial dissection and washing of the tissue. In a recent analysis of several hundred CVS samples in the author's laboratory, in which maternal RFLPs were sought which should not have been present in the fetal DNA, it was found that less than 5 per cent of samples were contaminated, and even in those that were it was at a level which would have not interfered with analysis of the fetal DNA. However, extensive contamination can lead to mis-diagnoses. Non-paternity may also cause difficulties in prenatal diagnosis and it is becoming apparent that it will be necessary to carry out a paternity test by DNA fingerprinting as a routine part of fetal DNA analysis. There are also a number of technical problems in the actual analysis of DNA in the laboratory which may give rise to errors, notably difficulty with DNA digestion and plasmid contamination.

The most difficult problem with RFLP linkage analysis for prenatal diagnosis is recombination. The value of using flanking markers and the importance of including sex difference in recombination into an analysis of the risk in any particular family was alluded to earlier in this chapter. Similarly, it was pointed out in the section on the haemoglobin disorders that there is a 'hot spot' for recombination within the β globin genes; ideally RFLPs that are downstream from the β globin gene and hence on the same side of the genes as the recombinational 'hot spot' should be used for diagnostic purposes. Unfortunately, however, the most valuable RFLPs are upstream from the 'hot spot' in the β globin genes (see Fig. 38, page 109), that is they are separated from the gene by a region of frequent recombination. Therefore there is approximately a 1 in 500 chance of recombination between these loci and a mutant β globin gene. Undoubtedly similar 'hot spots' for recombination will turn up in other parts of the genome.

● The future

● Bringing DNA diagnosis into day-to-day clinical practice

As more loci for single gene disorders are assigned, the underlying mutations determined, and RFLPs established, carrier and prenatal detection of monogenic disorders will become increasingly available. Enough is already known to suggest that CVS is likely to be safe and acceptable and that the techniques of fetal DNA analysis work in practice. As PCR becomes routine, and non-radioactive labelling techniques more reliable, it should be possible to simplfy the detection of point mutations so that most of them can be diagnosed by dot blot analysis. Even for conditions as heterogeneous as β thalassaemia it may be possible to use this approach for the majority of cases, retaining either RFLP linkage or rapid sequence analysis for the rare mutations. It seems likely that many, if not all, the steps involved will be automated.

For the immediate future it seems unlikely that we shall embark on widespread screening programmes for single gene disorders unless they are very common; cystic fibrosis and β thalassaemia in appropriate populations, for example. Whether more widespread screening with a battery of probes will become a routine part of prenatal care remains to be seen.

How then are we to transfer these sophisticated techniques into day-to-day clinical practice? Before we do there is no doubt that, in these days of the application of market-place economy to health care, the first question that will be asked is whether the cost of any of the potential applications is justified at all. Here we are in difficulty straight away. There have been very few adequate cost–benefit analyses carried out with respect to the carrier detection and prenatal diagnosis of major chromosome abnormalities or monogenic disorders. In other words we have very little idea about the relative costs of screening and prenatal detection compared with that of allowing affected children to be born and looked after in the community for many years. Early studies that tried to assess these questions in the case of Down syndrome came up with rather equivocal answers. A more recent pilot study of our own, which attempted to assess the costs of running a DNA diagnosis service compared with that of maintaining β thalassaemic children in the community, suggested that the prenatal diagnosis programme was extremely cost-effective. We know even less about the presumed beneficial effects of allowing families at high risk for having children with serious genetic disorders the possibility of having normal children. Similarly, there have been few studies of the long-term psychological effects that may follow a termination of pregnancy for disease of this kind.

Given this level of ignorance about the basic economics and pastoral aspects of prenatal detection of disease what should we advise those who administer our health services? First, it is clear that carrier detection and prenatal diagnosis of monogenic disease is effective and will become increasingly available over the next few years. It is essential that pilot studies are carried out by competent centres to monitor the costs and efficiency of these programmes. Just as there have been enormous pressures by immigrant populations for screening for the haemoglobin disorders, it seems likely that now that the molecular basis of cystic fibrosis has been determined there will be considerable enthusiasm for incorporating screening tests for this disease into antenatal care programmes. Thus it is going to be very important to try to work out the costs of integrating screening of this type into our present antenatal care services and hence to work out our priorities for preventative genetics.

A reasonable working approach, given our current state of knowledge, might be along the following lines. There is little doubt that within a year or two we will be able to identify many monogenic diseases in pregnant women by the use of PCR and dot blot analysis which may well be automated for routine screening. Initially, these methods should be used only for common diseases in particular communities, cystic fibrosis and β thalassaemia for example. In this context it will be important to continue to look for cheaper biochemical tests for screening for these conditions. The haemoglobinopathies are a prime example. Most of them can be identified in heterozygotes from data that are derived from a standard haematological work-up in the antenatal clinic; only abnormal blood counts need be followed up by DNA screening. Provided that adequate counselling services can be developed it should be possible to move quickly towards prenatal detection of these common diseases in the community. As for the less common monogenic disorders it seems likely that their prenatal detection will be restricted to families in which there is already a history of an affected child. As automated dot blot technology becomes simpler and cheaper it may be possible to expand the number of monogenic diseases that can be screened for in the antenatal clinic.

These developments depend, of course, on a well-informed population. For chorion villus sampling to be effective women will have to be educated to present early in pregnancy. It will be essential for them to know precisely for what they are being screened and for them to decide whether they want to be part of the programme. In many countries excellent screening programmes are already established and DNA technology can be easily incorporated into them; but if this is to succeed it is absolutely essential that some solid cost-benefit analyses are set up. These are never easy and because of the rapidly changing and developing technology of DNA analysis the question of when to embark on such analyses could pose difficulties, especially at the present time. This makes it even more important that adequate data collection and costing should be incorporated into pilot programmes.

● Future technical advances

Another technical advance that seems to be 'just round the corner' is the possibility of combining *in vitro* fertilization with prenatal diagnosis of genetic disease (Fig. 89). Here the idea would be to obtain a number of fertilized ova and analyse them for a particular genetic disease before replacing one of the unaffected ova into the uterus. Couples with a 1 in 4 or 1 in 2 chance of producing a baby with a serious genetic disorder might prefer this approach, particularly if they find abortion unacceptable. Furthermore, many women who are undergoing *in vitro* fertilization for infertility are in an older age-group, when Down

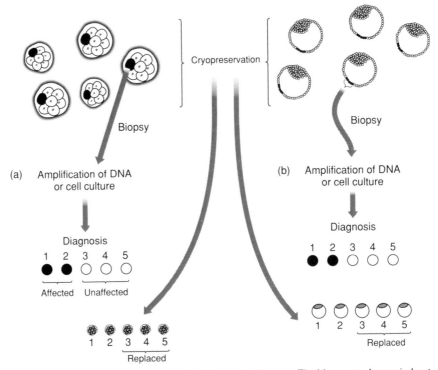

Figure 89. Pre-implantation diagnosis of genetic disease. The biopsy can be carried out either at the 8-cell or blastocyst state. In either case the eggs would be frozen and the diagnosis carried out by PCR.

syndrome becomes a significant problem. Women who have had repeated prenatal diagnoses and who have been unfortunate enough to have a series of affected fetuses become disheartened; the possibility of *in vitro* fertilization with reimplantation of an unaffected pre-embryo offers a more certain way of producing a normal child.

The advent of PCR together with the development of methods for biopsying pre-embryos raises the possibility that it will be possible to combine IVF with detection of genetic disease. Since it is now possible to amplify DNA from a single cell for genetic diagnosis the major technical problem is how safely to biopsy the pre-embryo.

After fertilization the egg divides repeatedly to give two, four, eight, and so on, cells. Animal experiments have shown that all eight cells are equivalent to one another so that if one or two are removed or destroyed the numbers can be reconstituted by further cell divisions, and normal young are born. A few cell divisions later the outer layer of cells changes in appearance; eventually it will go on to form part of the placenta. At this stage fluid accumulates in the centre of the fertilized egg. This stage of development is called a blastocyst. Implantation of the blastocyst in the wall of the uterus begins about a week after fertilization. By the end of 2 weeks most of the tissues derived from the fertilized egg have specialized to form the life-support systems that will form the future placenta. A small group of unspecialized cells in the central embryonic plate accumulate around a groove called the primitive streak and begin to form the outlines of the embryo which, over the next few weeks, will gradually acquire a head and tail, a nervous system and heart, and so on. In addition to the 8-cell stage it is also technically possible to obtain a few cells from the outer layer of the blastocyst, the trophectoderm.

There are two general approaches to pre-implantation diagnosis (Fig. 89). First, the eggs could be recovered from the woman's ovaries, fertilized *in vitro*, and allowed to develop to the 8- or 16-cell stage for a biopsy of one or two cells. Second, the woman could have normal intercourse with her partner so that fertilization would take place *in vivo*. A few days later the resulting blastocysts could be washed out of her uterus and then biopsied; at this stage it would be possible to obtain 5–10 cells for biopsy because the blastocyte would contain about 100 cells. In either case the eggs would be frozen while the genetic analyses were being carried out.

How would this work in practice? First, the woman's ovaries would be stimulated to produce more eggs than one by a hormone injection. After this there would be a clinic visit to recover the eggs. If the second option had been chosen, washing the blastocysts out of the uterus, no anaesthetic would be required. After the diagnostic tests the one or two of the conceptuses now known to be unaffected would be thawed and replaced in the uterus, on a second clinic visit. If she did not become pregnant this procedure could be repeated later.

Obviously this novel approach to the detection of genetic disease requires extensive study to determine the safety of pre-implantation biopsy and to ensure that the production of human chorionic gonadotrophin, the hormone required for implantation, is not depressed after blastocyst biopsy.

At first sight all this sounds rather unlikely and, even if it is technically feasible, it smacks of a further intrusion of technology into the natural processes of reproduction. However, if it does become possible it may be much more acceptable than current prenatal diagnosis practices for many couples. After all, replacement of a fertilized egg that has been shown to be clear of a particular genetic disease means that the couple can embark on a completely normal pregnancy without the prospect of abortion, early or late.

There is no doubt that this area of human genetic research will be actively pursued over the next few years. Because of the technical difficulties involved its use may always be restricted to couples with particular reproductive problems or who, for one reason or another, find more conventional forms of prenatal detection distasteful. But we already have sufficient information about the value of DNA technology for the avoidance of monogenic disease to suggest that prenatal diagnosis will remain the centrepoint of preventative genetics, at least until gene therapy becomes developed to the stage where it can be widely applied for the correction of these conditions.

● Further reading

Antonarakis, S.E. (1989). Diagnosis of genetic disorders at the DNA level. *New Engl. J. Med.*, **320**, 153–63.

Ballabio, A., Gibbs, R.A., and Caskey, C.T. (1990). PCR test for cystic fibrosis deletion. *Nature*, **343**, 220.

Canadian Collaborative CVS-Amniocentesis Clinical Trial Group (1989). Multicentre randomised clinical trial of chorion villus sampling and amniocentesis. *Lancet*, **i**, 1–6.

Chamberlain, J.S., Gibbs, R.A., Ranier, J.E., Nguyen, P.N., and Caskey, C.T. (1988). Deletion screening of the Duchenne muscular dystrophy locus via multiplex DNA amplification. *Nucl. Acids Res.*, **16**, 11141–56.

Chehab, F.F., Doherty, M., Cai, S.P., Kan, Y.W., Cooper, S., and Rubin, E.M. (1987). Detection of sickle cell anaemia and thalassaemias. *Nature*, **329**, 293–4.

Chehab, F.F. and Kan, Y.W. (1990). Detection of sickle cell anaemia mutation by colour DNA amplification. *Lancet*, **335**, 15–17.

Cooper, D.N. and Schmidtke, J. (1986). Diagnosis of genetic disease using recombinant DNA. *Hum. Genet.*, **73**, 1–11.

Crawfurd, M.d'A. (1988). Prenatal diagnosis of common genetic disorders. *Br. Med. J.*, **297**, 502–6.

Galjaard, H. (1987). Worldwide experience with first-trimester fetal diagnoses by molecular analysis. In *Human genetics*, (ed. F. Vogel and K. Sperling), pp. 611–21. Springer-Verlag, Berlin.

Handyside, A.H., Pattinson, J.K., Penketh, R.J.A., Delhanty, J.D.A., Winston, R.M.L., and Tuddenham, E.G.D. (1989). Biopsy of human preimplantation embryos and sexing by DNA amplification. *Lancet*, **i**, 347–9.

Handyside, A.M., Kontogianni, E.M., Hardy, K., and Winston, R.M.L. (1990). Pregnancies from biopsied human preimplantation embryos sexed by γ-specific DNA amplification. *Nature*, **344**, 768–70.

Harper, P.S., Quarrell, O.W.J., and Youngman, S. (1988). Huntington's disease: Prediction and prevention. *Phil. Trans. R. Soc. Lond. B.*, **319**, 285–98.

Kerem, B-S., Rommens, J.M., Buchanan, J.A., Markiewicz, D., Cox, T.K., Chakravarti, A., Buchwald, M., and Tsui, L.-C. (1989). Identification of the cystic fibrosis gene. *Science*, **245**, 1073–80.

Kogan, S.C., Doherty, M., and Gitschier, J. (1987). An improved method for prenatal diagnosis of genetic diseases by analysis of amplified DNA sequences. *New Engl. J. Med.*, **317**, 985–90.

Lancet (1990). Cystic fibrosis: prospects for screening and therapy. **335**, 79–80.

McLaren, A. (1987). Can we diagnose genetic disease in pre-embryos? *New Scientist*, **116**, 42–7.

Meredith, A.L., Upadhyaya, M., and Harper, P.S. (1988). Molecular genetics in clinical practice: evolution of a DNA diagnostic service. *Br. Med. J.*, **297**, 843–6.

Miles, J.H. and Kaback, M. (1978). Prenatal diagnosis of hereditary disease. *Pediat. Clin. N. America*, **25**, 593–618.

Old, J.M., Thein, S.L., Weatherall, D.J., Cao, A., and Loukopoulos, D. (1989). Prenatal diagnosis of the major haemoglobin disorders. *Mol. Biol. Med.*, **6**, 55–63.

Prenatal Diagnosis and Genetic Screening (1989). Report of the Royal College of Physicians, London.

Rhoads, G.G., *et al.* (1989). The safety and efficacy of chorionic villus sampling for early prenatal diagnosis of cytogenetic abnormalities. *New Engl. J. Med.*, **320**, 609–17.

Saiki, R.K., Chang, C.-A., Levenson, C.H., Warren, T.C., Boehm, C.D., Kazazian, H.H., and Erlich, H.A. (1988). Diagnosis of sickle cell anemia and β-thalassemia with enzymatically amplified DNA and nonradioactive allele-specific oligonucleotide probes. *New Engl. J. Med.*, **319**, 537–41.

Weatherall, D.J. (1985). Prenatal diagnosis of inherited blood diseases. *Clin. Haematol.*, **14**, 747–74.

Weatherall, D.J., Old, J.M., Thein, S.L., and Wainscoat, J.S. (1988). The role of cloned genes in the prevention of genetic disease. *Phil. Trans. R. Soc. Lond. B.*, **319**, 249–61.

Gene therapy

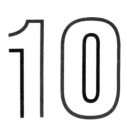

Since it is now possible to isolate human genes it should be feasible, at least in theory, to replace defective genes and hence to cure genetic diseases. Before discussing this important problem it is worth considering the more conventional methods that are currently available for the treatment of these disorders. The reader can then decide whether it is justifiable to meddle with our genomes in this way.

● Current methods for treatment of genetic disease

Very few genetic diseases can be cured. Certain congenital abnormalities can be fully corrected by surgery. However, for the majority of conditions there is no form of treatment other than symptomatic. There are many varieties of symptomatic treatment for genetic diseases, which vary in expense for the health services and discomfort for patients. Examples include replacement therapy for the missing coagulation factor in haemophilia, long-term transfusion therapy for thalassaemia, replacement with immunoglobulin for children with inherited forms of hypogammaglobulinaemia, growth hormone therapy for some forms of genetic dwarfism, and so on. Such treatment is costly and may be only partly successful. Granted, life for a haemophiliac child has been revolutionized by the use of factor VIII concentrate which can be given at home, but this treatment is particularly expensive and is still not without the risk of causing liver damage due to virus hepatitis. Furthermore, the recent appearance on the scene of the acquired immune deficiency syndrome (AIDS) has caused concern about the dangers of repeated administration of blood products. Some of these problems may be overcome when it becomes possible to make these missing factors in bacteria using recombinant DNA technology.

Thalassaemic children, many of whom can be kept alive only by regular blood transfusion, grow and develop normally only to die in the second or third decades from the effects of iron-loading derived from the transfused blood. This is a particularly distressing problem because the children are often extremely well for the first 10 or 15 years of their lives, during which time both they and their parents live under the continual cloud of the knowledge that they are likely to die before they reach the age of 20. Recently, some of these problems have been overcome to some extent by the introduction of methods for removing the iron that accumulates as the consequence of transfusion, but these are painful, time-consuming, and expensive. Generally speaking, a life of continuous replacement therapy for a genetic disease is extremely difficult for both patients and their families.

It is possible to correct the defect that underlies some genetic diseases by designing diets that prevent the accumulation of toxic metabolites. Phenylketonuria is a good example, and requires strict adherence to the diet throughout childhood and hence close surveillance by the patients' parents and physicians. Pregnant women who have phenylketonuria, and who do not stick to their diet, are liable to have infants with intrauterine growth retardation, microcephaly, and various congenital abnormalities. Other genetic metabolic disorders that have been treated by dietary modification with variable success include galactosaemia, fructose intolerance, and inborn errors of essential amino acid metabolism, e.g. maple syrup urine disease. Dietary restriction is not effective when the particular toxic substance is produced endogenously. For example, ammonium produced by the breakdown of nitrogenous compounds is normally eliminated via the urea cycle, a complex pathway involving a number of enzymes, each of which may be genetically defective. Disorders of this pathway were first treated by limitation of nitrogen intake but the results were disappointing. More recently, attempts have been made to provide alternative metabolic pathways for ammonium metabolism.

Efforts have been made to replace missing enzymes in metabolic disorders in which a specific deficiency has been demonstrated. Much of this work has been directed at correcting some of the storage diseases, Gaucher's disease for example. The missing enzymes have been delivered by intravenous infusion, packaged in liposomes, or dispatched directly to the reticuloendothelial system in a variety of other ingenious ways, including the use of red cell ghosts. The results have been extremely disappointing. Thus, while it is sometimes possible to correct enzyme deficiencies in tissue culture, or even in experimental animals, this approach has not yet been successful when applied to patients.

More recently, attempts have been made to correct genetic blood diseases or metabolic disorders by bone marrow transplantation. The idea is to completely eradicate the patient's bone marrow, including the stem cells, and to replace it with HLA identical marrow. Ideally, this is obtained from a sibling; there is a 1 in 4 chance that any sibling will be compatible. Though non-related donor transplants have been carried out, this procedure is still at an early stage of development and so far is not very successful. Even when a sibling of appropriate HLA type is available, there may be difficulties with bone marrow transplantation. The marrow may be rejected, but even worse the donor lymphocytes may cause what is called a 'graft-versus-host' reaction which may lead to an illness ranging from an acute fever with skin rashes and diarrhoea to a chronic disorder resembling scleroderma. Based on the observation that graft-versus-host disease is very uncommon if transplantation is carried out early in life, recent work in this field has been directed to correction of genetic diseases as soon as possible after birth.

The general principles of marrow transplantation in the context of genetic disease are that the error should be expressed by the stem cells of the marrow, that the donor marrow will produce the missing component in the host, that in the case of an enzyme deficiency the missing enzyme will be spilled into tissue spaces or delivered cell-to-cell and gain entry into cells by pinocytosis, and that the recipient must be tolerant to the missing component. Marrow transplantation has been used successfully to treat thalassaemia and a number of genetic disorders of lymphocyte function, in particular severe combined immunodeficiency. It has also been used to correct genetic disorders of phagocyte function and a number of inborn errors, particularly the lysosomal storage diseases. Lysosomes are subcellular cytoplasmic particles that contain hydrolytic enzymes. As described in Chapter 6 the latter are involved in the breakdown of complex molecules derived either from macromolecules entering cells by endocytosis, or from within the cell itself. These diseases are due to inborn errors of metabolism affecting specific lysosomal enzymes so that either undegraded or partially degraded macromolecules accumulate in lysosomes. Nearly 50 genetic disorders have been treated by bone marrow transplantation with varying success. A partial list of these conditions is shown in Table 35.

How successful is the symptomatic treatment of genetic disease? In 1985 a joint research programme was developed between McGill and Johns Hopkins Universities. Altogether 351 monogenic disorders were assembled and the effects of treatment were assessed on three variables: lifespan, reproductive capability, and social adaptation. They found that such therapy as is available produced a normal lifespan in 15 per cent of the conditions, allowed reproduction in 11 per cent, and social adaptation in only 6 per cent. Even in diseases that were well

Table 35. *Some genetic disorders which have been corrected by marrow transplantation*

Lymphocyte function
    X linked severe combined immunodeficiency (SCID)
    Swiss type SCID
    Adenine-deaminase deficiency
    Wiskott–Aldridge syndrome

Red cell
    β thalassaemia
    Sickle cell anaemia

Storage disorders
    Hurler's disease
    Gaucher's disease (types I and III)
    Metachromic leukodystrophy

Other
    Osteopetrosis

understood the results were not much more encouraging. In summarizing their study the group reported that treatment was only completely successful in 8 diseases (12 per cent of the total), moderately effective in another 26 (40 per cent), and completely useless in the remainder (48 per cent). It is clear that our current ability to treat inherited diseases is very limited. It is not surprising, therefore, that thoughts have turned to the possibility of gene replacement therapy.

● Gene replacement or corrective therapy

The replacement of defective genes, or forms of corrective manipulation of genetic defects, must be a major goal in the application of genetic engineering technology to human disease. It is now possible to isolate genes together with their flanking regions which contain at least some of the important regulatory sequences. It is not difficult to insert these genes into foreign cells; the surgery of gene replacement therapy is feasible, at least in the test-tube. We shall examine briefly some of the problems involved and the approaches that are being investigated to overcome them.

Before discussing the different approaches to gene therapy we should be clear about what we are trying to achieve. In replacement therapy we would try to insert a defective gene somewhere in the genome so that its product could replace that of a defective gene. This approach would be most suitable for recessive disorders where, in the homozygous or compound heterozygous state, there is a deficiency of an enzyme or other proteins. Theoretically it would not matter where our gene was functioning in the genome provided that we gave it the appropriate regulatory sequences to that it would be expressed in the right issues. Clearly this would not be a useful approach to treating dominant disorders associated with the production of an abnormal gene product which interfered with the product of a normal gene. Corrective gene therapy, on the other hand, would require that we somehow replaced a mutant gene or part of it with a normal sequence. This could only be done by some form of induced recombination events. Another form of corrective therapy would be the suppression of a particular mutation by a transfer RNA that was introduced into a cell. Finally, we might try to bypass a particular mutant gene by stimulating the production of a similar gene that was normally functional at a different developmental stage.

● The problems of gene replacement therapy

Since so much is known about the haemoglobin genes and their disorders, we shall examine the problems that might be encountered in attempting to correct a single gene disorder like β thalassaemia. The object would be to replace the product of a defective or missing β globin gene with that of a normal β gene.

What is our target cell for insertion of the normal gene? Nearly all the recognizable blood cell precursors that haematologists can identify in the bone marrow are already terminally differentiated, that is they will go through cycles of division and maturation to form mature red cells, white cells, and platelets which will survive in the circulation for a limited time before they are destroyed. It follows that to cure a genetic blood disease like thalassaemia a 'good' gene must be inserted into haemopoietic stem cells, the self-sustaining cell population from which are derived all the formed elements of the blood, red cells, white cells, and platelets. This approach presents some serious difficulties. First, we can't identify human stem cells; they can only be assayed in murine systems which are not suitable for human experimentation. At best we can make semi-educated guesses about how many there are in a volume of bone marrow and hence the number of cells into which we might be able to introduce our globin genes. Furthermore, until very recently methods for introducing foreign DNA into cells were highly inefficient and thus we could only introduce our gene into a very small proportion of stem cells. For example, it seems likely that there is 1 stem cell for every 1000 to 10 000 human bone marrow cells; even this may be an optimistic guess. Using the standard calcium microprecipitation method for gene transfer (see below) we would need 10^9 marrow cells to transfer one new gene into one stem cell. As we shall see later, the development of more efficient methods of transferring foreign genes into cells may solve this particular problem.

If we have only been able to introduce our gene into a proportion of stem cells, there is no reason why these particular cells should flourish at the expense of the remainder. Certainly, if β gene function improved in the erythroid cells to which the treated stem cells gave rise, these progeny cells would be at a selective advantage; but selection would not occur at the *stem cell* level. In fact the stem cells containing a 'foreign' gene might be disadvantaged. Thus as well as our globin gene we might have to introduce another gene or genes giving a proliferative advantage to the cells into which they were placed. A less attractive alternative would be to ablate the bulk of the stem cells, that is, after taking a marrow sample for insertion of the new genes, to pretreat our patients in the same way as before a marrow transplant.

There are other problems that we may have to face given our rather primitive knowledge about the properties of haemopoietic stem cells. From such data as are available it appears that, certainly in adults, the bulk of the stem cell population is out of cycle at any one time; the cells are resting rather than actively dividing. Since, as we shall see later, most of the methods that have been developed for inserting genes into cells require that they are in the active stages of the cell cycle this may make it even more difficult to correct the defect in a useful number of stem cells. Furthermore, if these cells are moving in and out of the cell division cycle it could be that a proportion of the cells into which we have successfully transferred our gene will then move out of cycle and hence our gene product will not be expressed in the blood of our recipient. Or it may be expressed intermittently as the transfected stem cells move in and out of the phases of the cycle.

Would the 'new' genes function properly in recipient cells? It is known that genes introduced into foreign cells can become integrated into the genome and that they may function, albeit inefficiently. We shall return later to the experimental evidence for these observations. In fact there is no *a priori* reason why genes that have been inserted into stem cells would not function in the progeny cells, but the really important question is whether they will come under the same control as their normal counterparts in these populations. Unfortunately, nothing is known about the differentiation step whereby a stem cell produces a daughter cell which will then enter the red cell, white cell, or platelet 'compartments' of the marrow. During normal haemopoiesis the globin genes remain 'switched off' in the white cell and platelet precursors. Since we have no idea how this type of regulation and differentiation occurs, we have no guarantee that our inserted genes will behave themselves in this way. The repeated commitment and differentiation steps may themselves interfere with the function of the foreign gene. It is quite possible, for example, that the white cell precursors derived from stem cells containing the foreign globin gene could synthesize globin chains; so might the megakaryocytes. Would this matter? Any unusual protein in a white cell might be immediately degraded and digested; thus it might not matter if the globin genes are expressed although it is difficult to be sure what effect this might have on white cell function. The effect of haemoglobin production in megakaryocytes or platelets is anybody's guess. These particular problems could be overcome if we knew more about the DNA sequences involved in the tissue specificity of gene expression. As we shall see later, there has been some recent progress in this area.

If by some lucky chance the haemoglobin genes came under normal regulation they might be activated at the appropriate stage of erythroid cell maturation. If, on the other hand, haemoglobin synthesis was prematurely switched on, and there was asynchronous production of α and β chains, this would produce an excess of one type of globin chain. An excess of β globin chains in early red cell precursors might well lead to their premature destruction; in effect we might convert β to α thalassaemia! In addition, we are asking a great deal of our inserted genes; to correct a homozygous thalassaemic defect a single β gene would have to produce 20 pg of β chains, or more. This is at least twice the amount of normal gene product; at best we might have to settle for the conversion of a homozygous to a heterozygous phenotype.

Another major worry about transferring genes into foreign cells is the safety of the procedure. Since many of the methods that are used for gene transfer are unable to determine where the inserted gene ends up in the recipient genome there are obvious possibilities for accidents to occur. For example, our inserted gene might land in a site that interferes with the function of a gene that is critical for the normal function and survival of a particular cell population. Even more worrying is the possibility that the 'new' gene might activate an oncogene and give rise to a neoplastic change in a particular cell population. These possibilities, though unlikely given the size of the human genome, suggest that it would be desirable to develop a way of inserting our gene so that we had at least some idea of where it was going. Finally, it is possible that in the case of the globin genes, and other gene families, regulation may not be restricted to individual genes but may require an intact gene complex. This would raise several problems for replacement therapy, particularly if the size of the complex is large; for example, it might lead to the duplication of other genes in the complex.

It is possible, of course, that in selecting globin as our model for discussing gene replacement therapy we have picked a particularly daunting problem. Perhaps it might be better to concentrate first on the replacement of genes that do not require such tight regulation, either in terms of the tissues in which they are expressed or in their level of expression. For example, there are a number of diseases due to deficiencies of so-called 'housekeeping' genes, i.e. genes that are expressed at a relatively low level in most cells; and, of course, we might pick a less specialized and more accessible target cell than the haemopoietic stem cell. Fibroblasts, for example, undergo little differentiation or specialization as they divide and it might be easier to start with a less demanding cell population of this type. On the other hand the very specialized nature of the globin system has certain advantages. If we consider the problem of replacing the defective gene in a disorder like cystic fibrosis, which must be expressed in several tissues including the lungs and pancreas, the problems become even more daunting.

Over the last few years the focus of research into gene therapy has shifted on a number of occasions, mainly because of the problems outlined in the previous sections. Globin was the first target, but more recently much work has been directed towards the transfer of housekeeping genes. Quite recently the field has gone full circle and globin is again a major candidate because of discoveries about important regulatory regions around its genes. In the sections that follow we will examine the current state of research into gene therapy and see how some of these problems are being tackled.

● Pre-requisites for human gene therapy

It is essential that several prerequisites are fulfilled before patients are subjected to gene therapy. First, in order to fully counsel a prospective patient or their family it must be possible to give an accurate account of the clinical course of the illness and its response to more conventional therapy; genetic diseases vary widely in their severity and even when the underlying molecular lesions are understood the reasons for this clinical variability often remain unexplained. Second, it must be possible to isolate the appropriate gene and to define, at least in outline, its major regulatory regions. Third, we have to identify and harvest appropriate target cells and develop safe and efficient vectors with which to introduce our new gene. Finally, there must be clear evidence from extensive animal experiments that our inserted gene will function adequately, that the recipient cell population will have a reasonably long lifespan, and that the gene that we have inserted will produce no deleterious effects in its new home.

● Somatic versus germ cell gene transfer

There are two main approaches to gene therapy. First, genes may be inserted into somatic cells, that is any body cell other than a germ cell. This method raises no major ethical issues because it is essentially the same as organ transplantation; any changes in the genotype of a cell population will be confined to the recipient. The second, germ-line therapy, involves the introduction of genes into fertilized eggs. In this case the genes will be distributed in both somatic *and* germ cells and hence will be passed on to future generations. Here we are moving into completely different ethical territory because we are, in effect, altering the genetic makeup of future populations.

● Techniques for insertion of foreign genes into cells

The transfer of genes into foreign cells may be achieved either directly or using a form of delivery system.

Direct insertion

There are a variety of ways in which DNA can be inserted into another cell. One of the simplest is based on the principle of the uptake of calcium microprecipitates of DNA which can be used to insert cloned genes. This approach is very inefficient and the rate of stable transfection is probably only about 1 cell in 10^5. A number of variations on this theme have been attempted including transfection of cells in suspension, or following their treatment with dimethylsulphoxide (DMSO), glycerol, chloroquine, or sodium butyrate. Unfortunately the efficiency of transfection by these techniques varies widely between different cell lines and is often unacceptably low. Furthermore, even when a better level of efficiency is achieved it is often confined to a specific cell line and hence is not generally applicable. By and large these techniques seem unlikely to be suitable for use in human gene therapy.

Another direct approach is to microinject DNA into the nucleus of cells. This requires considerable expertise, and because it involves treating one cell at a time is unlikely to have any practical application in gene therapy. Automated methods for injection may improve matters however.

A more recent method for direct insertion of genes involves the exposure of cells to a pulsed electric field, a technique called electroporation. It is believed that cells treated in this way open up pores in their plasma membranes. Although when it was first developed this approach also gave a low efficiency of transfection there have been some recent improvements. For example, a modification has been described which has resulted in more than 1 per cent of the viable cells showing stable expression of a selectable marker gene. To date there is no information about the long-term viability of cells that have been treated in this way or about the possibility of genetic damage caused by exposure to a strong electrical field.

Finally, there has been a recent description of a relatively efficient method of DNA transfer using laser micropuncture of cell membranes.

RNA viruses (retroviruses)

Retroviruses are adapted by evolution for the efficient delivery of their genome into cells, with integration into the host genome and a high level of expression of their internal sequences. There are several reasons why the use of retroviral vectors seems to be a promising approach to gene therapy. In particular, the efficiency of integration is high in dividing cells, and only single copy inserts are incorporated into the host genome.

Retroviruses have a complicated structure and lifestyle (Fig. 90). The virion particle consists of a dimer of viral RNA within a protein coat surrounded by a lipid bilayer containing viral-specific glycoproteins which attach themselves to cells during infection. The virion contains the virus-coded enzyme, reverse transcriptase. After entering cells the coat is shed and the RNA genome is copied into DNA by reverse transcriptase. A double-stranded DNA circle is formed and specific retroviral sequences direct the integration of viral DNA into the host genome. After integration viral sequences transcribe full-length and spliced RNAs. The spliced RNAs are translated to generate glycoproteins while the full-length RNA is either translated into internal structural proteins of the virion core and reverse transcriptase or packaged into virion particles as new genomic RNA. The subsequent assembly and budding of virion particles from infected cells is non-lytic.

The main features of the genome of a typical retrovirus are shown in Fig. 91. A variety of recombinant retrovirus vectors have been constructed. The viral genome needed for the infection, integration, and transcriptional control of the genome is all contained in the long terminal repeat sequences (LTRs), which are preserved together with the packaging sequence (*Psi*), but viral sequences of which the function can be supplied in *trans*, are taken out. Thus the *gag* sequences which encode internal structural proteins of the virion core, *pol* genes which encode reverse transcriptase, and *env* genes which encode the envelope glycoproteins are all deleted and replaced by a dominant selectable marker and the gene that we wish to transfer (Fig. 91).

The recombinant and now defective retroviral genome in the form of plasmid DNA is then introduced by transfection into murine fibroblasts to generate cell lines that produce the recombinant retrovirus. Simultaneous infection with wild-type helper viruses which have had their packaging sequences removed (Fig. 91) can provide the required packaging proteins, although it is now possible to achieve the same result by the use of specialized packaging cell lines that contain helper virus sequences within their genomes. In essence the engineered vector retrovirus uses its packaging sequences to package its RNA into proteins produced by the helper virus which, because it lacks these sequences, cannot

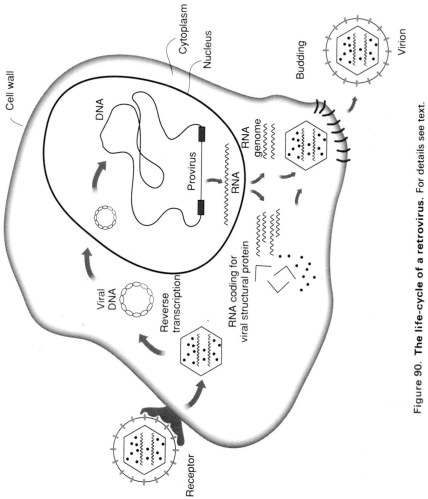

Figure 90. **The life-cycle of a retrovirus.** For details see text.

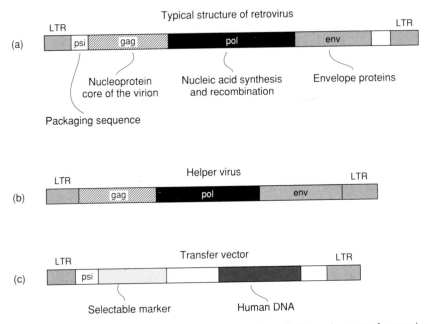

Figure 91. **Modifying retroviruses for gene transfer.** **A** The main genes of a retrovirus. **B** Helper virus. **C** A transfer vector construction.

transmit its own RNA and remains trapped in the cells (see Fig. 92). Vector virus particles are shed into the surrounding medium which can then be harvested and used to infect the recipient cells, or the latter can be incubated directly with the cells that are budding off the viral particles.

Experiments using recombinant retroviruses of this type have demonstrated that gene transfer can be achieved. For example, murine bone marrow has been cultivated with packaging cell lines that produce recombinant retrovirus, collected, and injected into lethally irradiated recipient mice. Since injected stem cells colonize the spleen it is possible to follow the fate of the transfected genes by analysis of the DNA of colonies formed in the spleen or, subsequently, in the blood of the animal. Studies of this kind have shown that genes have been transferred into pluripotential haemopoietic stem cells and that the transfected cells appear to be long-lived, at least for up to 4 months after transplantation. Furthermore they are multipotential, i.e. they give rise to both lymphoid and myeloid progeny.

A variety of genes have been transferred into intact mice using retroviral vectors including a neomycin resistance gene (G418), hypoxanthine phosphoribosyl transferase (HPRT), dihydrofolate reductase (DHFR), human globin, and human adenosine deaminase (ADA). In addition to murine stem cells, retrovirus-mediated transfer and expression of drug resistance genes has also been achieved using human haemopoietic progenitors in culture, and the human

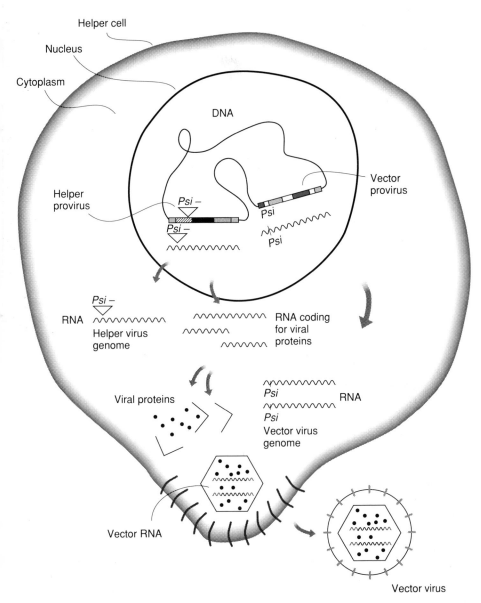

Figure 92. **Producing a vector for gene transfer with the use of a helper virus.** The transfer vector provirus contains the Psi sequence and hence the genome is automatically encapsulated by viral proteins produced by helper virus DNA. The resulting particles are released by budding from the helper cell. But the vector virus is capable of only one infection because it lacks the information needed to make virus proteins. Modified from Nicholls (1988).

ADA gene has been transferred into and expressed in diploid skin fibroblasts obtained from an ADA-deficient human.

While these results are encouraging, the level of expression of many of these transferred genes has been extremely variable. Retrovirus-mediated transfer of genes into cultured haemopoietic cells has often resulted in their expression at levels similar to or even higher than that of the endogenous genes. For example, a Lesch–Nyhan lymphoblast line, deficient in HPRT, was used to determine whether the defect could be corrected by a retroviral vector containing a functional HPRT gene. This turned out to be the case and the metabolic derangements caused by HPRT deficiency were almost completely corrected. On the other hand, transplantation of transfected haemopoietic cells into mice has often resulted in low or almost undetectable expression of the inserted genes although encouraging improvements have been reported recently. Similarly, although expression of human ADA or neomycin-resistant genes has been demonstrated in monkeys after transfection of their bone marrow the expression was confined to a very small proportion of white blood cells.

It is not yet clear why the expression of transferred genes is so low in these *in vivo* experiments. One problem is that retroviruses only infect cells in cycle, and most haemopoietic stem cells are out of cycle in the adult marrow. Furthermore, it is possible that the genes may be inactivated or rearranged during haemopoietic differentiation. In this context it has been possible to obtain expression of the genes for factor VIII and HPRT in human or mouse skin fibroblasts. It will be interesting to see whether these cells are able to maintain more persistent expression of transferred genes, particularly as they undergo very little differentiation after engraftment. Retrovirus-mediated gene transfer has also been achieved using primary cultures of mouse or rat hepatocytes.

Many problems remain, in particular the level of expression using retroviral vectors for gene transfer. A number of ingenious attempts have been made to improve the situation. For example, some encouraging results have been obtained by inserting the sequence for rat growth hormone together with 237 bases of genomic 5′ flanking sequence into a retroviral vector. The growth hormone genes were regulated in fibroblasts by their own promotor and regulatory sequences, as evidenced by stimulation by glucocorticoid and thyroid hormones. However, there are still enormous problems to be overcome concerning the level and stability of expression using retroviral vector systems. Whether it will be possible to improve the situation by the incorporation of internal enhancer sequences into these vectors remains to be seen. Retroviruses have their own enhancers immediately upstream from their promotors in the long terminal repeat (LTR) sequence, but the species- and tissue-specificity of enhancers, as mentioned earlier, may be of particular importance in determining the appropriate expression of inserted genes.

The recent discovery of sequences upstream from the human α and β-like globin gene clusters which have strong tissue-specific and positional-independence properties is very encouraging. These sequences, called dominant control regions (DCRs), have been found to direct high level, copy-number-dependent expression of human α and β-globin in transgenic mice. Interestingly, the human α genes are also fully active in transgenic animals if 'driven' by the β globin DCR. This is a particularly important advance because, if the precise regions of DNA that comprise the DCR can be defined, and included in constructions containing human globin genes within retroviral vectors, it may be possible to overcome some of the problems of low-level expression of inserted genes.

Another encouraging development over the last few years has been the improvement in methods for manipulating human haemopoietic stem cells, both *in vitro* and *in vivo*. For example, using long-term culture it is possible to subject the marrow cells to repeated rounds of transfection, and hence to transduce up to 50 per cent of the progenitors. Furthermore, transfection efficiency has been improved by the use of mixtures of haemopoietic growth factors. Whichever method of gene transfer turns out to be the most effective, it seems likely that further improvements will be required in manipulating stem cells before it is possible to move to somatic gene therapy in patients.

Finally, as mentioned earlier, it should be emphasized that very little is known about the safety of retroviral delivery systems. There is no doubt that they can rearrange their own structure and also exchange sequences with other retroviruses including helper viruses. There is still the possibility that a retroviral vector might recombine with an endogenous viral sequence to produce an infectious recombinant virus. Although the properties of a virus of this type are difficult to anticipate the outside possibility remains that they might be oncogenic; recently, 'self-destructing' retroviruses have been engineered to try to solve this problem. Another potential hazard relates to the site of integration; because this is random it is possible that inserted retroviral sequences might end up next to an oncogene and cause its uncontrolled activation. Although, the size of the human genome means that the latter type of event is highly unlikely it remains a potential problem.

● Targeted modification of human genes

Targeted modification of genes by exogenous DNA has been possible in yeast for many years. However it is only recently that preliminary studies of this approach to the alteration of the human genome have been attempted.

In principle, this approach to the replacement of defective genes has many attractions. In particular, it is site-directed and hence should not cause the problems of random integration. The idea is that the exogenous DNA should contain a region with the same nucleotide sequence as the target gene so that homologous recombination can occur between the regions of sequence identity. In other words the method uses nature's way of gene mixing. Depending on the arrangement of the incoming sequences relative to the target, the recombination event could either introduce new sequences into the recipient chromosome by a single crossover, or substitute sequences by gene conversion or double crossover events (Fig. 93).

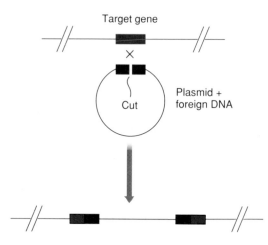

Figure 93. Site-directed recombination.

Several advances in site-directed gene replacement have been made recently. Plasmids have been linearized with restriction enzymes to produce a double strand break within the region homologous to the gene target. These have tended to be much more efficient than closed circular molecules which are also capable of generating recombination; it is presumed that the ends of the DNA molecules are more active in recombination. Although there have been some spectacular successes with this approach many problems remain. In particular the efficiency is low and there is a worrying tendency to induce new mutations after recombination with the 'foreign' DNA. However, because of its potential specificity it is very important that work continues in this promising area.

● Specific correction of genetic defects with suppressor tRNA genes

Many single gene disorders result from nonsense mutations, i.e. single base changes which produce premature stop codons in the middle of exons and hence which make it impossible for the affected genes to produce full-length protein products. It is possible to correct these defects by the use of suppressor transfer RNAs that can insert amino acids into the altered codons. Recent work has suggested that functional suppressor genes of this type can be constructed by site-specific mutagenesis. Unfortunately these molecules mediate only low levels of suppression. Thus a major question is whether it would be possible to achieve a level of suppression at which the appropriate genes could function in such a way as to produce adequate amounts of gene product. Current work in this field is directed towards constructing retrovirus vectors containing the suppressor transfer RNA genes which can be inserted with high efficiency into bone marrow cells.

● Transgenic approaches

The introduction of DNA into fertilized eggs and subsequent integration into both somatic cells and germ cells has been achieved successfully in a variety of species (see Chapter 3). These experiments have been carried out with the object of developing the transgenic animal as a model for studying gene regulation. DNA has been injected directly into fertilized eggs or transferred using retroviral vectors.

There is no doubt that foreign DNA introduced either by microinjection or retroviral transfection integrates into chromosomal DNA, is carried in germ cells and is then transmitted to subsequent generations. Some remarkable results have been obtained. For example, the introduction of metallothionine/growth hormone fusion genes into mice stimulates the production of growth hormone in tissues that normally synthesize metallothionine. Induction of the metallothionine promoters with metals has caused treated mice to grow to about twice their normal size. Tissue-specific expression of a variety of human genes has been obtained and a number of genetic diseases of mice, including thalassaemia, have been corrected. This model is also extremely useful for studying the effects of oncogene expression and for the analysis of defective embryonic development by insertional mutagenesis.

Currently, transgenic correction of human disease is not being contemplated. I shall return to this topic in Chapter 12 when we consider the practical and ethical issues involved.

● Immunological problems following gene therapy

One of the major unresolved problems of human gene transfer therapy is whether the donated genes, regardless of the route that is used for their transfer, will cause an immune response in the recipient. After all, their products represent completely new proteins as far as the patient is concerned.

Surprisingly perhaps, there is very little information about the antigenic properties of 'foreign' proteins of this type. As mentioned earlier, bone marrow transplantation has been used successfully to correct a number of genetic disorders, but this is nearly always followed by the administration of drugs to suppress the immune system and therefore the antigenic properties of the newly introduced protein may well have been masked. There is no doubt, however, that an immune response can be mounted against proteins that are given to patients as part of replacement therapy. For example, about 15 per cent of patients with haemophilia A develop inhibitors, antibodies against factor VIII. Curiously, only about 1 per cent of patients who receive blood products to correct the defect in haemophilia B make antibodies. On the other hand, there is no evidence that thalassaemic patients make antibodies against α or β globin chains.

There are probably many reasons why the mounting of an immunological response against a missing gene product varies both from patient to patient with a particular disease and between diseases. One factor may be the type of cell in which the foreign antigen is presented to the patient. Another important determinant may be the underlying mutation. For example, if a patient had a complete deletion of a particular gene it might be expected that they would be much more likely to mount an immunological response to its product than if they had had a point mutation which meant that they had produced some product, albeit abnormal. In the latter case there would have been a good chance that they would have become tolerant to the product.

Recent studies suggest that in patients with Christmas disease there is a strong correlation between the underlying molecular defect and the likelihood of producing antibodies against factor IX. In 18 out of 21 patients with major deletions of the factor IX gene, antibodies were produced, whereas only 1 out of 16 patients with point mutations of the gene reacted in this way. The position regarding haemophilia A is less clear although by and large it appears as though patients with large deletions of the factor VIII gene are more likely to make antibodies against factor VIII.

Thus from the scanty information that is available it is clear that the likelihood of developing antibodies against a newly introduced gene product will be very difficult to assess. It will depend on many factors including the molecular pathology of the disorder and the particular tissue in which the gene is expressed. But enough is known already to suggest that this is going to be a major problem for gene therapy and may well mean that patients will have to receive some kind of immunosuppressive treatment both before and after gene transfer. It may not be possible to anticipate which conditions will be associated with this problem and we may have to learn by experience.

● Likely candidate diseases for gene therapy

It seems likely that the best candidates for gene therapy in the immediate future are disorders such as Lesch–Nyhan disease which is due to a deficiency of hypoxanthine phosphoribosyl transferase (HPRT), purine nucleoside phosphorylase deficiency (PNP), or adenine deaminase (ADA) deficiency. These diseases are due to deficiencies of enzymes produced by so-called housekeeping genes, which are 'on' in most cells and do not require very precise regulation. All three conditions are severely disabling and it is hoped that a low level expression of inserted genes into deficient cells will correct at least some of their functional abnormalities. The limited experience with HPRT deficiency suggests that this is the case. However, even in these disorders there are enormous difficulties to be overcome. In particular, although the defect in each of these conditions is expressed in cells of bone marrow origin, at least in the case of the Lesch–Nyhan syndrome there is deficiency of HPRT in brain cells which could probably not be corrected by current technology. If it proves possible to obtain prolonged and relatively high levels of production of factor IX in skin fibroblasts, Christmas disease might be another condition for early consideration for gene therapy of this type.

Other single gene disorders will be even more difficult to correct. For example, although a great deal is known about the molecular defects in thalassaemia and some of the structural haemoglobin disorders, it seems unlikely that it will be possible to insert normal globin genes in the immediate future. These genes have to be under extremely tight regulation. As mentioned earlier, it would be no good inserting a β gene into the haemopoietic stem cells of a patient with β thalassaemia only to see it over-expressed in their progeny with the production of the clinical phenotype of α thalassaemia!

One encouraging fact for the future of gene therapy is that ADA deficiency can be corrected by bone marrow transplantation, as can a number of other single gene disorders that affect haemopoietic stem cells, β thalassaemia for example (see Table 35). Hence there is no reason why these conditions should not be cured by somatic gene therapy once the difficulties of transfection and expression are overcome. Until it becomes possible to transfect a sufficient number of stem cells it may still be necessary to attempt to provide the treated population with some form of selective advantage; cells must be in cycle to be infected with retroviruses and since the majority of haemopoietic stem cells are out of cycle the efficiency of transfection will remain a serious problem. However, it is conceivable that, by the use of genetically engineered haemopoietic growth factors, at least some of which are said to act at the stem cell level, it may be possible to encourage a greater number of stem cells into cycle. This possibility, together with recent progress in the identification of major regulatory sequences in the human globin gene clusters and the development of methods for isolating stem cells, suggests that somatic gene therapy will ultimately be successful.

● Other approaches to the correction of genetic diseases

Many serious genetic diseases, and indeed some of the commonest acquired diseases of old age, involve the central nervous system. At first sight the brain does not look like a very promising organ to attack by gene therapy. One approach to this problem which is being investigated is the possibility of using a combination of *in vitro* gene transfer together with autologous cell grafting into specific regions of the brain as a way of restoring local function. For example, in an experiment of this type rat fibroblasts were transfected with a vector containing mouse nerve growth factor and then implanted into a rat brain; cholinergic neurons were protected from degeneration and death after injury to the particular region of the brain. Whether developments of this type will have any relevance to the treatment of genetic disorders of the nervous system, or to some important acquired conditions such as Alzheimer's or Parkinson's disease, remains to be determined.

Another and completely different approach to the correction of single gene disorders is to try to replace the activity of a defective gene by activating a gene with a similar function, which was used at an earlier stage of development and subsequently switched off. The idea of reactivating genes that are normally used only in early development to take the place of defective adult genes is attractive, if rather esoteric. For an example we must turn again to the globin genes.

As we saw in Chapter 3, the important haemoglobin disorders, sickle cell anaemia and β thalassaemia, are characterized by defective adult haemoglobin synthesis, i.e. they result from mutations of the β globin genes. In fetal life the β globin genes are only active at a very low level and the bulk of the haemoglobin is of the fetal variety. The switch from Hb F ($\alpha_2\gamma_2$) to Hb A ($\alpha_2\beta_2$) reflects a change from γ to β globin chain synthesis, which occurs late in gestation. Of course, this is why infants who have sickle cell anaemia or β thalassaemia, which affect the structure or synthesis of the β globin chains, are normal at birth and only become symptomatic when β chain production is fully established at the age of about 6 months. Were these children not to switch over from fetal to adult haemoglobin production, that is γ to β chain synthesis, the defective β genes would not be expressed and the clinical disorder would not develop.

Would it matter if a baby went on producing fetal haemoglobin into adult life? Some elegant experiments of nature have answered this question for us. Individuals with sickle cell anaemia or β thalassaemia who have also inherited genes for hereditary persistence of fetal haemoglobin are protected from the effects of the sickle cell or β thalassaemia genes. Fetal haemoglobin is a perfectly good oxygen carrier in adult life and a number of adults with 100 per cent Hb F are leading a completely normal life!

There is another interesting and encouraging facet to this story. It is quite clear that the γ globin genes are not irrevocably turned off after birth; there are many conditions in which they are reactivated, albeit at a low level. These include severe bone marrow stress caused by bleeding or after periods of depression due to drug therapy or radiation. It follows, therefore, that all we need to do is to find out how to encourage γ chain synthesis to persist in children with β globin gene disorders or, failing that, how to reactivate γ chain production once it has been switched off. These facts have been known to workers in the haemoglobin field for at least a quarter of a century and yet we still don't know how to tackle this problem. This is not surprising when it is remembered that we don't have the faintest idea how the developmental switch from fetal to adult haemoglobin production is regulated.

Undaunted by our total ignorance of the way in which our genes are regulated during development, several research groups have attempted to stimulate fetal haemoglobin production in patients with β thalassaemia and sickle cell anaemia. The rather optimistic reasoning behind these efforts goes along the following lines. Active genes are demethylated, whereas inactive genes are methylated. It has been known for many years that if baboons are made anaemic by bleeding they tend to increase their fetal haemoglobin production, at least a little. So, it has been argued, why not see if this effect can be enhanced by an agent that might demethylate γ globin genes? Surprisingly perhaps, the administration of

5-azacytidine, a potent demethylating agent, causes these anaemic animals to produce large quantities of fetal haemoglobin.

These observations led to the administration of 5-azacytidine to groups of patients with sickle cell anaemia or β thalassaemia and there was a small, but significant, increase in Hb F production in some of them. While many doubt the ethics of these experiments, particularly in view of the well-known cytotoxic and carcinogenic properties of 5-azacytidine, the fact remains that this agent is capable of augmenting γ chain production. It has been fiercely debated as to whether this effect is due to an alteration in the methylation state of the γ chain genes or whether it is mediated by a perturbation of haemopoiesis. Assuming the latter to be true, a number of workers have fed hydroxyurea, a drug used in the treatment of leukaemia, to patients with sickle cell anaemia. Again, this agent causes a modest increase in the production of Hb F in some patients with sickle cell anaemia; clinical trials are underway to see whether the long-term administration of this agent has any beneficial effects on the clinical course of this disease.

These are extremely crude approaches to the manipulation of the production of fetal haemoglobin and, to date, have not been particularly successful. However, it is encouraging to know that it is possible to 'manipulate' these genes at all, and these preliminary results suggest that it may well be worthwhile continuing work in this field. Whether gene manipulation of this kind has more general relevance to the management of genetic diseases is doubtful however. There are a few other examples of proteins which, like haemoglobin, change during development, but this may be a very specialized adaptive mechanism which is not required for the bulk of enzymes and structural proteins.

● A start at human gene therapy

Given the preceding account of some of the difficulties that may be involved in initiating human gene therapy the reader may be slightly surprised to see that this chapter is ending with an account of the first attempts at this *tour de force*. Strictly speaking this is not true of course, because two abortive attempts at gene therapy were attempted over 10 years ago, but very recently the first efforts at a procedure of this type using some of the techniques outlined in this chapter have been reported.

The background to this recent attempt at human gene transfer is quite complicated. For the last few years efforts have been made to treat patients with advanced cancer using cyclophosphamide combined with immunotherapy with interleukin 2 (IL-2) and autologous tumour infiltrating lymphocytes (TIL). This programme, pioneered at the National Cancer Institute in the United States, appears to have produced some remissions in patients with advanced malignant disease. The American investigators decided that they would like to have more information about the properties of TIL. In particular they felt it necessary to study the *in vivo* distribution of these cells and wanted to know if there was a correlation between the clinical response and the presence of TIL at the tumour site, in adjacent lymph nodes, or in the circulation. The problem was that there was no way of distinguishing TIL at these sites.

It was decided, therefore, to insert a selectable marker gene via retroviral-mediated gene transfer into TIL and to follow the fate of the transfected cells in patients who were being treated for advanced cancer. Not surprisingly, it took a considerable time before the various monitoring committees of the National Institutes of Health accepted the protocol for this experiment, but eventually permission was given at the beginning of 1989 and the first gene transfer experiments took place in May 1989. As of December 1989 five patients had been studied. Apparently the protocol had gone well, there were no side effects attributed to the gene transfer procedure, all safety studies had been satisfactory, and the gene-marked TIL had been successfully identified in blood samples and in tumour biopsy specimens from the patients examined. Of course it is a long road from the studies of this type in terminal cancer patients to the correction of genetic diseases but these experiments suggest that at least a few of the problems that have been outlined in this chapter may be amenable to solution.

As this book goes to press reports are starting to appear of an unexpected development in the field of gene therapy. Several groups have reported independently that they have been able to demonstrate dystrophin production after the transfer of cultured myoblasts (muscle cells) into the muscles of patients with Duchenne muscular dystrophy who, prior to transfer, had no detectable dystrophin. Clearly there are other options for the management of genetic disease which can now be analysed more effectively following the results of recombinant DNA studies on the basic molecular defects. This is another and totally unexpected fallout from molecular medicine, and one for which further results will be awaited with great excitement.

● Summary

The gene replacement field has been intensely active over the last few years. Indeed it has been suggested, rather irreverently, that there may be more research workers trying to correct ADA deficiency in this way than there are affected children in the countries where this type of work is being carried out. So far, the results are rather disappointing, but there are some encouraging signs. Much more is being learnt about the properties of haemopoietic and other stem cells, transfection vectors are becoming more efficient with time, and there are hints that site-directed recombination may be feasible as a more logical approach to the correction of genetic diseases. Much of this activity is being regarded with some trepidation by the general public, who wonder where it is all going to stop. We shall return to this theme when we consider the ethical issues arising from gene transfer experiments in the final chapter.

● Further reading

Anderson, G.L. and Ebans, G.A. (1988). Introduction and expression of DNA molecules in eukaryotic cells by electroporation. *Biotechniques*, **6**, 650–61.

Anderson, W.F. (1984). Prospects for human gene therapy. *Science*, **226**, 401–9.

Anonymous (1990). The N2-TIL human gene transfer clinical protocol. *Human Gene Therapy*, **1**, 73–92.

Bordignon, C., Sheu-Fung, Yu, Smith, C.A., *et al.* (1989). Retroviral vector-mediated high-efficiency expression of adenosine deaminase (ADA) in hemopoietic long-term cultures of ADA-deficient marrow cells. *Proc. Natl. Acad. Sci. USA*, **86**, 6748–52.

Capecchi, M.R. (1989). The new mouse genetics: altering the genome by gene targetting. *Trends Genet.*, **5**, 70–6.

Doetschman, T., Maeda, N., and Smithies, O. (1988). Targeted mutation of the *Hprt* gene in mouse embryonic stem cells. *Proc. Natl. Acad. Sci. USA*, **85**, 8583–7.

Dzierzak, E.A., Papayannopoulou, T., and Mulligan, R.C. (1988). Lineage-specific expression of a human β-globin gene in murine bone marrow transplant recipients reconstituted with retrovirus-transduced stem cells. *Nature*, **331**, 35–41.

Eglitis, M.A. and Anderson, W.F. (1988). Retroviral vectors for introduction of genes into mammalian cells. *Biotechniques*, **6**, 608–14.

European Medical Research Councils (1988). Gene therapy in man. *Lancet*, **i**, 1271–2.

Friedmann, T. (1989). Progress toward human gene therapy. *Science*, **244**, 1275–81.

Friedmann, T. (1990). The evolving concept of gene therapy. *Human Gene Therapy*, **1**, 175–81.

Hobbs, J.R. (1988). Displacement bone marrow transplantation and immunoprophylaxis for genetic diseases. *Adv. Intern. Med.*, **33**, 81–118.

Law, P.K., *et al.* (1990). Dystrophin production induced by myoblast transfer therapy in Duchenne muscular dystrophy. *Lancet*, **336**, 114–15.

McCune, J.M., Namikawa, R., Kaneshima, H., Shultz, L.D., Lieverman, M., and Weissman, I.L. (1988). The SCID-hy mouse: murine model for the analysis of human hematolymphoid differentiation and function. *Science*, **241**, 1632–9.

McLaren, A. (1987). Can we diagnose genetic disease in pre-embryos? *New Scientist*, **116**, 42–7.

Mannino, R.J. and Gould-Fogerite, S.C. (1988). Liposome mediated gene transfer. *Biotechniques*, **6**, 682–91.

Miller, A.D. (1990). Retrovirus packaging cells. *Human Gene Therapy*, **1**, 5–14.

Miller, A.D., Palmer, T.D., and Hock, R.A. (1986). Transfer of genes into human somatic cells using retrovirus vectors. *Cold Spring Harbor Symp. Quant. Biol.*, **51**, 1013–20.

Nichols, E.K. (1988). *Human gene therapy*. Harvard University Press, Cambridge, MA.

Spangrude, G.J., Heimfeld, S., and Weissman, I.L. (1988). Purification and characterization of mouse hematopoietic stem cells. *Science*, **241**, 58–62.

Temin, H.M. (1990). Safety considerations in somatic gene therapy of human disease with retrovirus vectors. *Human Gene Therapy*, **1**, 111–23.

Valle, D. (1987). Genetic disease: an overview of current therapy. *Hosp. Pract.*, **22**, 167–82.

Weatherall, D.J. (1989). Somatic gene therapy. In *Fetal medicine* 1, (ed. C. Rodeck), pp. 289–306. Blackwell Scientific, Oxford.

Williams, D.A. and Orkin, S.H. (1986). Somatic gene therapy. Current status and future prospects. *J. Clin. Invest.*, **77**, 1053–6.

Wilson, J.M., Jeferson, D.M., Chowdhury, J.R., Novikoff, P.M., Johnston, D.E., and Mulligan, R.C. (1988). Retrovirus-mediated transduction of adult hepatocytes. *Proc. Natl. Acad. Sci. USA*, **85**, 3014–18.

Yee, J.-K., Moores, J.C., Jolly, D.J., Wolff, J.A., Respess, J.G., and Friedmann, T. (1987). Gene expression from transcriptionally disabled retroviral vectors. *Proc. Natl. Acad. Sci. USA*, **84**, 5197–201.

Some broader implications of the new genetics for clinical practice in the future

11

The sophisticated tools of molecular and cell biology will be used to study many diseases over the next few years. What practical benefits will result? Almost certainly we shall learn a lot about human molecular pathology. In addition, we can reasonably expect to see the development of increasingly successful methods for the diagnosis and avoidance of many common genetic diseases. As mentioned in the previous chapter, the potential for a radical cure of some of these conditions is also on the horizon. However, while we are waiting for the benefits of improvements to gene therapy the main efforts of clinical geneticists will be directed towards the avoidance of inherited diseases.

As already intimated in earlier chapters, recombinant DNA technology has much more to offer than simply improving the diagnosis, avoidance, and management of single gene disorders. It should start to yield some insights into the molecular pathology of some of the common disorders of western society although this will certainly not happen overnight. Furthermore, recombinant DNA technology provides us with the opportunity to study human development and the ways in which this can go wrong in the genesis of congenital malformation and mental retardation. In short, these remarkable technological advances should lead to new methods of diagnosis and treatment across the whole spectrum of clinical practice. It seems likely that our new found technology will make a major impact on broader areas of human biology, including such complex topics as evolution, ageing, and human behaviour.

In this chapter we shall summarize the likely effects of recombinant DNA technology on clinical genetics, and then examine a few areas of clinical practice that seem particularly likely to benefit from its application in the future.

● Mapping the human genome

In Chapter 5 we outlined how it should be possible to build up both genetic and physical maps of the genome. Just the idea of sequencing the whole of the human genome has been the subject of heated debate over the last few years. While much of the argument has centred round expense, priority compared with more pressing problems in medical research, and the best way to proceed, there is no doubt that the debate has also been clouded by institutional and national pride, commercial concerns, and the usual parochial attitudes that tend to colour international collaborative activities in science. Numerous national and international committees have been established and programmes have come and gone. The lack of productivity of much of this activity has resulted, at least in part, from attempts to plan an ambitious project during a period when new technical advances were coming so rapidly that decisions taken a few months earlier became completely redundant!

Apart from the formidable organizational and methodological problems posed by a project of this magnitude there is still considerable debate about priorities. Should, for example, the first priority be a genetic or a physical map, and how far should sequencing of vast regions of uncharted and conceivably uninteresting DNA be encouraged. Given the fact that most of the information that will be of immediate interest to medical science will be in expressed sequences should we not be tackling a cDNA map first?

Quite recently a proposal has been made which promises to take much of the heat out of the debate and which, if followed through, could provide a genuine solution to the problem of integrating the activities of laboratories throughout the world towards producing a physical map of the human genome, a goal which few doubt would be of enormous value for medical research. The idea is as follows. As pointed out in Chapter 5 it should be possible to obtain a contig map, that is sets of overlapping clones covering most of the genome. These could be combined with restriction enzyme site maps showing the order and distance between cleavage sites, though contig maps are difficult to construct and leave gaps, and the value of restriction enzyme mapping varies widely in different parts of the genome. The new idea is to 'mark' all these different landmarks, whether contigs, segments with unusual restriction sites, probes that define mapped DNA polymorphisms, sequences that hybridize to particular chromosome bands, and so on. The markers would be sequence-tagged sites (STSs), that is about 200–500 bp of sequence of the particular piece of DNA. This would be achieved by making two short primers complementary to the opposite strands and ends of the particular sequence track and then, using the polymerase chain reaction as described in Chapter 3, by synthesizing STSs. The latter would then be assimilated into a central data base.

The beauty of the above approach is that it would provide a common language with which to store data from widely diverse sources. Two laboratories could instantly compare contigs, and the material would be of equal value however it was derived, provided these simple procedures were carried out. The field would not be restricted to large laboratories; any worker with appropriate sequence data, however modest, could contribute using the same 'language'.

Given the increasing size of fragments that can be cloned, up to several hundred kilobase pairs in yeast artificial chromosomes, it has been estimated that in 5 years it might be possible to produce an STS map with an average spacing of 100 kb, representing 30 000 STSs. It is likely that a start could be made immediately; perhaps 2000 to 3000 useful probes are already available.

There is nothing fundamentally new about this concept. It is simply the idea of converting the vast amount of mapping data that is already available into the common language of DNA sequence that is so appealing. If the international scientific community takes it up the whole thing may be feasible provided that the formidable difficulties of data storage and dissemination can be overcome. If this *tour de force* is achieved many of the possibilities outlined in the remainder of this chapter may become realities.

Recently, the National Institutes of Health have set out a 5-year plan for the Human Genome Project. Essentially it involves the construction of a genetic map with markers spaced on average 2–5 centimorgans apart, the development of a physical map consisting of overlapping sets of clones DNA or closely spaced unambiguously ordered markers with continuity over lengths of 2 million basepairs, and the discovery of better methods for DNA sequencing that will allow large-scale sequencing of DNA at a cost of $0.50 per basepair. During the evolution of better methods for sequencing it is hoped that an aggregate of 10 million basepairs of human DNA in large continuous stretches will be obtained. In addition, it is planned to sequence about 20 million basepairs of DNA from a variety of model organisms, particularly the mouse, and to develop effective software and database designs to support these large-scale mapping and sequencing projects. Whether or not these goals are achieved there seems little doubt that the human genome project is on the road.

● Molecular pathology

● Single gene disorders

As appropriate gene probes are developed, and as we gradually fill in the map of the human genome, it will be increasingly easy to analyse the fine structure of human genes and their flanking regions. In this way we shall obtain a detailed picture of the molecular pathology of many single gene disorders.

In an earlier chapter we described what is already known about the molecular basis for the common disorders of haemoglobin synthesis and other single gene conditions. In the relatively short time since this work started, a remarkable picture of the molecular diversity of these diseases has emerged. Almost every genetic lesion that has been described by microbial geneticists, including many that were never even dreamt of, have turned up. We already have examples of single base changes, deletions of one or more bases or entire genes, insertions, inversions, unequal crossing-over, nonsense mutations, initiation or termination mutations, mutations involving the regulatory boxes in the flanking regions of structural genes, and a whole family of more subtle mutations involving the processing of messenger RNA. Since there must be a limited number of things that can go wrong with a gene, it is tempting to speculate that what we have learnt about thalassaemia may have pre-empted much of the molecular pathology of monogenic disease. In other words, as we analyse the defects in other single gene disorders we shall find abnormalities very similar to those that underlie the thalassaemias. No doubt there will be some surprises, but it is likely that we already have a reasonable idea of the repertoire of the mutations of single gene diseases.

As these studies are extended they will provide insights into the reasons why some single gene disorders have such a variable clinical phenotype. Terms such as 'variable expression' are used to describe differences in phenotypes which are found together with what appear to be the same genetic determinants. It has been suggested that this topic is too complex for any rational analysis; I doubt if this is true. In an earlier chapter we considered how the remarkable clinical diversity of what appears to be the 'homozygous state' for β thalassaemia can be explained on the basis of the heterogeneity of β thalassaemia mutations and by the interaction of different forms of α thalassaemia with the β thalassaemias. It seems likely that the variable expression of other single gene disorders will reflect heterogeneity of the mutations that cause them and the action of perhaps a few other genes that can modify the expression of the particular mutant gene. Indeed, as this book goes to press it is encouraging to hear that early results on the molecular pathology of cystic fibrosis are already suggesting that particular mutations may modify the expression of the CF locus with regard to the presence or absence of pancreatic insufficiency.

This is an extremely important aspect of human genetics because, as prenatal diagnosis becomes easier and more commonplace, and gene therapy becomes a reality, it will be increasingly important to be able to make accurate predictions of the phenotypes associated with different mutations.

● Chromosome disorders

It is very likely that there are subtle chromosome abnormalities that cannot be detected by the current techniques of cytogenetics, but which might be identified by restriction enzyme technology. For example, we have studied the interesting syndrome of mental retardation associated with α thalassaemia due to defects involving the α globin gene cluster on chromosome 16. Unlike the inherited α thalassaemias described in Chapter 6 this syndrome is not associated with a simple Mendelian form of inheritance, but results from a mutation acquired from the parental germ cells. This condition was identified only because the lesion on chromosome 16 happens to involve a region from which we could identify a gene product, i.e. the α chains of haemoglobin. In some of these cases there are long deletions involving this region of chromosome 16, while in others, although the α globin genes appear to be at least partly inactivated, no abnormalities can be found by gene mapping. Further analysis of this syndrome has shown that some of the deletions seem to be simple interstitial lesions whereas others are associated with different parental translocations involving chromosome 16. The reason for the association of defective α globin gene action in the non-deletion cases remains to be determined. It seems likely that, at least in the deletion cases, we are dealing with another example of a contiguous gene syndrome, as defined in Chapter 6 and also considered further later in this chapter, and that further analysis of this condition may reveal some important 'developmental' genes at the tip of chromosome 16.

These observations suggest that there may be many chromosome abnormalities, including submicroscopic deletions or insertions, which will be identified by restriction enzyme analysis or related techniques, once we know where to look and have developed the appropriate probes. Furthermore, it may well become feasible to define the molecular basis for the various syndromes of mental retardation associated with fragile chromosomal sites. It may also be possible to identify additional chromosomal material, trisomy 21 for example, using quantitative gene mapping. We can already identify the sex of a fetus by chorion villus sampling and mapping fetal DNA using probes for unique and repetitive sequences specific for the Y chromosome.

There are other reasons for optimism that molecular cytogenetics will have much to offer in the future. As mentioned in Chapter 5 the new techniques of confocal laser scanning microscopy, and the high resolution *in situ* hybridization methods that are being developed with non-radioactive probes, should provide ways of ordering cloned genes on regions of the chromosome, as well as defining deletions and insertions.

● Congenital malformations

Malformations due to defective embryogenesis may be single or multiple, and trivial or so serious as to be incompatible with life. About 14 per cent of newborn infants have a single minor malformation, 3 per cent have a major malformation and about 0.7 per cent have multiple major malformations. The frequency of serious malformations is even higher at conception, perhaps 10–15 per cent, but the majority of these fetuses are lost by spontaneous abortion.

As pointed out in Chapter 2, there is a strong genetic component to congenital malformation. Data derived from several sources suggests that about a third of congenital malformations of known cause are genetic in origin, with multifactorial inheritance as the commonest identifiable aetiology, followed by monogenic and chromosome disorders. It is interesting to note that only 7 per cent of congenital malformations can be traced back to definable environmental factors such as maternal illness, congenital virus infection, or exposure to drugs or alcohol. Over 60 per cent of cases of major congenital malformation have no obvious cause. While it is important to continue to look for underlying environmental agents and maternal factors, the fact that chromosomal abnormalities seem to play such a major role in cases of known aetiology suggests that this will be a particularly fruitful area of research in the future. Even if we can identify environmental factors it still has to be explained how they cause damage to the genome and malformation of the developing fetus.

One of the most interesting areas of research that directly links the new applications of recombinant DNA technology and molecular cytogenetics to an understanding of developmental abnormalities is the contiguous gene syndromes. This interesting group of disorders, already outlined in Chapter 6, includes syndromes that demonstrate recognizable and recurrent patterns of malformation, usually in association with mental retardation. They may be sporadic or familial. However, in the latter case they differ from typical monogenic disorders by their patterns of inheritance. They are also different from the classical chromosome syndromes caused by specific aneuploidy and detectable by routine cytogenetic examination. A partial list of some of the contiguous gene syndromes together with their chromosomal assignments is shown in Table 36.

Table 36. *Contiguous gene syndromes*

Disease or syndrome	Cytogenetic change
Retinoblastoma	Deletion 13q14
Wilms' tumour	Deletion 11p13
Lancer–Gideon syndrome	Deletion 8q24
Beckwith–Wiedemann syndrome	Duplication of 11p15
Prader–Willi syndrome	Various changes 15q11
Miller–Dieker syndrome	Deletion 17p13
Di George syndrome	Deletion 22q11
Hb H-mental retardation	Deletion 16p13.3

Clinical descriptions of these conditions are given in the text.

Although many patients with contiguous gene syndromes show no abnormalities by standard cytogenetic analysis, small deletions or insertions can be demonstrated by gene mapping or by the use of RFLPs. The lesions involved in some of these syndromes are summarized in Table 36. For example in the Prader–Willi syndrome, characterized by neonatal hypotonia and difficulty in swallowing, deformities of the face and genitalia, and over-eating and obesity during later development, there is a small deletion on the long arm of chromosome 15 which is apparent either cytogenetically or by gene mapping. Similarly, the Di George syndrome, characterized by neonatal seizures, failure to thrive, abnormalities of the aortic arch and facial development, and an absent thymus and associated defects in cellular immunity, is usually found together with an interstitial deletion of chromosome 22 in the region 22q11. The fact that these and the other contiguous gene syndromes summarized in Table 36 are usually accompanied by a similar phenotype suggests that the associated deletions or insertions affect groups of genes, some of which may be involved in the regulation of the developmental pattern of specific anatomical areas. Although it will be extremely difficult to analyse these complex phenotype/genotype relationships it is becoming clear that the identification and characterization of these disorders offers a very promising approach to our understanding of human development and its abnormalities.

Another extremely active research field in developmental biology may have important implications for our understanding of congenital malformations. As with so much of the 'new biology', the basic concepts are not new but the availability of powerful analytical tools has allowed them to be explored in a novel fashion. In 1894, Bateson suggested that the study of chance deviations in normal developmental patterns might provide clues about the rules that govern the regulation of development. This opened up a new field, the science of positioning and body patterns. It has been found that the homeotic genes of the fruit fly *Drosophilia*, which regulate the development of whole body segments, have DNA sequences in common with many other species including annelid worms, frogs, birds, mice, and man. Homeotic mutations in insects result in major developmental abnormalities including substitutions of one or more segments normally found elsewhere along the body axis. All vertebrate embryos go through a stage of development at which the body is composed of a linear series of segmental units, or somites, from which the skeleton, nervous system, and other systems are ultimately developed. It has been found that humans have an equivalent of the homeotic genes, possibly related in the distant evolutionary past to those of insects. Furthermore, there is increasing evidence that the products of these genes are DNA-binding proteins that play an important role in gene expression during development. These observations may have important implications for the study of the molecular basis of congenital malformation.

The transgenic animal model, outlined in Chapter 4, provides another valuable tool to dissect developmental abnormalities. It will be recalled that this experimental system was developed primarily for studying the factors that control the expression of genes. However, the 'foreign' DNA can cause mutations by inserting itself near or into the recipient's genes. Some of these insertions cause developmental abnormalities. The injected DNA can thus serve as a 'label' for defining genes that may be involved in early development. For example it has been found that inbreeding transgenic animals, in which the *myc* oncogene is inserted into the genome, produce offspring with deformities of their limbs. These deformities, and those of other strains of inbred mice, have changes reminiscent of certain homeotic mutations in *Drosophila*. The limb deformity gene in mice is on chromosome 2 and, of particular interest, is the finding that the *myc* insert in the transgenic mice with limb deformities is very close to this locus. It should be possible to isolate DNA fragments from segments flanking the *myc* gene insert and determine their nucleotide sequences. With luck this may provide information about the limb deformity genes and, more importantly, the nature of their products.

Another recent series of intriguing experiments in transgenic mice also emphasize the potential value of this system for studying the genesis of congenital malformation. In an attempt to express a c-*myc* gene in the erythroid cells of developing mice, and hence to perturb the normal processes of blood cell development, the gene was inserted by the transgenic route in a genetically engineered construction in which it was 'driven' by an adult globin gene promotor. Although there was no effect whatever on erythroid differentiation the newborn mice developed cystic disease of the kidney and died of renal failure. The researchers obtained convincing evidence that these remarkable cystic changes were due to overexpression of the c-*myc* gene. Although this experimentally produced disorder is not entirely the same as human adult polycystic disease, these interesting observations provide further confirmation of the value of the transgenic animal model for studying the mechanisms of abnormal development.

Other lethal developmental mutations have been caused by introducing viruses into early embryos. One defect that was analysed in detail causes the death of embryos at about the 12th day of gestation. It turns out that this is due to the integration of the viral genome into the gene for collagen.

Although it is apparent that most congenital abnormalities, if they have a genetic basis at all, are polygenic in origin there are a few conditions that appear to follow a monogenic inheritance. For example there is a form of cleft palate that follows an X-linked pattern of inheritance. By using a number of X chromosome probes it has been possible to define the approximate region of the X chromosome that contains the gene involved. Although monogenic inheritance of congenital anomalies of this type is rare, analyses of the affected families provide another valuable approach to defining genes that play a major role in development. It is clear, therefore, that we now have some useful leads about how to go about studying developmental mutations and thereby learning more about the genes that regulate normal development and the types of mutational events that may underlie some forms of congenital malformation.

● Common polygenic diseases

In Chapters 7 and 8 we considered how recombinant DNA technology can be applied to the study of common polygenic disease, including cancer. It is particularly difficult to anticipate how fast things will move or what practical applications will arise from this work over the next few years. Except for a few exceptional cases it seems unlikely that a major impact on day to day clinical practice will ensue although the long-term potential may be enormous.

The major goal for the study of the genetic aspects of heart disease, autoimmune disease, and the major psychoses will be to try to determine which genes are of particular importance in the polygenic systems that underlie these conditions. Having done so it should be possible to determine how these particular genes in affected individuals differ from their wild-type alleles in the normal population. Once this is known we should be able to relate these structural variations to the function of their products and hence to start to understand the pathogenesis of these disorders. This, in turn, should lead to better forms of prevention and treatment. For example, it may enable us to define subsets of individuals who are at particular risk from exposure to environmental agents and thus to apply preventative medicine in a more focused way. Also, we should be enabled to develop more rational strategies for the management of the conditions involved.

The difficulties in applying RFLP linkage analysis to polygenic disease should not, however, be underestimated. As pointed out in Chapter 5, there are some very promising developments in this field, particularly the discovery of new families of highly polymorphic loci which should be of particular value for linkage studies of that type. Although we have these powerful new mapping techniques, the problems of ascertainment and, in particular, the difficulties in handling the mathematics of the vast amount of data that will be generated from work of this kind suggest that we should not expect dramatic results too quickly. It is quite likely that we will go through a long period of uncertainty during which we will obtain inconsistent results, rather like those described in Chapter 7 for schizophrenia and Alzheimer's disease. Nevertheless our new technology is so powerful that in the long term it should be possible to straighten out these problems and obtain some solid information about the chromosomal location of genes that are involved in the pathogenesis of common disorders.

It will be apparent from the brief analysis of the current state of knowledge on the pathogenesis of cancer, as outlined in Chapter 8, that neoplastic transformation almost certainly involves the acquisition of different mutations in particular cell populations. In some cases at least one of these mutations may be inherited. It will be particularly important to try to define the frequency of the recessive cancer genes. It is also apparent that at least some of the genetic events that occur during one or other of the stages in neoplastic transformation involve the activation of cellular oncogenes. In short, these remarkable studies are telling us that the genetic route to the neoplastic phenotype is extremely variable; a particular malignancy may be generated from a number of different mutations during the course of its evolution.

Epidemiological studies carried out over the past 20 years have provided uncontrovertable evidence that environmental factors play an important role in the genesis of cancer. It seems very likely that the effects of these agents are mediated through their action on the genome of susceptible cell populations and that, in the case of many cancers, this will represent the first step in the development of the neoplastic phenotype. It may well turn out that there is considerable individual genetic variation in the ability to deal with environmental carcinogens. Thus one practical outcome of the genetic approach to cancer should be the definition of individuals at particularly high risk from exposure to carcinogens. It may also be possible to develop new preventative approaches to cancer by neutralizing the effects of environmental agents. Examples may include the development of vaccination programmes against Epstein–Barr (EB) virus, which seems to be involved in the pathogenesis of nasopharyngeal carcinoma in Chinese populations, and against hepatitis B virus, the causative agent of hepatomas (liver cancers) in many populations in which the infection is endemic. Another approach to the prevention of cancer which may be facilitated by DNA technology is in testing food additives and other agents of this type for their mutagenic properties.

How far it will be possible to reverse the effect of the multiple mutations that underlie the malignant phenotype remains to be determined. We shall consider this important question, and the possibilities of developing more powerful diagnostic agents for the identification of malignant disease, in the following sections.

● Diagnostic uses of recombinant DNA

We have seen how gene probes have revolutionized carrier detection and prenatal diagnosis of monogenic disorders. Their place in clinical genetics is now firmly established. However, the diagnostic possibilities of recombinant DNA technology do not stop at inherited diseases. It seems likely that these methods will be used across the whole spectrum of clinical practice over the next few years.

● Diagnostic pathology

DNA analysis is starting to play an important role in diagnostic pathology. The techniques that are of most value include Southern blotting, Northern blotting, *in situ* hybridization and, more recently, the polymerase chain reaction (PCR).

DNA technology is proving valuable for the diagnosis of different forms of leukaemia and lymphoma. For example, it is possible to identify the cells of origin in acute leukaemia using probes for the immunoglobulin and T cell receptor genes. As described in Chapter 3 these genes undergo rearrangements during B and T cell ontogeny. Hence it is feasible not only to identify the cells of origin of lymphoid cancers but to confirm their clonality. The latter is of particular value for studying tissue biopsies in which it is not clear whether a population of lymphocytes is part of the neoplastic process, and therefore clonal, or whether it reflects a reactive infiltration of polyclonal lymphocytes. DNA analysis is also valuable for diagnosing other complex types of leukaemia, for example, chronic myeloid ukaemia in which there is no demonstrable Philadelphia chromosome. In such cases it has become possible to identify products of the *bcr* region (see Chapter 8), even in cases in which a typical Philadelphia chromosome is not present. Gene mapping is also being used, with or without PCR, to identify small populations of residual leukaemic cells, particularly after bone marrow transplantation or ablation therapy for leukaemia.

Another very promising application of DNA screening techniques for the detection of cancer comes from the field of human papillomaviruses. It is now believed that some of this heterogeneous family of viruses play a direct role in the generation of human cancers. For example, epidemiological studies have suggested that specific virus types HPV15 and 18 are present in many squamous cancers of the genital tract. One particularly important area of research in this field is the relationship of human papillomavirus (HPV) to genital cancer. Cancer of the cervix is one of the commonest and most distressing human cancers and is almost certainly preventable. A very high prevalence of HPV16 has been found in cervical cancer biopsy specimens in many parts of the world. Recently, PCR has been used to increase the sensitivity of these studies. Initial analyses of cervical material by PCR suggest that HPV type 16b sequences are found predominantly in women with normal cervices, whereas HPV type 16a has a strong association with malignant transformation. If these observations are confirmed on larger series, subtype-specific HPV DNA screening by PCR may become a valuable adjuvant to cytological examination of cervical smears, and could provide both valuable epidemiological data and, even more importantly, prognostic information.

As the significance of abnormal oncogene activity is clarified, DNA technology will be used increasingly for both the diagnosis of tumours and for determining their prognosis. As described in Chapter 8 it has already been possible to relate the prognosis of certain tumours, e.g. neuroblastoma and breast cancer, to the level of oncogene activation as determined by Northern blotting. Similarly, as more is understood about recessive cancer genes it should be possible to extend this technology to the definition of individuals with a particularly high likelihood of developing such cancers; families with cases of retinoblastoma have already been studied for this purpose. As more is learned about the genes involved in drug resistance it should become easier to develop more logical protocols for cancer chemotherapy.

Quite recently another novel approach to the early detection of cancer has been described. The dominant disorder, multiple endocrine neoplasia type 2a has been assigned to chromosome 10 and RFLPs have been identified which lie close to the gene. It is now possible to identify at risk individuals early in life, which is particularly important as the thyroid cancers associated with the condition are curable. This type of analysis should be applicable to any familial cancer.

● Forensic pathology

The development of mini-satellite DNA probes which hybridize to many hypervariable regions scattered throughout the genome, and which produce DNA fingerprints, was described in Chapter 4. It turns out that these patterns are specific to any one individual. Hence this approach is applicable to paternity testing and for identifying individuals from traces of DNA prepared from blood, hair, or semen obtained at the site of crimes.

There are many ways in which DNA fingerprinting can be adapted for forensic purposes. A number of highly polymorphic sequences can be analysed, or single copy probes or mixtures of single copy probes for such regions can be prepared. Furthermore, it is possible to design individual probes for specific forensic requirements. For example, a Y-specific sequence can be used for sex determination and, even more interestingly, probes can be designed which contain population-specific polymorphisms. Quite recently it has been possible to use the polymerase chain reaction to study polymorphic regions and hence the speed and sensitivity of analysis can be greatly increased. Even more discouragingly for the criminal community, it is now clear that the sources of biological material from which DNA can be extracted are extremely flexible. As well as blood, semen, and any body tissue including bone, adequate amounts of DNA can be obtained from saliva and even from hair roots. Furthermore, DNA is remarkably tough and can be extracted from extremely unpromising material a long time after it has been deposited.

● Infectious disease

DNA probes are already being used widely for the detection of bacteria, viruses, and parasites. This technology can be rendered more sensitive by the use of PCR and, like the use of gene probes for monogenic disorders, can be simplified by the development of dot blot technology. These methods can be also extended, by the use of *in situ* hybridization, to detect specific viral genomes, as for example in infected cell cultures or paraffin-embedded tissue sections. Probe kits are already available for legionella, *Mycoplasma pneumoniae*, *Mycobacterium tuberculosis*, *M. avian*, *M. intracellulare*, *Neisseria gonorrhoeae*, and herpes simplex virus. Over the next few years it will be necessary to test these probes for micro-organisms in clinical practice, and to compare the results in terms of speed, reliability, and cost with more conventional microbiological techniques. By combining automated methods for DNA extraction, PCR, and non-radioactive labelling, it may be possible to automate most of the steps in identifying pathogens.

PCR is also being used for more subtle studies of infectious disease, for example for the detection of the human immunodeficiency virus (HIV) in individuals who could not be determined to be HIV-positive by serological studies, as in infants born to HIV-infected mothers. PCR has also been used to analyse the relationship between retroviruses such as human T cell leukaemia virus type 1 (HTLV 1) and chronic neurological disorders such as tropical spastic paraplegia, and to investigate the association between HTLV 1 or different papillomaviruses with cancer.

Recombinant DNA technology is also being applied to the study of the epidemiology of antibiotic resistance. The pathogenecity and antibiotic sensi-tivity of bacteria is transferred by particular plasmids or bacteriophage. Resistance to some antibiotics arises by the spontaneous mutation of single DNA bases in bacterial chromosomes. For example, reduced sensitivity to streptomy-cin or nalidixic acid results from abnormal function of a DNA gyrase or the 30S ribosomal subunit, respectively. However, most antibiotic resistance is due to the production of variant proteins, usually enzymes, and is associated with the presence of particular plasmids. Although these observations have yet to find clinical application it seems likely that in the future it should be possible, by understanding these mechanisms, to utilize much more logical antibiotic regimes and to monitor patients for the emergence of resistant strains during treatment.

There are many potential advantages in being able to speed up the diagnosis of bacterial, viral, and parasitic illnesses by DNA technology. Currently available culture and biochemical techniques often leave a considerable gap between the onset of an infective illness and its precise diagnosis. The possibility of being able to identify the organisms, or their products, by the extremely sensitive techniques of recombinant DNA technology should provide a solution to at least some of these problems. This will include not only the direct identification of infectious agents, but, as described later in this chapter, the many cytokines and other molecules through which the pathological changes associated with severe infection are generated.

● The treatment of disease

Recombinant DNA technology has already opened up a large biotechnology industry which holds considerable promise for the future. While many of the companies involved have found it difficult to produce agents of immediate clinical benefit as quickly as they would have liked, enough progress has been made over the last few years to suggest that, in the long term, we should expect the generation of many valuable therapeutic agents.

● Human proteins

The most obvious application of recombinant DNA technology in the therapeutic field is the production of human proteins in micro-organisms. The first success in this field was the production of human insulin. This product, made available through fermentation of *E. coli*, is now being used to treat insulin-dependent diabetes. Similarly, human growth hormone produced in micro-organisms is being used to treat the various forms of growth hormone deficiency. The latter treatment came into its own when suspicions were aroused that a few patients who had received growth hormone of animal origin might have developed a clinical picture similar to Jakob–Creutzfeldt disease, a dementing disorder that is thought to result from infection with a slow virus.

Because of the development of AIDS following the use of infected blood there has been great interest in the genesis of blood products by recombinant DNA technology. Human clotting factor VIII, a deficiency of which causes haemophilia, has been produced successfully in this way. A number of other blood proteins have also been manufactured in micro-organisms, notably tissue plasminogen activator which is used for the treatment of myocardial infarction and other conditions associated with intravascular thrombosis.

One of the most spectacular success stories is the commercial development of recombinant erythropoietin. This hormone is normally produced in the kidney in response to hypoxia and is necessary for red cell production. A deficiency of this agent in patients with chronic renal disease produces severe anaemia. Patients with the anaemia of renal disease who receive recombinant erythropoietin show a rapid rise in their haemoglobin level. So far this treatment has been associated with very few side-effects and has transformed the lives of many patients receiving renal dialysis who, before it was available, survived only on regular blood transfusion. It remains to be seen whether erythropoietin will find a role in treating other forms of anaemia.

Another early success story in the use of recombinant DNA for the generation of therapeutic agents has been in the field of thrombolytic therapy. One of the major fail-safe systems to deal with unwanted thrombosis is the activation of plasminogen to an active enzyme plasmin which breaks down fibrin to soluble degradation products. There are a number of activators of plasminogen. The naturally occurring activator, called streptokinase, has been found to be a valuable agent for the treatment of myocardial infarction and pulmonary embolus following deep vein thrombosis. Because it is produced by streptococci it is antigenic and hence may cause reactions when it is used for the first time to treat patients, and it is very difficult to use it on a second occasion. There is a human protein, called tissue-type plasminogen activator (t-PA), which is a trypsin-like serine protease. t-PA is a poor plasminogen activator in the absence of fibrin, but it binds specifically to fibrin and activates plasminogen at the fibrin surface several hundred-fold more efficiently than in the circulation. Human t-PA has been made by recombinant DNA technology and large-scale trials are under way to compare its efficiency with that of streptokinase in the treatment of coronary thrombosis and venous thrombosis. There seems little doubt that in the future other human antithrombotic or thrombolytic agents will be prepared by recombinant DNA technology.

Several of the other haemopoietic growth factors described later in this chapter were developed for therapeutic trial using recombinant DNA technology. The rationale behind these studies is to attempt to shorten the period of neutropenia, and hence susceptibility to infection, following cancer chemotherapy with drugs that damage the bone marrow. G-CSF has been given to patients with malignant disease with a resulting rise in the neutrophil count; there have been very few side-effects in initial trials. Similarly, patients who had received GM-CSF for a variety of clinical indications have had a variable increase in neutrophils, monocytes, and eosinophils. At high doses this agent produces more side-effects. There have already been several trials of the use of G-CSF and GM-CSF in the haematological malignancies although their role in treating these conditions is not yet fully worked out; there is always the danger of stimulating leukaemic cell populations.

Currently, the place of the various colony stimulating factors in clinical practice has to be defined. It may well be that used in combination they may increase haemopoietic recovery after cancer chemotherapy or bone marrow transplantation, and they may have a limited role in treating some of the hypoplastic disorders of the bone marrow. For example, recent studies suggest that some forms of congenital neutropenia may respond to G-CSF.

There is also considerable interest in the potential therapeutic value of some of the immune mediators that are described later in this chapter. For example, the observation that interleukin-2 (IL-2) receptors are expressed solely by antigen-activated T cells has suggested that immunosuppression might be mediated using antibodies against part of the receptor. Indeed, it has been possible to improve the survival of cardiac allografts using this approach. Even more encouragingly, the development of experimental autoimmune diabetes mellitus and systemic lupus erythematosus has been suppressed in the same way. Il-2 has also been used to generate large numbers of tumour antigen-specific cytotoxic lymphocytes as an approach to adaptive immunotherapy. Stimulation of an immune response via the IL-2 receptor is also under clinical investigation as a potential form of immunotherapy for cancer; IL-2 has also been used as an adjuvant for stimulation of the immune response to vaccines.

At the time of writing all these studies on the potential therapeutic actions of IL-2 are very much at a preliminary stage, but already enough has been learnt to suggest that this will be a very profitable area for the development of novel immunosuppressive and immunoenhancing technologies in the future.

In Chapter 7 we saw how autoimmune disease is the result of persistent activation of T cells by self-antigens. Like all antigens recognized by T cells they consist of small peptide fragments held in the presenting sites of HLA class I or II molecules. We also saw how, because of the apparent homogeneity of the T cell receptors that generate some autoimmune diseases, it is possible to treat experimental autoimmune disease by immunizing animals with peptides based on the sequence of these receptors. Another approach is to provide substitute peptides which will remove the stimulus to the particular T cell populations. No doubt as more is learnt about these complex interactions it may be possible to develop approaches to the management of autoimmune disease.

Another family of regulatory proteins that have been obtained by recombinant DNA technology and which, despite our ignorance of their precise physiological role, have been given to patients in preliminary trials are the interferons. We shall describe current research in this field later in this chapter. The therapeutic possibilities that have been studied mainly concern their potential as inhibitors of the growth of human cancers. Although preliminary trials with many of the common cancers have been disappointing a few success stories are emerging. It turns out, for example, that human interferon α (IFN-α) can produce remissions in a high proportion of patients with hairy-cell leukaemia, a B-cell tumour in which there is massive enlargement of the spleen together with morphologically distinct lymphocytes in the peripheral blood. The interferons may have other uses in haematological malignancies, although so far these are less well defined. Another quite remarkable chance observation is that human IFN-γ seems to be active in overcoming the genetic defect in neutrophil function which underlies at least some cases of chronic granulomatous disease (see Chapter 6).

In this section we have touched briefly on just a few of the therapeutic agents that have been produced by recombinant DNA technology and which seem to have a promise for use in clinical practice. With a few exceptions, where the true physiological role of agents was understood, this field seems to have tried to run before it could walk. In other words the functions of many of the genetically engineered mediators that have been given to patients in preliminary trials are not fully understood. In a later section we will review briefly the state of play of research directed towards a better understanding of the physiological and pathological activities of some of these proteins.

● Vaccine production

The development of antibiotics and the extraordinary success stories following the vaccination programmes for smallpox and poliomyelitis have tended to lull us into the idea that infectious disease is no longer a serious problem. This is not helped by the fact that the problems of the developing world do not loom high on the curricula of many Western medical schools. Globally, however, infectious disease remains the major killer and the emergence of new epidemics like AIDS is a reminder that novel agents are always just around the corner. Respiratory infections are still the major killer in childhood, both in the developed and developing world. Rotavirus infection and its resultant diarrhoeal illnesses kills millions of children each year. Other major killers of the third world include hepatitis, malaria, schistosomiasis, and leishmaniasis, to mention only a few. In addition to AIDS there is a worrying resurgence of other sexually transmitted diseases. It is clear, therefore, that infectious diseases present a major challenge for the future.

Recently, there has been considerable interest in the development of vaccines, stemming mainly from advances in recombinant DNA technology and protein engineering. These techniques have made it possible to analyse the genomes of pathogens as a major step in defining important aspects of antigen structure and heterogeneity. They have also facilitated the expression of proteins from different pathogens in heterologous systems such as *E. coli* and yeast and have raised the possibility that we may be able to develop new generations of live vaccines by genetic engineering directed towards attenuation of strains.

Recombinant DNA technology provides a number of approaches to vaccine production. Having defined good candidate antigens it is possible to clone the appropriate genes and express them in animal or insect cells or in yeast. One of the early successes has been the production of a vaccine against hepatitis B. This has enormous implications for world health because the virus, as well as causing liver damage in many populations, plays a major role in the development of liver cancer, or hepatoma. Initially it was impossible to grow this small DNA virus but the problem was solved by cloning the gene for the appropriate antigen into yeast. So far, the vaccine appears to be safe and effective. The engineered yeast cell contains the information for only one viral gene and hence there is no way that a complete virus or any other infectious agent can arise during the production of the vaccine. No doubt many other agents will be produced using yeast cloning vectors.

Other approaches to the development of vaccines, which involve a combination of recombinant DNA technology and protein engineering, are summarized in Table 37. They include the synthesis of antigens or fusion products by bacteria, the production of anti-idiotypes, and the generation of small peptides which, up to a certain size, involves chemical or enzymic synthesis. Synthetic peptide vaccines offer many potential advantages. First, they should be safer to use than vaccines produced in other ways. Second, the best vaccines of this type would contain only those sequences of a particular protein which would stimulate the most desirable immune response. Finally, they should be particularly stable. The main question, of course, is how to define the particular amino acid sequence that will provide these properties. Although in some cases we may be able to make an educated guess this will not always be possible. One way round this problem is to prepare a monoclonal antibody with the desired property, viral neutralization for example, and then to synthesize the peptide to which it binds most tightly. A number of other approaches including crystallographic analysis of the protein and computer modelling may be feasible.

Table 37. *Approaches to vaccine production*

Live (attenuated)
Inactivated (killed)
Genetically engineered proteins
Synthetic peptides
Anti-idiotype antibodies
Genetically engineered attenuation

When we consider the problems of developing vaccines against some of the world's major killers, for example, trypanosomiasis and malaria, the difficulties are quite staggering. For example, trypanosomes show enormous antigenic variation which seems to reflect the presence in its genome of hundreds of different genes, each encoding a different surface glycoprotein and each with a different primary protein structure. Clearly this parasite is perfectly designed to escape the host's immune defences. Interestingly, although even natural resistance to malaria is not very effective, this particular parasite does not seem to have developed a system akin to that of the trypanosome to avoid immune defences. Thus although is has many different antigens that are expressed at different stages of its life cycle, most of the genes that have been studied so far are only present in one copy.

Many different malarial antigens have been defined at different stages of the parasite life-cycle and their genes have been cloned and the structure of their products determined. Interestingly, many of the secreted antigens of the malarial parasite contain blocks of repeated amino acid sequences. It has been suggested that these molecules act as 'immunological decoys' to overburden the immune defence system and that the repeat sequences might therefore act as immuno-stimulators. A variety of antigens have been genetically engineered or developed as peptide fragments in the hope of producing a vaccine against either the invasive or blood stages of the malarial parasite, so far without much success.

● Combining recombinant DNA technology with protein engineering

It seems very likely that major therapeutic advances will stem from combining recombinant DNA technology with protein engineering. For example, there is much interest in trying to design tumour-specific antibodies with the objective of either killing tumours directly or attaching diagnostic markers or chemothera-peutic agents to them so that they can be targeted directly at cancer cells. Already, a variety of monoclonal antibodies have been generated with this aim in mind.

One of the major technical problems in using rodent monoclonal antibodies as 'magic bullets' to kill or image tumours is that the foreign immunoglobulin can elicit an antiglobulin response which may interfere with therapy or cause allergic or immune-complex hypersensitivity reactions. Ideally, human antibodies should be used and it would be particularly advantageous to be able to manufacture human monoclonal antibodies of the desired specificity. However, it has proved very difficult to make such antibodies by the conventional route of immortalization of human antibody-producing cells. Recently a novel approach to this problem has been developed which combines elements of recombinant DNA technology and protein engineering; in essence, 'humanizing' of monoclon-al antibodies is involved.

This remarkable *tour de force* has been carried out in the following way. Antibody genes have been transfected into lymphoid cells, and the encoded antibodies expressed and secreted. By some ingenious genetic engineering, genomic exons have been shuffled and simple chimeric antibodies with mouse or rat variable regions and human constant regions have been made. Such 'mixed' molecules have at least two advantages over mouse antibodies. First, the effector functions can be tailored as desired. For example, it turns out that human IgG1 and IgG3 are the most effective IgG isotypes for complement and cell-mediated lysis, and therefore for killing tumour cells. Second, the use of human rather than mouse isotypes should minimize the antiglobulin responses during therapy by avoiding the production of anti-isotypic antibodies.

These principles have been used to reshape human heavy and light chains towards binding the Campath-1 antigen, which is expressed on most lympho-cytes and monocytes but not on other blood cells, including haemopoietic stem cells. The idea was to reshape a human IgG1 antibody by introducing hypervariable regions from the heavy and light chain variable domains of a rat antibody directed against human lymphocytes. It turns out that this reshaped human antibody was as effective as the rat antibody in complement lysis and more effective in cell mediated lysis of human lymphocytes. The anti-Campath-1 antibody has been already subjected to limited clinical trial and shown to cause a reduction of tumour size in patients with lymphoid malignancies. This ingenious approach has a variety of other applications including the development of anti-idiotype vaccines and, by incorporating toxins or their subunits, engineering specific immunotoxins.

The 'humanizing' of monoclonal antibodies is just one example of the way in which the development of therapeutic agents is likely to go in the future. There is no doubt that as the structure and regulation of surface molecules including receptors becomes better understood at the molecular level it should be possible to tailor-make a variety of pharmaceutical agents. With the increasingly sophisticated approaches for analysing protein structure and the functional properties of receptors and their ligands by computer graphics modelling, it seems likely that more new classes of therapeutic agents will be developed. So far the use of protein engineering has been restricted largely to modifying specific interactions as the way of studying the mechanisms of enzyme action. Techniques for site-directed mutagenesis are well advanced and it is becoming increasingly easy to construct mutant proteins for analysing structure/function relationships. It should not be long before altered proteins will be used for providing enzymes with novel properties and for use as highly specific therapeutic agents.

● Other areas of research in human molecular and cell biology of future clinical relevance

There are many other applications of recombinant DNA technology which, while currently confined to basic biological research, may have important implications for medical practice in the future. In this final section we will examine just a few of them.

● The regulation of cell growth, differentiation, and function

The idea that the regulation of the production and differentiation of cells is controlled by specific molecules is not new. As long ago as 1906 Paul Carnot suggested that a humoral factor might control the production of red blood cells, but it was another 70 years before the hormone involved, erythropoietin, was finally isolated. During the 1920s attempts were made to isolate growth-promoting factors from the pituitary gland, and at about the same time Alexis Carrel recognized that cells in culture grow more rapidly in the presence of tissue extract. It was natural, therefore, that the cancer field would concentrate much of its efforts on studies of the regulation of growth, and by the 1940s there was considerable interest in the relationship of the neuronal regulation of tumour growth. In the early 1950s it was discovered that certain tumours secrete a substance that stimulates nerve growth, and that the mouse salivary gland is a very rich source of this factor and another that stimulates the growth of epidermal cells, later called epidermal growth factor. By the 1970s the amino acid sequence of these two factors had been determined.

Work carried out between the late 1920s and 1970s led to the characterization of at least one class of serum growth factors which seemed to be derived mainly from platelets. The purification of platelet-derived growth factor (PDGF) was finally achieved in the late 1970s and in the early 1980s this work was linked up with the oncogene field following the discovery that PDGF and v-*sis* are essentially the same molecule.

The story of the discovery and isolation of other growth factors also covers many years of slow progress. For example, it has been known since 1924 that some serum proteins have insulin-like growth activity. Eventually it was found that there is a family of proteins, now known as insulin-like growth factors or somatomedins, which are stronger mitogens than insulin, although not such powerful activators of cellular metabolism. Similarly, a powerful mitogenic substance was isolated from brain in the late 1930s but it was not until the late 1970s that fibroblast growth factor (FGF) was isolated and purified from neuronal tissue.

One of the most remarkable recent achievements in the analysis of the regulation of growth and differentiation of cells has been the isolation, purification, cloning, and functional characterization of a family of proteins, or cytokines, which are the products of the cells of the haemopoietic system, including granulocytes, lymphocytes, monocytes, and macrophages. Because these regulatory molecules have diverse effects that often involve a wide variety of cell types of the haemopoietic system, a complex and constantly changing nomenclature has grown up round them. A partial list of these cytokines is shown in Table 38. Some of these molecules have a clearly defined role in the regulation of red cell or granulocyte production. Others, lymphokines, are polypeptide products of activated lymphocytes which participate in a variety of cellular responses, in particular the regulation of the immune system. Again, several lymphokines have been named according to their biological effect, B-cell differentiating factor for example. However, many of them have more than one biological role and therefore a nomenclature has been developed that uses the term 'interleukin' followed by a particular number. To complicate matters further, some lymphokines have retained their original name, the interferons for example. Enough is known already to suggest that these families of regulatory molecules will have important medical applications in the future. In the sections that follow we shall briefly examine some of the better defined haemopoietic growth factors and interleukins as likely candidates.

Haemopoietic growth factors

The different cells of the blood are the products of multipotential, self-generating stem cells. It turns out that the regulation of proliferation and differentiation of blood cells is controlled by a family of specific glycoproteins which can be

Table 38. *Some regulatory proteins of the haemopoietic/macrophage system*

Protein	Action
Erythropoietin	Red cell production
GM-CSF	Promotes granulocyte and macrophage colonies
G-CSF	Promotes granulocyte colonies
M-CSF	Promotes macrophage colonies
Interleukin 1	Activates resting T cells. Cofactor for haemopoietic growth factors. Many others
Interleukin 2	Growth factor for activated T cells
Interleukin 3 (multi-CSF)	Promotes multi-lineage haemopoietic progenitors
Interleukin 4	Growth factor for activated B cells
Interleukin 5	Stimulates proliferation of eosinophil precursors
Interleukin 6	Many actions including interferon-like, B-cell stimulation, hepatocyte stimulation. . . .
Interferon (α and β)	Antiviral. Class I antigen expression. Antiproliferation etc.
Interferon (γ)	Induces class I and II antigens, macrophage-activation etc.
Tumour necrosis factor	Wide range (see text)
Transforming growth factor (β)	See text

identified and monitored by their ability to form colonies of maturing progeny cells of a particular type in semi-solid culture media. Because of this property these glycoproteins are called colony stimulating factors (CSFs). The CSFs are involved in the control of the granulocyte-macrophage lineages. For historical reasons the humoral regulator of red cell production is called erythropoietin.

Over the last few years it has been possible to isolate and purify a number of haemopoietic growth factors, to clone and sequence their genes and pin-point their chromosomal locations and, most recently, to isolate and characterize the specific receptors with which they interact. A partial list of the haemopoietic growth factors, together with their functions, is given in Table 38.

A simplified model of the developmental pattern of the haemopoietic cells, starting from the pluripotential haemopoietic stem cell, is shown in Fig. 94. It might be helpful to readers not versed in the arcane nomenclature of experimental haematology if I digress briefly to (hopefully) clarify it for them. When haematologists examine blood or marrow they see mature red or white blood cells or their immediate precursors. It turns out, however, that this is only the tip of the iceberg. Once it became possible to grow haemopoietic progenitors in semi-solid culture media it soon became apparent that there are families or earlier progenitors which are already committed to becoming white or red blood cells. These can be defined by their ability to form colonies and hence are called colony

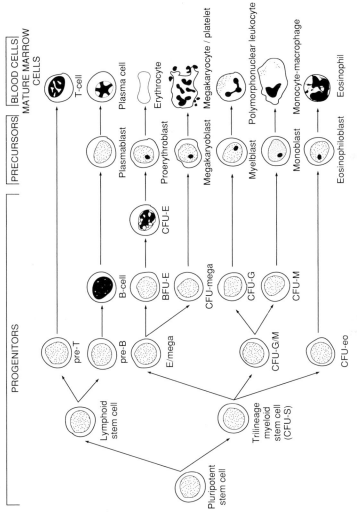

Figure 94. The maturation sequence of progenitor cells that give rise to different mature blood cells.
The properties of the different progenitors are described in the text.

forming units, CFU; they are further characterized by the type of cell to which they are destined to become. For example, CFU-G is a cell that is already committed to the extent that it will produce only granulocytes; similarly CFU-E is the designation given to a cell in the earlier stages of the erythroid series. However it turns out that there are cells that are less committed; for example, CFU-GM is the designation given to cells that still have the capacity to form either granulocytes or macrophages. It follows, therefore, that haemopoiesis is a stepwise process during which the progeny of pluripotential stem cells pass through a series of stages of commitment and differentiation towards becoming the mature cells of the peripheral blood. The new techniques of cell culture allow us, albeit rather artifically, to study the different stages in this pathway and the various regulatory molecules involved.

As indicated in Table 38, the different haemopoietic growth factors have variable degrees of specificity with regard to their target cells. For example, IL-3 acts on all progenitors whereas G-CSF and M-CSF seem to be more specific for CFU-G and CFU-M, that is pure granulocyte and macrophage colonies respectively; GM-CSF is active against all progenitors. Erythropoietin stimulates primarily the different erythroid progenitors although it seems to have some action on platelet precursors. Three of the haemopoietic growth factors are the products of genes that form a tight cluster on the long arm of chromosome 5, whereas that for G-CSF is on chromosome 17.

It appears that the CSFs have multiple biological functions; as well as their proliferative capacity they seem to mediate at least three other activities which may involve intracellular signalling pathways. They are involved in the maintenance of membrane integrity and cell viability and in the commitment to irreversible differentiation. Furthermore, they cause functional stimulation of mature granulocytes and macrophages as measured by increased phagocytosis, superoxide production and, in the case of macrophages, cytotoxicity, and the production of a number of other molecules including interleukins, interferon, tumour necrosis factor, and plasminogen activator. Of course, many of these actions may well be 'downstream' from the primary action of these molecules but it is quite clear that their action results in functional differentiation of various haemopoietic cells in addition to stimulation of their proliferation.

Haemopoiesis is, therefore, regulated by a family of molecules with varying degrees of specificity and cross-reactivity. This must allow for maximum flexibility of proliferative response, although the precise way in which this hierarchy of molecules functions to control blood production remains to be described. Similarly, although there is increasing evidence for the existence of molecules that may inhibit haemopoiesis, and thus function in negative feedback loops for the regulation of blood cell production, they have not yet been fully characterized. Valuable information will undoubtedly come from further study of the CSF receptors. For example, although the CSFs do not show cross competition for receptor binding it turns out that there is a remarkable hierarchical sequence of down modulation of receptors in this system; the occupancy of IL-3 receptors seems to down modulate all other receptors.

Similarly, GM-CSF receptor occupancy down modulates G-CSF and M-CSF receptors. Interestingly, the M-CSF receptor is structurally related and probably identical to the c-*fms* cellular oncogene product, a situation with intriguing similarities to the v-*erbB* cellular oncogene which encodes a protein that is a truncated form of the epidermal growth factor receptor.

Lymphokines and related mediators

The identification of this family of molecules, which subserve a wide variety of activities involving the cellular immune and haemopoetic systems, has been a saga of conflicting nomenclature. However, the structure of several of these molecules has been clearly defined and some of their important activities characterized (Table 38). For example, interleukin I (IL-1) is involved in T cell activation including the production of IL-2 receptors and the synthesis of IL-2. In addition, it appears to be a pyrogen, induces the synthesis of acute phase proteins in liver cells, and enhances collagen synthesis and cell division. It also acts synergistically with haemopoietic growth factors, possibly by enhancing the expression of their receptors.

T cell growth and activation requires the production of another molecule of this class, called IL-2. The synthesis of IL-2 seems to require actual cell-to-cell contact between monocytes and T cells. Following the interaction of IL-2 with its receptor, T cells divide and secrete a number of other soluble lymphokines including gamma interferon, B-cell growth factors, and IL-3, all of which are important for the regulation of the activity of both the immune and haemopoietic systems. The discovery of IL-2 has had an enormous impact on immunology because it has made it possible to grow antigen-specific T cell lines.

Recent studies on the mechanisms of interaction of IL-2 with its receptor have started to throw some light on the regulation of the T cell immune response. Resting T cells do not produce IL-2, nor, incidentally, are they able to respond to IL-2 when it is added exogenously. This suggests that signals coming from the T cell antigen-receptor complex somehow co-ordinate the transcriptional activation of both the IL-2 gene and the genes encoding the IL-2 receptors. If this notion is correct, it follows that the concentration of IL-2 and the expression of functional IL-2 receptors are the variables that ultimately determine how long clonal expansion occurs after antigen stimulation. It appears that IL-2 receptor synthesis continues while antigen is present and declines after it is cleared.

As mentioned earlier, IL-3 plays an important role in the regulation of haemopoietic stem cell division and differentiation; its former name, multi-CSF, reflects this particular activity. Interleukins 4 and 5 were identified by their ability to potentiate the production of mast cells and eosinophils or B lymphocyte precursors. It now seems likely that IL-5 has at least two major functions, the activation of mature eosinophils and the induction of B cell maturation. Interleukin 6 was initially characterized by its effect on cells of B lymphoid lineage but more recently IL-6 was found to have effects on the self-renewal of haemopoietic stem cells, at least *in vitro* and in combination with IL-3. It is now clear that IL-6 plays a central role in mediating the 'acute phase' response to a wide range of infections.

The cloning and sequencing of the genes for the different interleukins, and the ability to obtain pure molecules in large quantities, offers a number of therapeutic possibilities for the future, some of which were considered earlier in this chapter. However, it should be remembered that their broad biological activities against many different cell types will always have to be borne in mind when attempting to define therapeutic indications.

Tumour necrosis factor

The extraordinary diversity of activity of some of these regulatory molecules is well exemplified by recent studies of another macrophage-produced mediator called tumour necrosis factor (TNF), or cachectin. This molecule has a remarkable history because its broad range of activity led to its discovery by two completely different routes. On the one hand, as TNF, it was isolated during attempts to understand the haemorrhagic necrosis of tumours which may occur in association with acute bacterial infections. On the other, as cachectin, it was discovered quite independently as part of research into the basis of the progressive wasting, or cachexia, which occurs in cattle with trypanosomal infection. The molecule was purified independently from these two routes; when a mouse TNF cDNA was cloned it turned out to have exactly the same predicted amino acid sequence as cachectin!

It turns out that TNF has an enormously wide range of biological activities. Macrophages are the main source, and TNF production is evoked by bacterial and virus infection; the main inducers are lipopolysaccharides. Among its many effects TNF stimulates the activation of neutrophils and promotes the production of IL-1 from endothelial cells. It also causes leucocytes to adhere to these cells and augments the expression of the IL-2 receptor on lymphocytes. Like IL-1 it also promotes the production and release of various acute phase proteins from liver cells. In short, it seems to be a general mediator of inflammatory responses.

There is increasing evidence that the production of TNF may have some deleterious effects. Its wasting action is probably mediated through suppression of the enzyme lipoprotein lipase. TNF may also be involved in generating some of the manifestations of endotoxic shock including the initiation of intravascular coagulation and promotion of the adherence of activated leucocytes to endothelial cells, and in causing the anaemia associated with a wide range of infections. There is some experimental evidence that the administration of monoclonal antibodies against TNF can protect animals against many of the clinical manifestations of endotoxaemia.

Interferons (INFs)

This family of cytokines has also had a chequered career. It was discovered in

1957; the term interferon was used to describe the fact that these molecules are produced by cells in response to viral infection and can protect other cells from attack by a wide range of viruses. The early years of interferon research were bedevilled by difficulties with production and purification, a problem that was overcome finally by the use of recombinant DNA technology.

The interferons are a multigene family, the products of which can be divided into three main types, INF-α, INF-β, and INF-γ. They are the products of macrophages; specific receptors for each type are widely distributed throughout the body. They have a remarkably wide series of effects on cellular function including conferring resistance to infection by many DNA and RNA viruses, modulation of the immune response by affecting both B and T cell proliferation and growth, fever induction, and the inhibition of growth of certain tumours. Indeed, the scope of their cellular activities is only just starting to be appreciated and very little is known about how they mediate many of the cellular responses that they produce. The therapeutic possibilities of interferons were outlined earlier in this chapter.

Transforming growth factors

Transforming growth factors (TGFs) are small peptides which were discovered initially because of their ability to induce transformation of non-neoplastic cells in culture. Subsequently they were found to be heterogeneous and at least two types, TGF-α and TGF-β, were identified both in normal and in neoplastic tissue. They are distinct peptides with their own unique receptor systems.

More recently it has been found that the TGFs are not restricted in function to promoting cell growth. Rather, they appear to play a much broader role in regulating inflammatory responses, the immune system, and tissue repair. For example it has been found that TGF-β, or rather a subtype named TGF-β1, is generated by haemopoietic cells. The TGFs seem to follow the general rule of many of the cytokines in that their activities are remarkably pleiotropic. However, they are of particular interest in that their ability to cause proliferation of fibrous tissue in the process of wound healing could, if it occurred in an uncontrolled way, provide the basis for a number of diseases that are characterized by pathological fibrosis.

Summary

It is clear that the cytokine families represent an extraordinarily diverse series of regulatory molecules which must have evolved with the increasing specialization of cells of the haemopoietic and immune systems. Many have extremely pleiotropic actions, although how much of this is primary and how much secondary and 'downstream' from their central mode of action remains to be worked out.

Recombinant DNA technology has raised the expectation that clinicians will, in a few years time, have many of these molecules in the hospital pharmacy. As mentioned earlier in this chapter, a few of them have already been given to patients, not always for very logical reasons. A great deal more knowledge is required of their primary functions, and how they interact with each other, before their place in clinical practice can be defined.

● Clinical neurology and the neurosciences

Chronic neurological diseases are among the most intractable in clinical practice and very little is known about their aetiology. Some of them are single gene disorders and are described elsewhere in this book. Over the next few years it is likely that many of these genes will be isolated and their function determined. As well as providing us with valuable information about the pathogenesis of these disorders it is likely that, as we come to understand how they are mediated, we shall learn a great deal about the normal function of the nervous system. As described in Chapter 7, the methods of recombinant DNA have much to offer in the field of dementia and other degenerative disorders of the nervous system.

The application of recombinant DNA technology to the neurosciences does not stop here. Undoubtedly this will be one of the most rewarding areas in human biology over the next few years. Already considerable progress has been made; for example it has been possible to construct cDNA libraries derived from brain mRNAs. Studies along these lines, and in which brain mRNAs have been compared with those of other organs, suggest that about 50 per cent of rat brain mRNAs are expressed exclusively in the brain. These data suggest that approximately 30 000 genes are expressed in the rat brain, and a start has been made in identifying the functions and products of at least some of them.

Neurotransmitters and neural receptors

Considerable progress has been made in understanding the genetic regulation of some of the important neurotransmitters and other mediators in the brain. Most of these molecules are peptides, many of which are derived from large precursor proteins. Several of the genes for these proteins have been analysed. It turns out that alternative RNA processing is a common mechanism for determining tissue specificity of patterns of peptide synthesis in the nervous system. For example, the calcitonin gene generates two messenger RNAs, one encoding the precursor of a novel neuropeptide, the other the precursor of the hormone calcitonin; the neuropeptide predominates in the nervous system.

Progress has also been made towards an understanding of neural receptors and their various ligands. For example, much is now known about the structure and the genetic control of the acetylcholine receptor and a start has been made in determining its allosteric activities and the sensitive transcriptional controls that underlie its function. Similar information is becoming available about the closely related muscarinic acetylcholine receptor, found in neurons and in cardiac and smooth muscle. The genes for the endogenous opioid peptides and their receptors have been cloned and their structure determined, and progress has been made in understanding the diverse family of molecules exemplified by sustance P and its related peptides. This family of neurotransmitters, or modulators of neuro-transmission, are involved with an extremely diverse series of functions ranging from salivary secretion to the transmission of pain signals. It turns out that substance P peptide sequences are expressed in three different mRNAs which are generated from one gene by differential RNA splicing. Furthermore, as many as three other related peptides can be generated from these precursors by differential post-translational processing, thus providing another example of the principle that many mediators in the nervous system achieve their remarkable diversity by differential precursor RNA splicing and translation. The specificity of peptide responses appears to be the result of selective receptor subtype expression.

Transport systems

Equally rapid advances are being made in the definition of the various sodium co-transport systems which mediate the movement of sodium ions and one or more inorganic or organic solutes across plasma membranes. Such transport may be either in opposite directions (antiport) with ions such as H^+ and Ca^{2+}, or in the same direction (synport) as with the co-transport of sugars, amino acids, and neurotransmitters. Many of these transporter molecules are intrinsic membrane proteins and considerable progress has been made in isolating them and the genes that control their synthesis. This area of research has important possibilities for the study of diseases of the nervous system, as well as in many other clinical settings; the relationship between transport systems of this type and hypertension was considered in an earlier chapter.

Regulatory peptides

As is the case in the haemopoietic and immune systems, there has been a veritable explosion of information about the role of different peptide regulatory factors in the nervous system. There is now unequivocal evidence that nerve growth factor (NGF) plays an important role in neuronal maturation and regulation in both the central and peripheral nervous systems. Messenger RNA for the receptor for NGF is expressed at its highest levels in the forebrain, an observation of particular interest in view of the cholinergic neurons of this region and their projection targets in the frontal cortex and hippocampus, areas that appear to be a major focus of damage in Alzheimer's disease. A number of other specific regulatory peptides, including brain-derived neurotrophic factor and glial-derived nexin have also been isolated although their precise function remains to be determined. Similarly, it has been found that astrocytes produce several other regulatory proteins including insulin-like growth factors, platelet-derived growth factor, and epidermal growth factor. The precise functions of these molecules in the nervous system remain to be determined.

Developmental studies

Even more remarkably, some insights are being gained into the mechanisms of development of the nervous system, which is an area of great clinical potential. Some of the most valuable information in this field has come from studies of the glial progenitor cells. This work exemplifies the type of progress that is likely to be made in understanding the developmental biology of the nervous system in the near future.

It turns out that the development of the rat optic nerve is an extraordinarily valuable experimental system. The central player in this model, which involves cells forming the connective tissue scaffolding of the nervous system, is a cell called a type 1 astrocyte which has properties in common with fibroblasts. These cells develop in the optic nerve and appear to co-ordinate further proliferation and lineage induction of a number of other more specialized cells. One of these is known as the O-2A cell because it can differentiate into either an oligodendrocyte or a type 2 astrocyte, the latter being a more differentiated cell that has processes. It turns out that type 1 astrocytes stimulate the proliferation of O-2A cells by secreting platelet-derived growth factor. This in turn drives an intrinsic cellular clock that appears to count cell divisions and hence sets the timing of oligodendrocyte differentiation. Once this process is underway it continues in the absence of any other cells or external growth factors. On the other hand, the production of type 2 astrocytes requires the intervention of an exogenous factor from serum or developing optic nerve which has been found to be a small protein called ciliary neutrotrophic factor. These elegant studies show how regulatory molecules may fire cells into various steps of differentiation, after which they may go it alone, as it were, by means of an intrinsic regulatory time clock.

The ultimate questions in neurobiology, of course, concern the relationship between mental states and behavioural patterns, and the chemistry of the brain that must, in some way, generate them. Already some progress has been made in correlating molecular events with learning. For example, in fish or animals it has been possible to correlate learning activities with the increased production of specific sets of glycoproteins. Using appropriate antibodies it has been possible to define the sites of synthesis of these molecules. It turns out that they are probably identical to the so-called brain growth associated proteins. It follows, therefore, that learning may occur by the same mechanism as growth, that is by progressive elongation and branching of axons and dendrites. Studies of DNA synthesis have shown that most of the increase in human brain weight after the age of 2 years must be in the weight per neuron. The latter is mainly a function of the arbor of dendrites and axons. This suggests that increasing weight must reflect mainly an increased and altered arborization of existing neurons. Since there is a dramatic decline in DNA synthesis in the brain after the age of 2 years it follows that few new brain cells appear after that age. Therefore the structural basis for the development of intellectual skills must reflect alterations of the unprogrammed connections of neurons which occur during further development.

Work in nematodes has shown a remarkable degree of plasticity within the developing nervous system. For example, if certain neurons with defined connections are removed adjacent remaining neurons of the same class send out axons to supply the missing connections. This suggests that there must be signals instructing the remaining neurons to ramify to fill the roles of their missing fellows. This phenomenon does not occur in the adult nematodes. There is increasing evidence of the existence of molecules that inhibit brain growth by a process that is under genetic control. A start has been made in isolating and defining some of these regulatory factors.

Cellular oncogenes in the nervous system

Recent studies of the *fos* oncogene may have important implications for the neurosciences. This gene was first discovered as the oncogene of two closely related mouse viruses that cause osteogenic sarcoma, FBJ and FBR (the term *fos* is derived from FBJ or FBR osteogenic sarcoma viruses). This is a particularly interesting gene because it may well be involved in the regulation of cell division; a variety of growth factors have a stimulatory effect on *fos*. Recent studies suggest that *fos* activity elicits the passage of cells from a resting into an actively dividing phase of the cell cycle. However, the *fos* oncogene has a broader scope of action than this. In the present context it has been noted that the expression of the gene is stimulated by agents that trigger nerve cell activity; *fos* is induced when neuroactive agents open channels that allow calcium ions to move into nerve cells.

The activation of *fos* by nerve cell stimulation occurs *in vivo*. For example, there is a sharp increase in *fos* gene activity when mice are treated with metrazole, a drug that causes seizures similar to those of human epilepsy. Following exposure to this drug *fos* protein synthesis occurs in nerve tracks as a phenomenon that occurs more slowly than the seizures; it is detected about 15 minutes after metrazole treatment and persists for up to 3 hours, whereas the seizures begin within a minute or two and stop after 30 minutes. It has been suggested that *fos* protein is in some way involved in the mediation of long-term adaptation of nerve cells to metrazole stimulation. Even more interestingly, it has been found that a possible target for *fos* regulation is the gene encoding a receptor for the inhibitory neurotransmitter gamma amino butyric acid (GABA). There is also a possibility that *fos* gene expression may contribute to the changes that are necessary for memory function.

Slow viruses, prions, and degenerative diseases of the nervous system

This brief summary of a few areas of current excitement in the application of molecular biology to the study of the nervous system would not be complete without a brief mention of a particularly novel area of research that may have very important clinical implications in the future.

Many of the so-called degenerative disorders of the nervous system occur at particular times of life. For example, multiple sclerosis usually starts in the second or third decade while the Gerstmann–Sträussler syndrome (GSS), a condition characterized by widespread degeneration of the nervous system and dementia, occurs in slightly older people. The other major degenerative disorders such as motor neuron disease, Parkinson's disease, Creutzfeldt–Jakob disease (CJD), which is another condition associated with widespread degenerative changes of the nervous system, and Alzheimer's disease occur generally between the ages of 45 and 85 years of age. Over the last few years it has become clear that certain animal, and probably human, degenerative diseases of the nervous system are caused by infections that may take many years to produce clinical manifestations. The concept of 'slow infections' was first introduced by a pathologist working in Iceland on neurological diseases in animals. There is a growing consensus of opinion that some human degenerative disorders represent 'slow infections' that are caused by at least two different classes of infectious agents, viruses and prions.

The first work on prions came from the study of a disease of the nervous system of sheep called scrapie. This was found to be transmitted by a virus-like agent for which the term prion was coined. A prion has been defined as a small proteinaceous infectious particle which is resistant to inactivation by the usual procedures that modify nucleic acids. Indeed there is some evidence that prions consist only of proteins, although it is still possible that they contain nucleic acid of some kind which hitherto has been impossible to isolate. As well as three diseases of cattle there are at least three human disorders in which it seems likely that prions play a major role, kuru, CJD, and GSS. Indeed these conditions may be variants of the same disorder. They can all be transmitted to experimental animals by innoculation. Kuru, a degenerative disease of the nervous system found in Papua New Guinea, is thought to have spread exclusively via a slow infectious mechanism by ritual cannibalism. A few other examples have been described of the possible exogenous transmission of prions, including CJD contracted from contaminated human growth hormone, but overall it is quite unclear how these agents gain access to the nervous system. There is increasing evidence that these agents accumulate in the nervous system and lead to spongiform degeneration and gliosis (overgrowth of connective tissue of the brain).

Recent work suggests that prion protein is the product of a highly conserved gene found in organisms as diverse as fruit fly and man. It is a membrane-bound protein but its function is still unknown. The abnormal form of prion protein that is found in brain extracts from patients with spongiform encephalopathies, and which is the main constituent of the amyloid plaques found in the brain in these conditions, has, in a few cases, been traced back to primary mutations of the prion protein gene. Point mutations of this gene leading to amino acid substitutions have been found in affected individuals or in families with GSS or CJD. Thus we have the extraordinary situation of a family of diseases associated with the production of abnormal proteins due to mutations at a locus which, since it is so highly conserved through evolution, probably has an important function in the nervous system. At the same time there is good evidence that these disorders are transmissable, yet the prion proteins do not appear to contain any nucleic acid. If they are indeed infectious they represent a completely new class of agents of this type. Clearly this will be an extremely exciting field over the next few years and one in which the techniques of molecular biology will have direct application to the elucidation of important clinical disorders in man.

Summary

Even though it has been possible to mention only a few growth areas in the application of molecular and cell biology to the neurosciences, it should be apparent that this will be one of the most exciting areas of basic research over the next few years. It is too early to predict where all this will lead in the context of clinical practice. But the remarkable insights that have been gained into the developmental biology of the brain should find many applications in our further understanding of congenital abnormalities of the nervous system. Similarly, work on the regulatory molecules, the control and synthesis of neurotransmitters, and on slow viruses and prions, has obvious applications in the study of such intractable problems as Parkinson's disease and dementia and may, in the long term, provide insights into other degenerative disorders.

● Vision

Failure of vision and blindness are common and pose a major load on our health resources. Although environmental agents play an important role, it is clear that genetic factors are involved in many forms of blindness. We have already considered how it has been possible to dissect the molecular basis of colour blindness. There are many candidate genes involved in the control of vision, some of which have already been cloned. They include the genes for rod and cone pigments, and G proteins and phosphodiesterases which are expressed in photoreceptors. There also appear to be several ion channels that are specific to the eye.

Recent work has mapped the locus for a common genetic form of blindness, retinitis pigmentosa (RP), to chromosome 3 (see Chapter 6). It was known that the gene for 'rhodopsin' lies in the same region. When this gene was isolated from an affected patient it was found to contain a point mutation, a C to A transversion which leads to a histidine for proline substitution; the latter is a highly conserved residue in many mammalian opsins and related signal receptors. It is likely that the loss of proline alters the secondary structure of the receptor. It is clear that RP is a heterogeneous disorder for which other mutations will probably be found soon.

The work briefly described here is an encouraging start to the dissection of the genetic causes of blindness. Progress in this important field should be rapid.

● Ageing

Since most species seem to have a built-in survival programme it is tempting to speculate that the process of ageing is under some kind of genetic control. On the other hand, many of the theories that attempt to explain the mechanisms of ageing are based on the idea that as we get older we accumulate increasing numbers of mutations that involve DNA replication, repair, transcription, and translation. In other words, ageing may simply reflect stochastic damage to DNA.

The arguments for and against the existence of specific genes for ageing are often based on evolutionary grounds. For example although it has been suggested that such genes might have evolved specifically to prevent overcrowding of species, there is no evidence that ageing serves as a significant contributor to mortality in natural populations, an observation that is held to preclude an adaptive role for putative 'ageing genes'.

In a complex multicellular organism that is not programmed to allow complete cell renewal, death will occur once a critical number of somatic mutations have accumulated. Although a number of models have been designed to accommodate this mechanism for ageing all of them are fraught with difficulties. In particular, they require mutation rates that are far too high to fit observed lifespans, at least in experimental systems. Some of these problems can be resolved if it is assumed that the expressivity of the required mutations becomes greater with time due to their mutual interactions. Another way in which the frequency of somatic mutations might increase in a non-linear manner with age is if the mutations were induced as the result of a cyclic propagation of errors in transcription or translation.

A particularly intriguing question that follows from these ideas is how the germ-line remains free from progressive deleterious changes. Although germ cells do deteriorate, in that the frequency of genetic abnormalities increases with both maternal and paternal age, there is no evidence that, in general, the offspring of older parents start life more aged that the progeny of young parents! It is possible that certain germ-line abnormalities are selected against or that meiosis provides a special opportunity to remove mutations from the germ-line.

Thus, although there are many inconsistencies to be sorted out, it appears that there is a general association between genetic instability and ageing. There is no doubt that cell lines from individuals with inherited defects in DNA repair show significantly reduced growth potential. As mentioned in earlier chapters, recombinant DNA technology offers enormous potential for working out the mechanisms of DNA repair. Perhaps this will, in turn, help us to start to understand the basic mechanisms of ageing.

● Human evolution

Our evolutionary history is written in our DNA. It is now possible to make detailed comparisons of gene structure between different groups of organisms and hence to analyse the changes that have occurred during evolution. This new field, molecular evolution, offers a great opportunity to augment what has been learnt by the study of fossil remains and comparative studies of different proteins.

It is beyond the scope of this book to describe the many applications of DNA technology to evolutionary studies. For example, as a general approach to taxonomic analysis it is possible to determine the relatedness of different species by DNA/DNA hybridization; mismatching due to evolutionary divergence will reduce the binding strength between the two DNA molecules. It has been calculated that a lowering of the dissociation temperature of such hybrids by about one degree centigrade is equivalent to about 1 per cent difference in nucleotide sequence. This technique has been used extensively to measure genetic difference between taxonomic groups. Although some of the data are still controversial they have provided some extremely valuable indications of genetic distance.

As intimated in earlier chapters the discovery of restriction fragment length polymorphisms (RFLPs) offers another extremely valuable tool for analysing population genetics and evolution. It is apparent that the RFLP haplotypes in the human globin genes are quite ancient and thus it is possible to study the way in which the common mutations of these genes have arisen and become distributed among different populations. The patterns of mutations themselves can be compared between different racial groups; for example, it appears that most populations except Africans have rather similar RFLP haplotypes in their α and β globin genes. These observations have suggested an early emergence of a relatively small population from Africa, a finding that is quite compatible with similar studies carried out on mitochondrial DNA polymorphisms. Because the latter are inherited exclusively in maternal DNA, and because of its high mutation rate, mitochondrial DNA is particularly valuable for population and evolutionary studies; it is possible, for example, to construct a phylogeny of human races based on single site polymorphisms.

One of the problems that has bedevilled human population genetics is to distinguish between selection and founder effects when interpreting the distribution of genes in populations. This difficulty can now be overcome because of the existence of large numbers of neutral polymorphisms in the structure of DNA. For example, we have used this approach to define the reasons for the extremely high frequency of α thalassaemia in some populations. In the Pacific islands there is a clear-cut cline in the distribution of α thalassaemia between Papua New Guinea in the north, where there is a very high frequency, and New Caledonia in the south, where the condition is very uncommon. It turns out that this cline is mirrored by the distribution of malaria in this region; it is hyperendemic in the north and non-existent in New Caledonia. In other words its distribution mirrors exactly that of α thalassaemia. This suggests that α thalassaemia may have reached its high frequency by protecting against malaria. Alternatively, however, it is possible that a population with a high frequency of α thalassaemia moved into this region from the north and that the gene frequency was gradually diluted as they moved south. This problem has now been addressed by examining batteries of other DNA polymorphisms which, in this particular case, showed no difference whatever across the region under study. We can conclude, therefore, that the reason for the high frequency of α thalassaemia in the north is very likely to have been protection against severe malaria. There seems little doubt that DNA polymorphisms will be used increasingly in human population genetics over the next few years.

At first sight it is difficult to see how evolutionary studies at the molecular level could ever have any value for clinical practice. If we can start to understand how our genetic makeup has made us more resistant or susceptible to bacterial, viral, or parasitic infections, or to other important environmental hazards during our evolutionary history it may be possible to develop new strategies for the control of diseases due to these agents. What does a thalassaemic red cell have that makes it unattractive to a malarial parasite? Could we reproduce these changes in any way? Why did some individuals survive major epidemics; what made them different? Evolution has left many tantalizing clues for the medical profession; it is up to it to unravel them now that the tools are at hand.

● Further reading

Bock, G. and Marsh, J. (eds) (1988). *Novel infectious agents and the nervous system*. Ciba Foundation Symposium, No. **135**. Wiley, Chichester.

Beutler, B. and Cerami, A. (1988). Tumour necrosis factor: cachexia, shock and inflammation: a common mediator. *Annu. Rev. Biochem.* **57**, 505–18.

Changeux, J.-P. (1989). The acetylcholine receptor: its molecular biology and biotechnological prospects. *BioEssays*, **10**, 48–57.

Cole, W.G., Jaenisch, R., and Bateman, J.F. (1989). New insights into the molecular pathology of osteogenesis imperfecta. *Q. J. Med.*, **70**, 1–4.

Curran, T. and Morgan, J.I. (1987). Memories of *fos*. *BioEssays*, **7**, 253–8.

Dinarello, C.A. and Mier, J.W. (1987). Current concepts: lymphokines. *New Engl. J. Med.*, **317**, 940–5.

Dryja, T.P., McGee, T.I., Reichel, E., *et al.* (1990). A point of mutation of the rhodopsin gene in one form of retinitis pigmentosa. *Nature*, **343**, 364–6.

Eisenstein, B.I. (1990). The polymerase chain reaction: a new method of using molecular genetics for medical diagnosis. *New Engl. J. Med.*, **322**, 179–82.

Emanuel, B.S. (1988). Molecular cytogenetics: toward dissection of the contiguous gene syndromes. *Am. J. Hum. Genet.*, **43**, 575–8.

Epstein, H.T. (1889). The molecular biology of brain and mind development. *BioEssays*, **10**, 44–7.

Evered, D. and Whelan, J. (eds) (1985). *Growth factors in biology and medicine*. Ciba Foundation Symposium, No. **116**. Wiley, Chichester.

Evered, D. and Whelan, J. (eds) (1988). *Research and the ageing propulation*. Ciba Foundation Symposium, No. **134**. Wiley, Chichester.

Hanley, M.R. (1989). Peptide regulatory factors in the nervous system. *Lancet*, **i**, 1373–6.

Howard, R.J. (1989). Malaria: the search for vaccine antigens and new chemotherapeutic agents. *Blood*, **74**, 533–6.

Janeway, C.A. (1989). Immunotherapy by peptides? *Nature*, **341**, 482–3.

Lancet (1989). Editorial. DNA technology and rapid diagnosis of infection. **ii**, 897–8.

Lancet (1990). Editorial. Prion disease—spongiform encephalopathy is unveiled. **336**, 21–2.

Leatherbarrow, R.J. and Fersht, A.R. (1986). Protein engineering. *Prot. Engin.*, **1**, 7–16.

Locksley, R.M., Nilsen, T., and Parsons, M. (1989). Parasites: molecular biology, drug and vaccine design. *Parasitology Today*, **5**, 271–3.

Kirdwood, T.B.L. (1988). DNA, mutations and ageing. *Mutat. Res.*, **Pilot issue**, 7–13.

Krause, J.E., Macdonald, M.R., and Takeda, Y. (1989). The polyprotein nature of substance P precursors. *BioEssays*, **10**, 62–8.

Lamb, J., Wilkie, A.O.M., Harris, P.C., *et al.* (1989). Detection of breakpoints in submicroscopic chromosomal translocation, illustrating an important mechanism for genetic disease. *Lancet*, **ii**, 819–23.

Martin, J.B. (1987). Molecular genetics: applications to the clinical neurosciences. *Science*, **238**, 765–72.

Marx, J.L. (1987). The *fos* gene as 'master switch'. *Science*, **237**, 854–6.

Metcalf, D. (1989). Haemopoietic growth factor 1. *Lancet*, **i**, 825–7.

Metcalf, D. (1989). Haemopoietic growth factor 2: clinical applications. *Lancet*, **i**, 885–7.

Moore, G.E., Ivens, A., Chambers, J., Farrall, M., Williamson, R., Page, D.C., Bjornsson A., Arnason, A., and Jensson, O. (1987). Linkage of an X-chromosome cleft palate gene. *Nature*, **326**, 91–2.

Nelson, T.J. and Alkon, D.L. (1989). Specific protein changes during memory acquisition and storage. *BioEssays*, **10**, 75–8.

O'Brien, S.J., Sevanez, H.C., and Womack, J.E. (1988). Mammalian genome organisation: an evolutionary view. *Annu. Rev. Genet.*, **22**, 323–52.

O'Garra, A. (1989). Interleukins and the immune system 1. *Lancet*, **i**, 943–7.

Olson, M., Hood, L., Cantor, C., and Botstein, D. (1989). A common language for physical mapping of the human genome. *Science*, **245**, 1434–5.

Paul, W.E. (1988). Lymphokine nomenclature. *Immunology Today*, **9**, 366–7.

Pays, E. Steinert. M. (1988). Control of antigen expression in African trypanosomes. *Annu. Rev. Genet.*, **22**, 107–6.

Porter, R. and Whelan, J. (eds) (1986). *Synthetic peptides as antigens.* Ciba Foundation Symposium No. **119**, Wiley, Chichester.

Price, D.L., Koo, E.H. and Unterbeck, A. (1989). Cellular and molecular biology of Alzheimer's disease. *BioEssays*, **10**, 69–74.

Reichmann, L., Clark, M., Waldmann, H., and Winter, G. (1988). Reshaping human antibodies for therapy. *Nature*, **332**, 323–7.

Slack, J.M.W. (1989). Peptide regulatory factors in embryonic development. *Lancet*, **i**, 1312–15.

Smith, K.A. (1988). Interleukin-2: inception, impact, and implications. *Science*, **240**, 1169–76.

Sobol, H., Narod, S.A., Nakamura, Y., *et al.* (1989). Screening for multiple endocrine neoplasia type 2a with DNA-polymorphism analysis. *New Engl. J. Med.*, **321**, 996–1001.

Southern, E.M. (1988). Prospects for a complete molecular map of the human genome. *Phil. Trans. R. Soc. Lond. B.*, **319**, 299–307.

Taylor-Papadimitrious, J. (1985). *Interferons; their impact in biology and medicine.* Oxford University Press.

Tracey, K.J., Vlassara, H., and Cerami, A. (1989). Cachectin/tumour necrosis factor. *Lancet*, **i**, 1122–6.

Vitetta, E.S., Fulton, R.J., May, R.D., Till, M., and Uhr, J.W. (1987). Redesigning nature's poisons to create anti-tumour reagents. *Science*, **238**, 1098–104.

Weatherall, D.J., Bunch, C., Old, J.M., *et al.* (1981). Hemoglobin H disease and mental retardation: a new syndrome or a remarkable coincidence? *New Engl. J. Med.*, **305**, 607–12.

Ethical issues and related problems arising from the application of the new genetics to clinical practice

12

Our new found ability to tinker with genes is giving rise to a certain amount of public concern. In fact, the application of the techniques described in this book does not raise any fundamentally new ethical problems for clinicians; at least not yet. Genetic screening and prenatal diagnosis have been accepted procedures for many years; all that our new technology will do is to increase the number of diseases that can be avoided in this way. Somatic gene therapy, even if it becomes feasible is not a fundamental departure from current clinical practice. However, there are important questions about the control of genetic diseases which will be highlighted by the wider application of these practices. Furthermore, as we learn more about developmental and behavioural genetics and become increasingly adept at transferring genes, we may be tempted into areas of research that present genuine ethical problems.

According to the *Shorter Oxford English Dictionary* the usage of the word 'ethics' has taken on a much broader connotation over the years. While in the strict sense it means the science of morals, ethics has come to encompass 'the science of human duty in its widest extent, including, besides ethics proper, the science of law, whether civil, political, or international'. It may also be used to describe practices that are acceptable to particular groups such as the medical or legal profession. Ethical questions raised by human molecular genetics span a wide range of disciplines ranging from moral philosophy to comparative religion, many of which are not within the scope of this book. However it is becoming increasingly important that clinicians, health administrators, and the public appreciate some of the questions that may be raised by our new found ability to avoid and treat genetic disease and manipulate human genes. I shall briefly outline some of my concerns.

● Specific ethical problems posed by the new genetics

● Do we really want to avoid genetic disease?

The attitude of many doctors and others to the avoidance of genetic disease by screening and selective termination of pregnancy was eloquently summarized in

1984 in a letter to the British Medical Journal by a highly respected African physician, Felix Konotey-Ahulu. He wrote as follows: 'I was born in the Krobo tribe with extra digits—a Mendelian dominant condition with a 1% incidence at birth in Ghana. Had I been born a few miles southeast across the Volta river, there would have been great rejoicing because local tribesmen had it that I was destined to be rich. If my mother had given birth to me a few miles northwest beyond the hills, I would not be here to write to you—I would have been drowned soon after birth. Fortunately the Krobo's were neutral to extra digits but until the government forbade the practice some tribal elders took it on to themselves to decide which genes ought to be allowed to survive! My fellow Krobo tribesmen did not spend time debating details like the most humane way to drown me at birth to cause least hurt to my mother, nor did they ever ponder how my three siblings with sickle cell disease could have been identified *in utero* and got rid of. No, they got hold of the vital principle that I was literally more than 7 digits and my two brothers and sister with sickle cell disease had other genes which endeared them to my parents.' In the same letter the author voices the fear that history has shown that often a few pressure groups or even a single person can decide what is right for an entire society—Nazi Germany was the prime example; now, he argues, it is the turn of the molecular geneticists.

This attitude is extremely common among clinicians. After all they have been trained to preserve and value life; abortion, for whatever reason, is totally repugnant to many of them. They look blankly at me when I suggest that we now have methods for the prenatal diagnosis of haemophilia or phenylketonuria. Clearly that is of no interest to them. They have many patients with these conditions who live full lives and are able to cope with unpleasant treatment and complications. The idea of the medical profession, or any other group, pressuring parents with the potential for producing children with these diseases into prenatal diagnosis and selective termination of pregnancy is a complete anathema to them.

Wider objections are sometimes raised when the topic of selective termination of pregnancy is aired in cases of genetic or congenital disability. They centre round questions about whether it is appropriate for society to decide that physical disability is always a bad thing. Surely, it is argued, some of our greatest creative artists suffered from such afflictions. Can we be sure that their talents were not expressed as the result of their physical or mental disadvantage? Do we want to terminate a pregnancy and lose a Beethoven? However, it may not be very helpful to base our attitudes to the avoidance of genetic disease on such unusual individuals. After all, there are numerous examples of outstandingly creative people who have remained in rude health for the whole of their working lives. It is difficult to substantiate the argument that unusual talent, or even genius, is seen only in the context of serious genetic disability, or any other pathology for that matter.

It would be surprising if many of these attitudes were not common among doctors and thoughtful members of society, regardless of whether their views are based on religious or humanistic beliefs. Why, they ask, should not society be responsible for caring for its genetically abnormal children, however incapacitated they may be. On the other hand, equally caring physicians and others take the attitude that the potential parents of genetically abnormal children should have the right to decide what kind of children they bring into the world. Most clinicians who have to care for large numbers of genetically abnormal or otherwise handicapped children feel likewise. They will also point out that many early spontaneous abortions show major chromosomal abnormalities; if this is nature's way of dealing with genetic defects why should they not do the same. Furthermore, sad though it may be, it is clear from my own research field that many of the developing countries simply cannot provide the care required to make life tolerable for children with some of the common genetic diseases.

Since there are such strong arguments on both sides, what should be the role of the medical profession in this sensitive situation? Perhaps it should continue to do its best to develop more humane methods for genetic screening and prenatal diagnosis, educate the public about their availability, and then leave the decision to individual parents, without legislation or any other form of coercion. While at first sight this pragmatic approach is attractive, I doubt if it is possible for us to take a completely neutral stance. I shall try to explain why as I touch on some of the practical difficulties of genetic counselling.

In his 1981 Reith Lectures, Kennedy made a case for a reversion of decision making in medical practice so that the patient, as the consumer, plays the major role. But I wonder if he has ever sat in an outpatient clinic and talked with patients about their problems. While I entirely agree with him that parents, or potential parents, must make up their own minds about matters as sensitive as genetic screening and termination of pregnancy, I am certain that their decisions will be significantly coloured by the way in which the case is presented to them by their genetic counsellors. Furthermore, parents (and patients) come to doctors for help, and in order both to assist and to share in their decision making the counsellor must sometimes be prepared to offer positive advice. The sensitive clinician will often notice the relief that parents show when some of the burden of such onerous decisions is taken from them. This means that, with the increasing availability of prenatal diagnosis, a tremendous onus will be put on clinical geneticists and counsellors to become completely informed about the natural history of genetic disease. Take Huntington's disease for example. Will a healthy teenager want to know that he or she has a gene for a disease that is likely to produce a miserable lingering death sometime in adult life? Some will welcome the knowledge so that they can evaluate the potential risks for their own children; others will not. The role of the counsellor is extremely difficult in this situation; they will need to be experienced, sensitive, and, above all, willing to spend a lot of time with families. In other words they must be good doctors, not just well-informed technicians.

Clearly, we shall have to be very careful about our choice of counsellors in the future, and train them to present increasingly complex concepts in simple language. If the present state of communication with parents in genetic counselling clinics is anything like that throughout the rest of medical practice, I suspect that we have a long way to go in this critically important part of patient care.

I hope that what I have just written does not suggest that I believe that these ethical and pastoral aspects should be taken lightly. Prenatal diagnosis and selective abortion will always be an extremely sensitive subject. Curiously, there have been very few studies of womens' attitudes to prenatal diagnosis and termination of pregnancy for genetic disease. As the result of a questionnaire sent to university graduates aged 38 to 43 it was found that 17 per cent out of a total of 266 who were willing to commit themselves said that they would not accept an offer of amniocentesis in pregnancy to screen for Down syndrome, a decision based mainly on religious and moral grounds. A very similar result was obtained in a recent study using cystic fibrosis as the test case.

In this context it is interesting to consider current attitudes to prenatal diagnosis for the haemoglobin disorders in different countries. Surprisingly, these programmes have been widely accepted in predominantly Catholic countries such as Sardinia and Italy; I suspect that this reflects the emergence of a more secular society rather than any change of attitude by the Church. While ethnic and religious objections to prevention of genetic disease by direct intervention seem to be becoming less common in many western countries, the situation is not nearly so clear in other parts of the world, particularly those with large Islamic populations. Indeed, from personal discussions it appears that there may be serious difficulties in setting up major prenatal diagnosis programmes, at whatever age of gestation, in many Islamic countries. On the other hand, from experiences in Thailand, it seems that the largely Buddhist population will have less difficulty in accepting selective abortion, particularly if it is carried out early in pregnancy and if a good case for the mother's well-being can be made.

Clearly, we (society as a whole—not just doctors) should regularly re-evaluate what we mean by 'quality of life' for a handicapped child. Widescale abortion may reduce the load on our paediatric and social services; but is surely not the ultimate solution to the problem of genetic disease. The factors that underlie our attitudes to these sensitive problems are bound to change. What is acceptable for a modern industrialized western society may be quite inappropriate for a developing country. And much will depend on whether we can develop better forms of treatment for genetic disease.

● Genetic screening programmes

The ethical and pastoral problems of genetic screening and prenatal diagnosis have been reviewed by many experienced geneticists and others and the arguments need not be repeated here in detail. Readers who wish to consider them further are referred to several excellent discussions cited at the end of this chapter. Any form of screening of individuals or populations for disease is a sensitive matter and should not be embarked upon lightly. Unless carried out with the complete knowedge and understanding of the persons who are to be screened, it is an intolerable invasion of privacy, particularly if the screening programme is made mandatory by law. Indeed, some would argue that medical practice is becoming much too intrusive and that no form of screening is acceptable. When we remember the benefits of screening for cancer of the cervix, or mass miniature radiography to 'find' cases of tuberculosis, this view is difficult to uphold. However, genetic screening is particularly sensitive, involving as it does the danger of stigmatization and personal concern about the carriage of 'bad genes' and their potential effect on future generations. The object of public health measures should be to improve the lot of the community. Unfortunately, although we have a little information about the effects of screening programmes on the prevalence of particular genetic diseases, there have been no good studies of their potential deleterious effects on individuals or populations. As we shall see later, unless a genetic screening programme is extremely well designed, the potential for serious social and psychological damage is immense.

Several bodies have attempted to produce guidelines for genetic screening programmes. One of the most comprehensive, the President's Commission for the Study of Ethical Problems in Medicine and Biomedical and Behavioural Research, was published in the US in 1983. This report covers the ethical, social and legal implications of genetic screening, counselling, and education. It makes several important points. First, confidentiality is absolutely essential. Genetic information should never be given to unrelated third parties, although there may be exceptions in particularly sensitive situations such as adoption. Second, the place for mandatory genetic screening programmes must always be limited and only considered when voluntary testing proves inadequate to prevent serious harm to defenceless individuals such as newborn infants. Third, any decisions regarding the release of incidental findings, and particularly involving sensitive information such as non-paternity or the diagnosis of an XY female, should begin with a presumption in favour of disclosure. In other words, although there may be occasions when information discovered in a screening programme might be held back for the benefit of an individual, the first duty of those who run these programmes is for complete honesty with those who are being screened. Fourth, and particularly important, a large-scale population screening programme should not be undertaken until the screening test has first demonstrated its value in well-conducted small-scale pilot studies. Furthermore, no screening programme should be set up without the availability of follow-up services for the population including genetic counselling and appropriate medical care. Finally, access to screening should take account of the incidence of genetic diseases in various racial or ethnic groups within a population without violating the principles of equity, justice, and fairness. The report also underlines the great importance of preceding a population screening programme by a period of intense education at all levels of the community. These are sensible suggestions and the report is a useful framework on which to develop genetic screening programmes.

As emphasized by the American report, education of the public is absolutely essential for the success of genetic screening. The harm that can be done by an ill-devised programme is well illustrated by what happened when sickle cell anaemia was rediscovered as a major health problem in the US in the early 1970s. The Black population was told that many of them were suffering from this neglected disorder and a massive screening programme was set up, backed by heavy federal support. Local communities became involved, together will ill-assorted individuals of diverse background and training (or lack of), and the entire programme became a major political, racial, and social issue. Screening programmes were not backed up with appropriate provision of genetic counselling. In several states laws were passed which made screening mandatory, without any provision for education and counselling. Worst of all, nobody had decided beforehand what should be done with the information once the population had been screened! All this badly organized activity produced considerable public anxiety, stigmatization, job and health insurance discrimination, and a variety of other undesirable effects; the programme achieved nothing. This disastrous episode has to be compared with the major success story of the control of Tay–Sachs disease in the Washington–Baltimore Jewish population by Kaback and his colleagues in the 1970s, which is a good example of what can be achieved in a well-informed and highly motivated population.

The importance of educating a community about genetic diseases is also emphasized by studies in the UK which have analysed the acceptance rates for prenatal diagnosis of thalassaemia in different ethnic groups. It turns out that there is a major difference between Cypriot and Asian immigrant populations in, their response to prenatal diagnosis; the London Cypriots have taken up the programme with great enthusiasms whereas the same does not apply to the Asian populations. The reasons are complex, and religious and ethnic factors may have played a role. However, the major difference is the limited extent to which the Asian communities in the UK have been adequately educated in preparation for prenatal diagnosis. The disastrous results and associated racial overtones of the screening programme for sickle cell disease in the US stand as a constant reminder of the potential dangers of introducing this type of activity into an ill-prepared society. Ethnic minority groups are particularly sensitive. The success of the introduction of prenatal diagnosis of thalassaemia in the London Cypriot population is largely a result of the major effort that was put into educating the community by an enthusiastic clinician and her colleagues.

With the exception of these experiences in London, there have been no well-designed pilot studies that have examined the effects of a programme for the prevention of a genetic disease in a racial minority. Indeed, we know very little about the effect or acceptability of these programmes in any population. In one small but well-designed study in village populations in Greece, genetic screening backed up by adequate counselling caused considerable psychological stress and individual stigmatization; there was no effect on the prevalence of the diseases for which the programme was instigated. This subject needs urgent attention, particularly if we plan to develop national programmes for the avoidance of common genetic diseases.

● The scope of programmes for the prevention of genetic disease

The new techniques described in this monograph will simplify screening for genetic disease and will widen the spectrum of disorders that are amenable to prenatal diagnosis. There are dangers in this, however. Because it will be easier to identify the genotype in early fetal life, there may be a tendency for the indications for prenatal diagnosis and therapeutic abortion to become less stringent. Indeed, this is already happening in the haemoglobin field. For example, rather than restricting their activities to fetuses at risk of having a crippling form of thalassaemia, some clinicians are counselling for the possibility of having a pregnancy terminated which is at risk of carrying a much milder form of the condition. This philosophy of perfection opens up all sort of dangerous avenues and we will have to be extremely careful about the choice and education of genetic counsellors in the future. Of course, this has always been a major concern in the prevention of genetic illnesses; the increasing ease of intrauterine diagnosis simply highlights the problem.

Another concern about the widespread use of prenatal diagnosis arises from our current ignorance about the natural history of many genetic diseases. I have already referred to our potential for understanding why apparently similar genetic diseases have such a variable clinical course. Progress in this important area is still slow, however. In this sense, the medical sciences have walked before they could crawl! Almost unbelievably, we find ourselves in 1990 with the most sophisticated and reliable techniques for prenatal diagnosis of sickle cell anaemia using fetal DNA, and yet we have ony the flimsiest idea about the natural history of the disease in many populations. Perhaps not surprisingly, when vast federal support was given for research into sickle cell anaemia in the US in the 1970s there was a natural tendency to explore the more glamorous molecular aspects of the subject and to neglect the patient almost completely. The same criticism can be levelled at most research in sickle cell anaemia over the last 15 years; the problem is not confined to the US. It is only recently that a few groups have started to study the natural history of this disorder, an approach pioneered by Serjeant in Jamaica but, unfortunately, ignored by many other workers.

Finally, and perhaps most germaine to the new genetics, is the question of how we will deal with the increasing amount of genetic information about individuals which will be amassed as our technology for gene analysis increases in sophistication. We have already considered the problems arising from our ability to identify conditions like Huntington's disease in early life and of which the distressing symptoms will only be manifest many years later. Supposing that, as part of our efforts to define the major genes involved in vascular disease or the major psychoses, we happen to learn how to identify individuals with a high risk of having a heart attack or developing schizophrenia later in life. It is quite possible that we will have this information many years before we know how to prevent these diseases developing. What will we do with this information? And what will we do if we are able to identify individuals at genetic risk from their employment, sensitivity to carcinogens for example? Will we maintain confidentiality, or will we have to tell potential employers?

There are no easy answers to these questions. Like most advances in medicine the new genetics will pose many new problems for society; if they are the price that we have to pay to understand the cause of the common killers of developed societies, and to control genetic disease, they are worth tackling. None of the potential problems are fundamentally new, but simply extensions of our increasing understanding of why we are what we are.

● Testing children for 'adult' genetic diseases

We have discussed several conditions in which advances in DNA technology have allowed us to identify diseases early in life which are not manifest clinically until much later. While identification of disorders that require immediate treatment raises no ethical problems, the growing list of conditions that appear in middle age such as adult polycystic disease, Huntington's disease, colon cancer due to familial polyposis coli, myotonic dystrophy, retinitis pigmentosa, and the concept that we may be able to identify individuals at particular risk for common polygenic disorders in the future, is bound to raise new problems for those who look after children.

While there may be a very good case for identifying some of these conditions in childhood, decisions of this type will have to be made with extreme care and after long discussion with parents. In some cases there may be a good case for trying to exclude a particular disease. For example, ruling out the possibility of adult polycystic kidney disease might prevent children having close follow-up with regular blood pressure estimations. Similarly, if familial polyposis coli can be excluded children in affected families will not require careful surveillance with colonoscopy in case they develop adenomas and subsequent cancers of the colon. On the other hand, it may be much more difficult to make a decision about screening for Huntington's disease, as mentioned in Chapter 9. Obviously as the child gets older and approaches reproductive age, and advice about contraception and future marriage is needed, the situation may change, but there seems little reason for testing early in life for conditions of this type. Unfortunately, some parents wish to know one way or the other and the question of whether it is ethically justified to refuse to obtain this type of information will arise. Genetic counsellors who deal with these problems will have to act with particular sensitivity, somehow bridging the difficult decision of whether to go along with the parents wishes and yet on the other hand trying to protect the child.

● Avoidance or treatment?

Given that we may have a much easier approach to prenatal diagnosis and the avoidance of genetic disease, will the impetus for research into the management or cure of these diseases be reduced? There is a genuine danger that this will be the case. Few would argue that prevention is better than cure. However, prenatal diagnosis and selective abortion are directed only at the secondary prevention of genetic disease. It will be very important to maintain a balance of research in clinical genetics which encourages work on the therapy of genetic diseases as well as their avoidance; widespread selective abortion should not be the ultimate goal of this field.

● Dysgenic effects

Will the widespread use of prenatal diagnosis encourage reproduction in families with genetic diseases, and thus help to maintain or increase the frequency of these conditions in populations? This so-called dysgenic effect has worried geneticists for a long time. In this context it is interesting to examine the effect of introducing prenatal diagnosis of thalassaemia into the Cypriot community in London. When they first learnt about the effects of this disease, and before prenatal diagnosis was available, the birth rate fell in affected families. Since prenatal diagnosis has become established and accepted, the birth rate has returned to the national norm. I doubt if the potential dysgenic effect of a programme of this kind can be used as an argument against its adoption. After all, there is evidence that, in at least some populations with a high incidence of genetic disease, affected families produce more children to compensate for their handicapped child, a phenomenon that has been observed in some areas of Italy, for example. The problem needs watching but there is no evidence that a programme of prevention will have a major effect on the size of the pool of our less attractive genes. We may provide more work for our genetic counselling clinics, but in the long term it is hoped that we can learn how to treat the important genetic disorders.

● Gene therapy

In considering the potential ethical problems that arise from the application of gene therapy it is important to distinguish quite clearly between somatic and germ-line therapy. In somatic therapy, as was pointed out in Chapter 10, the idea is to insert genes into specific somatic cells where, if all goes well, they will function during the lifetime of an individual and hence correct a genetic disease. This new approach presents a number of practical problems that were set out in Chapter 10. However, it does not differ in any important way from any other form of organ transplantation. We are quite happy to transplant kidneys or hearts; once its safety has been determined there should be no major ethical difficulties arising from gene therapy of this type. On the other hand, the insertion of genes into germ cells, which in practice means injecting them into fertilized eggs, is another matter.

Germ-line gene therapy is fundamentally different from somatic cell therapy in that the inserted genes would be passed on to future generations and therefore we would be embarking on a completely new road. If we decided that we wish to indulge in germ-line therapy we would be altering the genomes of our great-grandchildren who will have taken no part in the decision. Here we would undoubtedly be playing with the evolution of the species.

There are several reasons why it seems quite inappropriate to consider germ-line gene therapy at the present time. First, it should be possible fairly soon to identify genetic diseases in fertilized human ova (see Chapter 10). If this is the case all we need to do to help parents who are at risk of producing children with a serious genetic disease is to obtain ova after *in vitro* fertilization, decide which carry the genetic defect, and then replace only those that do not. In this way the family can be assured of having normal children and there is no need to tamper with the genetic makeup of the future individuals.

There are a number of even more pragmatic reasons for not indulging in germ-line gene therapy. In particular, we have no idea about the stability over successive generations of genes inserted into fertilized eggs or about any long-term deleterious effect that they might have. For the moment there seems no reason to consider this approach in man. Whether there ever will be must remain for future generations to decide, but for the moment the majority of human geneticists are convinced that experiments in human germ-line gene transfer should not be carried out.

● Embryo research

As I have intimated several times in this book, the major challenge for human genetics in the next decade is to try to understand how genes are regulated during development. In other words, how does a fertilized egg with 3×10^9 nucleotide pairs make a human being? Until we start to understand some of the basic mechanisms of developmental genetics we shall not make much progress in sorting out many of the problems of congenital malformation and the mechanisms of chromosome damage that give rise to the various chromosomal defects. It is possible, therefore, to envisage a time when we may wish to apply the tools of the new genetics to study early fetal tissue or living embryos. Indeed, in Chapter 10 we saw that methods are being developed for removing a few cells from fertilized eggs for the purpose of genetic diagnosis; this problem is already with us.

In vitro fertilization (IVF) was developed originally to help infertile couples, particularly those in which the woman had blocked fallopian tubes, which may interfere with fertilization or passage of the conceptus to the womb. This technique, and more recent variations on this theme, has proved to be of great value in treating some cases of infertility. However, these approaches are not yet entirely successful and a lot more work needs doing before the majority of infertile couples who have the potential to be helped by IVF can have children. This, together with the great potential for medical research that would follow from understanding early human development and from the ability to identify genetic disease in the fertilized ovum constitute the main argument in favour of encouraging research on human embryos. Most of the methods that are used for IVF result in the production of a number of 'spare' embryos and hence the major problem that has to be faced is whether it is right to use them for experimental purposes.

Before considering the ethical problems of embryo research it is important to understand what such work might encompass. It is possible to make a strong argument for allowing a limited amount of restrictive research on human embryos up to the end of the fourth week of gestation, or even later, on medical grounds. Certainly we need to know more about the newly fertilized egg if we are to improve the lot of infertile couples and if we are to understand more about the origin of major chromosomal abnormalities such as Down's syndrome. As mentioned in Chapter 10 a great deal more work needs to be done at the blastocyst stage, that is when there are between 30 and 120 undifferentiated cells, if we are to be able to identify genetic disease with the objective of replacing unaffected conceptuses. A little later, perhaps from days 7 to 14, the fertilized ovum is implanted. Virtually nothing is known about the early interactions between a conceptus and the uterus at this stage. By day 15 the early embryo is starting to differentiate and the primitive streak appears; it is now possible to define the embryo proper as compared with the external membranes, placenta to be, and so on. It is at this critical stage that we should be able to learn more about the early development of the brain and spinal cord and start to understand some of the causes of such serious malformations as spina bifida and anencephaly. By the end of the fourth week of gestation there are the beginnings of organ development and it is here that studies of other more specific congenital anomalies such as heart disease would be particularly valuable.

Given that there are good medical arguments for a limited amount of research on embryos, the next question is whether there should be a developmental time limit set on it. This is an extremely difficult problem which has, as its underlying theme, the question of when an individual's life begins. The easy answer is, of course, at fertilization, or conception. But this won't do. Genetic individuality occurs during the process of meiosis in the formation of the gametes; why pick the moment of fertilization? Another important landmark, as already mentioned, is the formation of the primitive streak, at which time the developing fetus can be distinguished as something separate from its supporting tissues. Perhaps implantation is the critical time of the acquisition of individuality. Yet this poses problems for the many religions that hold that the soul cannot enter the fetus at this stage since it is still capable of division in the process of twinning; the soul, they teach, is unique and therefore indivisible. The first sign of 'life' is the development of the circulatory system and the first contractions of the heart muscle at about the 21st day. Responsiveness, at least in terms of a primitive nervous system, is acquired between the 5th and 6th week. By 7 or 8 weeks the tiny embryo is developing clearly recognizable features such as hands and feet, and by 12 weeks electrical activity can be detected in the brain. Some definitions of 'life' set the time even later; St. Thomas Aquinas taught that it occurs when the fetus can be felt to move and when the *animus* or soul takes up residence. At about 24 weeks the fetus is capable of surviving outside the womb, though only with assistance, and at 28 weeks achieves protection under British law from the infant life preservation act.

From these considerations it is clear that it is impossible to make a logical definition of when life actually starts. Thus if embryo research is to be allowed, and yet some kind of constraints are to be imposed, an arbitrary decision has to be made. One such attempt was set out by the Warnock Committee in the United Kingdom which took the line that the human embryo should be protected and that a reasonable time after which research should not be carried out was 14 days. But equally well-informed expert committees have suggested a later stage of gestation of up to 6 weeks.

At first sight, it seems strange that a society which, until recently had condoned abortion for the most trivial social reasons should suddenly become so concerned about the human rights of embryos, insisting that they must be protected by law. The reasons are complex. First, there has been much sensational journalism and ill-informed public debate that has lead to the idea of scientists creating monsters in test-tubes. Sadly, much of the debate is carried on at this primitive level, stirred up by various factions, some with genuine religious objections but many others that seem to follow a fanatical 'right-for-life' doctrine. At times it appears as if our society is regressing to the Dark Ages.

Of course, it can be argued that, unlike adults, embryos are not able to give informed consent, and must therefore be protected. However, young children cannot give informed consent and yet, under certain circumstances, they (with the consent of their parents) partake in clinical trials and act as subjects for medical research. Had this not happened, and had this type of work been banned, we would not have achieved our present ability to treat, and often cure, childhood leukaemia, one of the major successes of paediatric medicine.

As this book goes to press the British parliament has voted overwhelmingly for embryo research to continue. This was a very encouraging decision because it suggests that reason has prevailed and that society, as reflected by government, has come to the conclusion that given adequate mechanisms for control it is appropriate that medical scientists continue work in this sensitive area. This has been an extremely important debate because it may well be the forerunner of many similar discussions about scientific research in areas of public concern. The basic and clinical sciences have learnt a great deal from this episode, not the least about the importance of education and dissemination of information through the media about sensitive issues of this type. The problems of communication between the scientists and their public must have underlined more than ever the importance of trying to improve the level of science teaching in our schools. The debate was emotional and often illogical, but it has been a valuable start in an attempt to draw together scientists and society in discussions of matters of extreme sensitivity and importance.

● Who owns the human genome?

A while ago a chilling picture appeared in one of our leading scientific journals. It depicted a businessman looking rather pleased with himself, and carried the caption 'my company owns chromosome 7'. Although it should be self-evident that nobody 'owns' the human genome, or any part of it, there is increasing concern about the potential for commercial exploitation of human recombinant DNA technology. Patents are being slapped on to DNA sequences and already a number of actions have been fought in the courts. Also there is concern that if particular areas of human genetics become commercially attractive more pressures will be put on individuals to undergo screening procedures, and the like.

The patent problems that are developing as the result of recombinant DNA technology are ill-defined and are becoming an increasingly lucrative source of legal practice. It is to be hoped that some common sense will prevail. It should be self-evident that no particular piece of human DNA can be the sole property of anybody. Equally, there is no doubt that a particular method designed to isolate, analyse, or express a particular DNA sequence can be patentable and there seems no reason for major concern if companies wish to patent methods for producing human proteins by recombinant DNA technology. It will be important to monitor the exploitation of the human genome and to make sure that commercial pressures do not push human genetic manipulation in directions that are in any way foreign to the normal standards of good medical practice, or that interfere with medical research or the dissemination of its results.

● Crossing genetic and evolutionary boundaries

Evolution is often depicted in the form of a tree with diverging branches, representing increasing diversity and the way in which species have developed by mutation and natural selection. Studies of protein polymorphisms have shown that we are remarkably diverse and are heterozygous at many loci, which is a distinct evolutionary advantage in that it is possible for some members of a species to adapt quickly to specific environmental changes. It is a general rule that reproduction between different species is impossible in that it leads to infertility or fetal death. Although there may be some horizontal passage of genes, by retroviruses for example, nature's way seems to be the vertical transmission of genetic material with a major accent on continuous diversification of the species.

Our new found ability to transfer genes between species by genetic engineering poses the question of how far we are justified in changing evolution in this way. So far there has been no major concern about placing human genes into bacteria for the production of human protein products. A great deal is being learnt about both normal and abnormal gene actions by inserting human genes into mice by the transgenic route. Attempts are also being made to produce human proteins by inserting genes into larger animals by the same route, proteins that are secreted into milk for example. But where do we draw the line? By suitable manipulation of oncogenes, or by inserting the genes for specific haemopoietic growth factors, it is possible to create breeds of mice with a high probability of developing cancer or a clinical picture very reminiscent of leukaemia. Such experiments may well be justified in helping us to understand human cancers. On the other hand, mice guaranteed to develop malignant disease have been genetically engineered in this way and patented for commercial purposes, complete with a lurid trade name. Lack of sensitivity by the scientific community and industry of this kind is certain to bring the whole field into disrepute.

If we stop and consider the kinds of activities that animal and plant breeders have been about for centuries it is difficult to be too hard on genetic engineers who are doing exactly the same kinds of things by different methods. However, we need to monitor these activities with extreme care. If the insertion of genes from one species into another is being carried out for a specific purpose, with a view to learning more about how genes function, in health and disease for example, and if the experiments are carefully designed with minimum discomfort to the recipient animals, there may be genuine justification. But there is no reason to carry out this type of procedure just for curiosity to see 'what turns up'; on looking at the current scientific literature it is hard to believe that some of the reported experiments have a more rational basis. This is a highly sensitive area and one that must be monitored very carefully by both molecular biologists and the public.

● Broader issues arising from the new genetics

Apart from these specific concerns about the new genetics our increasing ability to manipulate the human genome raises a number of more general issues. Some of them are rather difficult to define, reflecting as they do a feeling of unease that human biology is tampering with the very basis of life. Others relate to what we might do with our new-found knowledge in the long-term future. In this last section I shall try to define a few of these problems and, hopefully, put them into some kind of perspective.

● A reductionist approach to human biology and medical practice

There is no doubt that medical research and clinical practice will change because of the application of recombinant DNA technology to the study of human disease. Partly because of the well-known difficulties of acquiring knowledge about anything new over the age of 35, the medical profession has already become polarized about the value of molecular biology. Many of those who are just starting their professional lives have an uneasy feeling that unless a large proportion of the research work of their medical school is 'molecular' it can't be up to much. At the other end of the spectrum there are many clinicians who are very sceptical about whether this new field will ever have any major impact on clinical practice. Perhaps if offers something for a few rare genetic diseases that they never see, but in the real world of heart attacks, high blood pressure, and varicose veins molecular biology still seems to be totally irrelevant. Even those who appreciate the potential of recombinant DNA see conflicts with patient care arising rom its clinical applications. In particular they perceive human molecular biology as the ultimate in reductionism; the last step in the process of dissecting their patients into disconnected pieces of chemistry. To appreciate this concern it is necessary to consider what has happened to clinical practice in recent years.

After the Second World War, and with the advent of powerful antibiotics and vaccines, many infectious diseases which hitherto had been major killers became a thing of the past, at least in western societies. It was assumed therefore that if medical science could bring off a *tour de force* of this kind, it could do the same for the common ailments of western society, heart disease, cancer, rheumatism, and the major psychiatric disorders. However, nearly half a century has gone by and the root cause of these conditions has not been discovered. During this time medical research has led to an increasingly spectacular series of high technology patch-up procedures which are enormously expensive, reflecting as they do our continuing inability to prevent these common diseases or to treat them rationally. This, in turn, has changed the character of our hospitals which are now seen as rather terrifyingly dehumanizing institutions. Our failure to make genuine progress in preventing or curing these common diseases has also led to the development of many forms of alternative medicine and to a major interest in so-called holistic practice, that is treating the whole patient rather than just their disease. Good doctors do this anyway but the pastoral aspects of patient care are perceived by many to have been lost in a welter of high technology.

It follows, therefore, that just as the clinical possibilities of recombinant DNA technology are starting to be appreciated, the medical profession is facing considerable criticism from its patients. At the same time as it is being asked to take a more holistic approach to clinical care it is facing what many see as the ultimate in reductionism. Meanwhile medical schools are worrying about how to teach their students to be better communicators and to become interested in ethics and the social sciences, and must now expect them to become molecular biologists into the bargain. And what will it cost? Is the 'new genetics' not just another piece of high technology to add to the list?

While it is clear that such problems exist I see no reason for taking a pessimistic view of the effect of molecular and cell biology on clinical practice. One of the effects of the post-war era of high technology medicine has been the division of clinical practice into ever smaller watertight specialist compartments. For the organization of medical research, and during the intense period of 'whole body' or 'whole organ' investigation which was so successful at the time, it was natural that such fragmentation would occur, and then spill over into clinical practice. As the emphasis of medical research changes to the study of disease mechanisms at the molecular and cellular levels there will be a tendency for the reunification of its activities; cardiologists, chest physicians, and the rest will all be using the same techniques to study disease and it should be much less tempting to carve up human beings into watertight compartments.

Furthermore, there is no *a priori* reason why an understanding of disease at the molecular level should generate bad doctors. Good clinical practice will always remain an art; the unique problems that each individual patient poses as the result of the interaction of intrinsic disease with their personality and social environment will not change. Provided we are willing to retain a balance between standards of excellence in clinical training, research in the clinic, bedside, and community, and the study of disease at the molecular level, there is no reason whatever why the better understanding of pathological mechanisms that will come from molecular and cell biology should have any deleterious effect on medical practice. Just the opposite in fact; it should enable us to prevent and treat disease more logically and hence to start to reduce our expensive, high-technology, and symptomatic approach to medical care.

There will, no doubt, be some changes in emphasis in the way we educate doctors of the future. The time spent studying molecular and cell biology will have to increase at the expense of whole-body anatomy and physiology. But there is no reason why medical students should have vast quantities of new information forced on them, so long as they gain a general understanding of the basic science on which much of future medical research and practice will depend. The majority of medical students will end up as practitioners, and medicine will remain an art based on a slow accumulation of scientific knowledge. Molecular biology will not change this, at least for the foreseeable future, and there is no reason why the pattern of medical training should change fundamentally.

Our clinical schools will have to decide how best to organize their research activities to incorporate the extraordinary possibilities that recombinant DNA technology have to offer for medical research. The work is expensive and requires an input from both clinical and non-clinical scientists. On the other hand the technology crosses all disciplines. It may be better, therefore, if rather than having each department fully equipped to do this kind of work, research facilities are developed such that scientists from all the clinical disciplines can be housed together so they can share expensive equipment and facilities, interact with each other, and provide a critical mass of workers in an environment where young clinicians can be trained in molecular biology and where molecular biologists can be exposed to the clinical world.

● How far should we go in manipulating the human genome?

As stated several times in this book, none of the current applications of molecular biology and genetic engineering for clinical practice raises fundamental ethical issues. Rather, they simply highlight issues that have been around for a long time. However, our new-found ability to manipulate the human genome is generating concerns about where this activity might end. Many of them are based on the 'slippery slope' argument.

Supposing that in a few years time it is possible to replace defective genes, and that somatic gene therapy becomes as routine as organ transplantation. Surely it might be tempting to indulge in germ-line gene therapy for a few serious diseases. Why, it is argued, should a family not rid themselves of a bad gene for good and all? And supposing this is practised widely, where might it end? Once we understand the genetic basis of musical talent, athleticism, various acceptable personality traits (whatever they might be) and so on, wouldn't it be tempting to dabble with a little 'enhancement' gene transfer. After all, the track record of *Homo sapiens* in the last few centuries is not all that attractive. A species that may have been selected for its aggressive capabilities, and which is capable of Hiroshima and Nagasaki, the Nazi deaths camps, the horrors of Vietnam, or, nearer home, the creation of the political climate of Northern Ireland, cannot be too proud of itself. Wouldn't it be tempting to move human evolution in a slightly different direction by a little genetic enhancement?

As philosophers like Jonathan Glover have pointed out it is wrong to develop an ostrich policy about such possibilities, however, scientifically improbable they seem at the present time. It is often said, though wrongly, that Lord Rutherford believed that it would never be possible to release energy from the atomic nucleus. Whatever the reason, it is clear that there was a singular lack of public interest and debate about what was going on in atomic physics in the 1930s. It is possible that, had this not been the case and had there been open discussion about the feasibility of the development of atomic energy, the tragedies of Hiroshima and Nagasaki would never have happened. Whether by opening up public debate about the long-term possibilities of genetic engineering we can prevent its gross misuse, either politically or in other ways, is for future generations to determine. But there is no reason for not trying.

One of the major concerns about human genetic manipulation is that our track record in the ethical aspects of human genetics is not entirely reassuring. This is highlighted in the excellent book *In the name of eugenics*, in which Daniel Kelves paints a disturbing picture of the development of the eugenics movement in the period leading up to and after the Second World War. The word 'eugenics' was invented by Francis Galton, a talented if eccentric Englishman who was born in the same year as Mendel, to describe the improvement of the species by selective breeding. Galton first published his eugenic thesis in 1865 in Macmillans Magazine and subsequently expanded his two-part article into a book called *Hereditary genius*. He had observed that distinguished people tend to come from distinguished families and thought, therefore, that heredity must determine not only physical features but also talent and character. In his first article he suggested a state-sponsored competitive examination for heredity merit; winners would be wedded to each other in a public ceremony at Westminster Abbey, after which they would be given financial encouragement to spawn numerous eugenically distinguished offspring!

In fact Galton was an extremely talented, self-taught scientist and one of the pioneers of quantitative genetics. His followers include many of the founders of the science of human genetics, Karl Pearson, R.A. Fisher, Lionel Penrose, and J.B.S. Haldane, all of whom became intensely interested in the eugenic movement. It is important to emphasize the quality of the men who formed this group; they were not cranks but some of the greatest names in human genetics.

Eugenics also took off in the US with the enthusiasm typical of any new movement. Under the auspices of John D. Rockefeller the Eugenics Record Office was developed to allow young men and women to come to Cold Spring Harbor for summer courses in training in human heredity and field research techniques. Once indoctrinated they were sent off into the community with a 'trait book'. The 'data' that they collected were returned to the Eugenics Record Office and duly catalogued. By the 1920s the eugenics movement was in full sway on both sides of the Atlantic. In Britain it attracted such radicals as Havelock Ellis, George Bernard Shaw, and the Webbs. The Eugenics Record Office in the US became extremely active and gave a considerable amount of political advice. The movement became closely affiliated to various bodies that were interested in differences in genetic makeup between racial groups and, in particular, in the growing belief that some races are genetically inferior. As the result of thinking along these lines various immigration laws were enacted in the US. For example, in 1924 an act based on these ideas was passed and signed into law by President Calvin Coolidge who, when Vice-President, had declared 'America must be kept American. Biological laws show . . . that Nordics deteriorate when mixed with other races.' A few years earlier in Britain a mental deficiency bill was introduced which allowed for segregation of the mentally feeble, although, to be fair, it was made mandatory to test for social capacity and did not demand legal segregation of all handicapped people, nor was sterilization demanded.

Things had moved ahead much more rapidly in the US. By 1914 at least 30 states had enacted new marriage laws, many of which declared void marriages of idiots and of the insane; others restricted marriage among the unfit of various types. The first state sterilization law was passed as early as 1907 and over the next 10 years similar laws were enacted by 15 or more states. These laws gave states power to compel the sterilization of habitual or confirmed criminals or individuals guilty of offences like rape. Although some members of the British eugenics movement looked on all this with admiration, this type of activity never really caught on in the UK to anything like the extent that it did in the US.

While there is no doubt that many of the more serious human geneticists were becoming increasingly disillusioned with the direction that the eugenics field was moving in the 1920s and 30s, it is equally clear that the politicians in Nazi Germany gained considerable encouragement from the movement. However, by the end of the Second World War, and the announcement to the world of the atrocities carried out in the cause of eugenics by Nazi Germany, the movement petered out. However, it reared its head again in the 1960s when a number of new eugenic issues were raised. For example, in 1969 Jensen published an article in the Harvard Education Review entitled, 'How much can we boost IQ and scholastic achievement'. Essentially, this article posed questions about genetic variation in intelligence among different racial groups and suggested that the lack of performance among the American black population might reflect an innate lack of intelligence. Environmental deprivation, which had hitherto been thought to be the main explanation for the differences in racial attainment, might, Jensen suggested, not be so important.

There were other reminders that the eugenics movement had not died in 1945. Herman Muller, a distinguished geneticist who had retained considerable enthusiasm for the eugenics movement, became interested in the possibility of improving the human race by artificial insemination. Indeed, 4 years after his death the Herman J. Muller Repository for Germinal Choice was built and housed in an office building in Escondido, California. The idea was to obtain donations of sperm exclusively from Nobel Prize winners and to use it for impregnation of healthy and intelligent female recipients. Unfortunately, at least for the repository, most Nobel Prize winners were not desperately keen on donating sperm for this purpose; more recently the Centre has relaxed its requirements and now looks beyond Stockholm for its stocks.

I have dwelt on Kelves' thought-provoking account of the eugenics movement because it reminds us that ever since the birth of the science of human genetics the idea of improving the human race in one way or another has never been far below the surface. Even now, despite the fact that the work of Jensen has been largely discredited, and much of the work of Cyril Burt on which many of our ideas about the inheritance of intelligence are based has turned out to be fraudulent, many find it difficult to escape the conclusion that geneticists will always have the improvement of the human stock in the back of their mind. It is not surprising, therefore, that there has been a lot of talk about genetic engineering directed at enhancement of the individual or race. Of course nobody is clear who should make the decisions about what enhancement actually means. Should it be doctors, a government committee, or even through the availability of a 'gene supermarket' where prospective parents can wander about stocking up traits that they would like to see expressed in their potential children. And there are concerns that gene manipulation of this kind could be used for political ends, and about what might happen if we attempt to alter human personality or equally subtle traits and get the whole thing wrong.

Of course these fears have not been helped by writers such as Aldous Huxley and George Orwell and the later generations of science fiction authors who have regaled us with stories of cloned human beings, the genesis of monsters in test-tubes, and a wide variety of more subtle disasters consequent on genetic engineering. And as human molecular biology has developed the press and television have tended to pick up its more sensational aspects. The human genome project has been pounced on by the media and presented as if its major goal was to produce a 'book of life' in which all our secrets will be revealed, stripped down to our last nucleotide base. What these presentations rarely do, perhaps understandably, is to point out the bewildering complexity of the whole thing. After all, we haven't the faintest idea how a simple structural gene is regulated. From our brief consideration of the nervous system in the previous chapter it is difficult to imagine that we will gain a level of understanding of the molecular basis of behaviour and other higher functions that will allow us to change human personality, at least for a very long time. It is important therefore that we put our current level of ignorance into context when we discuss the possibilities of genetic engineering.

Most of these concerns stem from a fear of the unknown. Indeed, some of the cries from both sides of the Atlantic, that research into any form of genetic manipulation should be banned, smack very much of the attitude to science in the dark ages. The same applies to much current political debate on the subject, and the problem is compounded by the exaggerated claims of some of the practitioners of molecular biology. Although all this suggests that we should take a pragmatic approach, and simply debate about what is possible today, there is no doubt that the extraordinary explosion of knowledge in this field requires us to be constantly looking to the future.

Surely it is quite impossible for one generation to lay down hard and fast rules about what may or may not be acceptable in, say two or three hundred years time. Each development, and how it should be controlled, should be widely debated when the state of the science becomes absolutely clear. For example, it is important that we set up national review bodies that can monitor the developments in gene therapy; they will be with us soon. Similarly, there is no reason why we should not place a moratorium on germ-line gene therapy, at least for the immediate future; it can always be changed by our great-grandchildren, if they so wish. The same might be advisable for any form of enhancement gene therapy. Remembering the lessons from atomic physicists earlier this century, it is essential that we develop a public debate on where we are going with human genetic manipulation. As highlighted by our brief survey of the eugenics movement, it is much too important a subject to be left to scientists and politicians.

To create an environment in which such a debate is possible we shall have to reconsider how we teach science in our schools. The current quality of debate, particularly in the British parliament, is disappointing, as evidenced by published accounts of the first round of discussions on the embryo bill. It is difficult to expect more of a society in which science accounts for only 5 per cent of the teaching time in many of its primary schools.

● Postscript

Medical research has moved into the most exciting period of its development. Unfortunately, at the same time the medical profession is going through a particularly daunting period. Largely because no political party or system has found a way of dealing with the escalating costs of medical care, governments in most developed societies are pressurizing their doctors to develop a market-place philosophy for the provision of health care. This is raising fundamental ethical issues about who sets priorities for medical practice. For although we have made little progress in understanding the basic cause of most of the major killers of western society, we have become extremely proficient at patching up the results of these diseases and in prolonging human life. The result is that medical practice has become an increasingly expensive, high-technological pastime, frightening for patients in its dehumanizing effect on their hospitals. This in turn has led to an increased interest in alternative medicine and an appeal to return to the holistic approach of patient care. It has been suggested that the profession is not concentrating sufficiently on educating its students and practitioners in the problem of ethics, communication, and the pastoral aspects of medical care. All these problems have left us confused, with more than enough to think about without having to take on the complex and often futuristic possibilities of genetic manipulation.

Where does the new genetics stand when viewed against this complex background? First it provides us with the potential for a much better approach to the avoidance and management of genetic disease. Second, it promises to open up areas of medical research that should enable us to understand the basic cause of many of the common diseases that are bankrupting our health services, and how better to prevent and manage them. This will not happen quickly but the long-term potential for success is enormous.

The question of timing in this new and rapidly expanding field is very important. Indeed, I already sense a certain disillusionment about the role of molecular biology in medicine. After all, gene therapy has now been 'just round the corner' for 10 years; why aren't the goods being delivered? And the proponents of molecular medicine have been promising wonderful things in the realms of a better understanding of common diseases such as vascular and psychiatric disorders for a long time; where is the practical fallout? Part of the difficulty is that molecular biology was rather over-sold to the clinical world during the period of its early development. This was partly due to over-enthusiasm but also reflects the fact that some of its proponents were not clinicians and did not always appreciate the enormous complexities of human disease and human beings! Indeed, as the single gene disorders are becoming better understood it is clear that there are levels of complexity of their interactions which could never have been guessed at 10 years ago. There is no doubt that polygenic disease will be many orders more complicated. The medical profession should not expect miracles overnight but rather should encourage a firm base of good science in this field as an insurance policy for future generations.

As clinical molecular genetics develops it should have the effect of unifying the medical specialities and clinical practice. What appears to be the ultimate in biological reductionism is, in reality, the beginning of a holistic approach to human pathology. As each new human DNA sequence appears, the uniqueness of each of us as an individual becomes increasingly apparent. There is no doubt that human molecular genetics will pose ethical problems for our great-grandchildren, and it is our responsibility to develop a well-informed public debate about the possibilities of this rapidly changing field, and where necessary, to control our scientists by appropriately constituted public bodies. If watched carefully in this way there is no basis for pessimism; the overall opportunities for improving the lot of our patients are enormous provided that it is never forgotten that medicine will always remain an art. Although two people with identical base changes in their DNA may have similar pathology, their reactions to it will always be different, depending on the interactions of the many other genes and environmental factors that have combined to make them the individuals that they are.

● Further reading

Austyn, J.M. (ed.) (1988). *New prospects for medicine.* Oxford University Press.

Committee of Inquiry into Human Fertilization and Embryology (1984). Her Majesty's Stationery Office, London.

Council for Science and Society (1984). *Human procreation. Ethical aspects of the new technique.* Oxford University Press.

Dunstan, G.R. and Seller, M.J. (eds) (1988), *The status of the human embryo.* King Edward's Hospital Fund for London, Oxford University Press.

Fletcher, J.C. (1982). *Coping with genetic disease.* Harper and Row, San Francisco, CA.

Harper, P.S. and Clarke, A. (1990). Should we test children for 'adult' genetic diseases? *Lancet,* **335,** 1205–6.

Holtzman, N.A. (1989). *Proceed with caution. Preventing genetic risks in the recombinant DNA era.* Johns Hopkins University Press, Baltimore, MD.

Kelves, D.J. (1985). *In the name of eugenics.* Alfred A. Knopf, New York.

Motulsky, A. (1983). Impact of genetic manipulation on society and medicine. *Science,* **219,** 135–40.

President's Commission for the Study of Ethical Problems in Medicine and Biomedical and Behavioural Research (1983). *Screening and counselling for genetic conditions. A report on the ethical, social, and legal implications of genetic screening. Counselling and education programs.* Government Printing Office, Washington DC.

Rose, S., Kamin, L.J., and Lewontin, R.C. (1984). *Not in our genes. Biology, ideology and human nature.* Penguin Books, Harmondsworth.

Rowley, P.T. (1984). Genetic screening: marvel or menace? *Science,* **225,** 138–44.

Suzuki, D. and Knudtson, P. (1989). *Genethics.* Harvard University Press, Cambridge, MA.

Weatherall, D.J. and Shelley, J. (eds) (1989). *Social consequences of genetic engineering.* Excerpta Medica, Amsterdam.

Yoxen, E. (1986). *Unnatural selection. Coming to terms with the new genetics.* Heinemann, London.

Index

abortion, spontaneous 23, 152–3
achondroplasia 13 (table), 158
acoustic neuroma 238
acquired immune deficiency syndrome (AIDS) 246
acute myeloblastic leukaemia 231–2, 234–5
adrenal hyperplasia 15 (table), 35 (table)
adrenogenital syndromes, racial difference 18 (table)
adult polycystic disease of the kidney 12 (table), 117–18, 281
  gene 117–18
  locus assigned by RFLP linkage 119 (table)
  prenatal diagnosis 281
afibrinogenaemia 153
agammaglobulinaemia, locus assigned by RFLP linkage 119 (table)
ageing 341–2
alcohol dehydrogenase 215
alcoholism 215
allergy 218
Alu I family 169
Alzheimer's disease 213–14, 340
  familial?, locus assigned by RFLP linkage 119 (table)
amelogenesis imperfecta 13 (table)
amino acids 4
  substitutions 148–50
    causing accumulation of abnormal metabolites 160–3
    in complex proteins 158–60
    involving post-translational modification of protein 157–8
amniotic fluid cells 256, 259
amplification refractory mutation system (ARMS) 93
amylin (islet amyloid polypeptide; diabetes-associated peptide) 198
angiotensin I 211
angiotensin II 211
antibodies
  IgA 59, 60, 70 (table)
  IgD 59, 60
  IgE 59, 60, 70 (table)
  IgG 59, 70 (table)
  IgM 59–60, 70 (table)
anti-Campath-1 antibody 328
anti-oncogenes 236, 239–42
anti-plasmin 153
antisense DNA 249
anti-thrombin III 153, 154
  deficiency 154, 166 (table), 172

α_1-antitrypsin 153
  deficiency 15 (table)
  PI-M 153
aortic aneurysm, abdominal 211
apoliproteins 202 (table), 207 (table)
arylamine *N*-acetyltransferase 217
arylsulphatase pseudodeficiency 181
Ashkenazi Jews 17, 18
asthma 218
ataxia telangiectasia 243–4
atopy 218
autocrine secretion 225
autocrine signalling 53
autoimmune diseases 198–200
autosomal dominant disorders 8–10, 11–14
autosomal loci mapping 134–5
autosomal recessive disorders 9 (fig.), 10, 14–16
5-azacytidine 306–7

bacteriophage 81–3
  λ 79, 83
  single stranded 79
balanced polymorphism 18
B cells 58, 59, 66, 70 (table)
  antibody production 59–73
Becker muscular disorder 173, 185
Beckwith–Wiedemann syndrome 240–1, 315 (table)
biotinylated nucleotides 95
bipolar affective (manic depressive) disorders 31
blindness
  childhood (X-linked) 16
  dominant 12 (table), 34 (table)
  recessive 15 (table), 35 (table)
Bloom syndrome 243
bone marrow transplantation 289–90
bovine papilloma virus genome 98
brain-derived neurotrophic factor 337
brittle bone syndrome, *see* osteogenesis imperfecta
Burkitt's lymphoma 228–31

cachectin (tumour necrosis factor) 330 (table), 332, 334
Campath-1 antigen 327
camptothecin 249
cancer 221–51
  cytogenetic changes 229 (table)
  genetic disorders predisposing 243–4
  immunology 246–7

cancer (*cont.*)
  loss of heterozygosity 238–9
  metastic 247
  mutations that produce cancer cell 242–3
  somatic cell genetics 32
  suppression 235
  treatment 307–8
cancer chemotherapy 247–9, 307–8
  drug resistance genes 247–8
  targeting against cancer cell products 249
  topoisomerases 248–9
cells
  differentiation 328–9
  function 328–9
  growth 328–9
  meiosis 5, 6 (fig.)
  mitosis 5, 6 (fig.)
cellular oncogenes (protooncogenes) 222,
    225–6
  in nervous system 339
centimorgan (map unit) 7
cerebellar ataxia 35 (table)
Charcot–Marie–Tooth disease 119 (table)
chorion villus sampling 259–61
  sources of error 281
chorioretinal degeneration 182
Christmas disease 157, 172, 180
  frameshift mutation 182
  nonsense mutation 182
chromatin 49, 101
chromosome(s) 5, 7, 22 (fig.)
  abnormalities 21–5
    frequency 23
  acrocentric 22
  autosomes 8
  centromere 22
  deletions used for finding genes 127–8
  direct transfer by cell fusion 98–9
  disorders 313–14
  fragile sites 25
  isolation by fluorescent-activated cell sorting
    112
  mapping 103–4
  metacentric 22
  metaphase 21
  normal male/female karyotypes 23
  reciprocal translocation 23, 25
  Robertsonian (centric fusion) translocation
    25
  sex 8
  sister chromatids 21–2
  terminal deletion 25
  trisomies 23–4
chromosome-mediated gene transfer 128
chromosome sorting 122
chromosome walking 123
chronic granulomatous disease 127
  gene 128
  reverse genetics 131–2
chronic myeloid leukaemia 231–4

cleft lip 27 (table), 28, 29 (fig.)
cleft palate 27 (table), 28, 29 (fig.)
  locus assigned by RFLP linkage 119 (table)
  X-linked inheritance 317
clotting factors, *see* factor VIII, IX
codons 40, 143
coeliac disease 199
collagen 158–9
  disorders 158–9
colon cancer 238, 241
colony-forming units 330–2
colony hybridization 85–6, 87 (fig.)
colony stimulating factors 330
colour blindness, red/green 103, 147, 166
    (table)
competitive *in situ* suppression hybridization
    121–2
congenital cyanosis 151
congenital malformations 26–8, 314–17
consensus sequence mutations 170–80
contiguous gene syndromes 315
cosmids 79
Creutzfeldt–Jakob disease 340
cryptic splice sites 177–80
3-5-cyclic adenosine monophosphate 54
cystic fibrosis 15 (table), 35 (table), 166
    (table)
  frequency 15, 27
  gene isolation 128
  locus assigned by RFLP linkage 119 (table)
  prenatal diagnosis 271, 278–9
  racial differences 18 (table)
  reverse genetics 132–3
cystinuria 15 (table)
cytokines 329
cytoplasmic inheritance 31–2

deafness
  adult onset (dominant) 34 (table)
  congential (recessive) 15 (table), 34 (table)
  dominant early childhood 12 (table)
debrisoquine 216
dementia 213–14
dentinogenesis imperfecta 13 (table)
deoxyribonucleic acid, *see* DNA
diabetes-associated peptide (amylin; islet
    amyloid polypeptide) 198
diabetes mellitus 31, 196–8
  type 1 196, 197
  type 2 196, 198
1,2-diacylglycerol 54
diaphyseal aclasia 13 (table)
Di George syndrome 315
DNA (deoxyribonucleic acid) 5, 40–2
  amplification 91–3
  analysis
    human genome mapping 2
    sources of error in prenatal diagnosis
      281–2
  binding proteins 51–3

cellular uptake of calcium microprecipitates 97
codons 40
complementary (cDNA) 126
diagnosis/clinical practice 282–4
'dot-blot' technology 95, 97
fetal
  analysis for single gene disorders 261–75
  sources 259–61
fingerprinting 320
fractionation 75–7
HTF islands 129
hypervariable regions 112–17
core sequence shared by mini-satellite families 116
inversion 175
loop basis for gene deletion 172, 173 (fig.)
mini-satellites 114, 116
mitochondrial 8, 32
polymerase 41
polymorphisms for genetic mapping 107–8
DNA ligase 81
DNA recombinant technology
  for diagnostic pathology 319–20
  for forensic pathology 320–1
  for infectious disease 321–2
  human protein production 332–5
  treatment of disease 322
  vaccine production 325–7
dominant control regions 185, 300–1
'dot-blot' technology 96, 97 (fig.)
Down syndrome (trisomy 21) 23, 24, 28, 35 (table)
  brain pathology 214
  maternal age 24
  screening of women 255
Duchenne muscular dystrophy 16–17, 34 (table), 166 (table), 167 (table), 185
  carriers 17
  clinical features 16 (table)
  frequency 16 (table)
  gene deletion 172, 173
  genetic marker 117
  locus assigned by RFLP linkage 119 (table)
  isolation of sequences 127–8
  new mutants 17
  partial gene deletions 264–6
  prenatal diagnosis 272, 277–8
  reverse genetics 129–30
Duffy blood groups 103
dysfibrinogenaemia 152
dystrophin 131, 185–6
  gene 265, 267 (fig.)

Edwards syndrome (trisomy 18) 23, 24 (fig.), 35 (table)
Ehlers–Danlos syndrome 13 (table), 58
electroporation 98, 295
elementary fibre 49
elliptocytosis 134

embryonic stem (ES) cells 100
embryo research 356–7
endocrine signalling 53
enhancer 51
epidermal growth factor 329
Epstein–Barr virus 199, 231, 318
erythropoietin 323, 330
ethical issues 347–68
etoposide 248–9
eugenics 363–6

factor VIII 166, 176, 322
factor IX 93, 166
familial adenomatous polyposis 238
familial amyloidotic polyneuropathy 162–3
familial hyperproinsulinaemia 157
familial polyposis coli, see polyposis coli
Fanconi syndrome 243
fetal blood sampling 2, 256–9
fetal haemoglobin, hereditary persistence 169, 171 (fig.)
fibrinogen 151–2
fibroblast growth factors 329
floppy mitral valve syndrome 158
fragile X syndrome 16 (table)
frameshift mutations 182–3
Friedreich ataxia 15 (table)
  locus assigned by RFLP linkage 119 (table)
fusion genes 174

galactosaemia 15 (table)
Galton, Francis (1822–1911) 363–4
gametes 5
Gaucher disease 162, 289
G-CSF 323, 330 (table)
gel retardation assays 101
gene(s) 4
  abnormal expression, types/levels 139–41
  activation 49–51
  analysis, see gene analysis techniques
  assigned by RFLP linkage 117–18
  β globin 109
  cis and trans 7–8
  co-ordinated expression 53–5
  deletions 169–73
  dominant 7
  fusion 174
  α-globin 169
  housekeeping 48, 294
  in in vivo systems 99
  intervening sequences (introns) 42
  linked 7
  methylated 49–50
  organization into families 55
  phase of linkage 7
  probes 73–5
  recessive 7
  regulation of expression 48–9
  regulatory sequences 51–3

gene(s) (*cont.*)
  single gene disorders, *see* single gene
      disorders
  structure 39, 42–3
  transfer, chromosome-mediated 128
  variation in number 169–73
gene analysis techniques 73–101
  gene probes 73–4
    non-radioactively labelled 94–5, 96 (fig.)
  oligonucleotide probes 75, 76, (fig.)
  molecular hybridization 73–7
  point mutation detection 93
gene cloning 79–84
  bacteriophage vectors 81–3
  larger DNA fragments 83–5
  plasmid vectors 80–1
gene finding 123–9
  jumping libraries 126–7
  pulsed-field gel electrophoresis 125
  yeast cloning 126
gene libraries 85
  screening to find particular gene 85–9
gene mapping (restriction endonuclease
      mapping) 79, 80 (fig.)
gene regulation 100–1
gene sequencing 89–91
  rapid 93
gene therapy 291–305
  candidate diseases 304–5
  correction with suppressor tRNA genes 302
  ethical issues 355–6
  immunological problems 303–4
  insertion techniques 295–301
    direct insertion 295
    RNA viruses (retroviruses) 296–301
  prerequisites 294
  somatic *vs* germ cell gene therapy 295
  targeted modification of human genes
      301–2
  transgenic approaches 303
genetic code 46
genetic counselling 255
genetic diseases 10–11
  avoidance 254–5
  current methods for treatment 288–9
  pre-implantation diagnosis 284–6
  prenatal diagnosis 269 (table)
  total burden 32–6
genetic fingerprint 115, 116
genome, human 103–35
  genetic mapping 104–7, 118–20, 133–5,
      319–12
  physical mapping techniques 120–3
    chromosome sorting 122
    high resolution 122–3
    in situ hybridization 121–2
    low resolution 120–2
    somatic cell hybridization 120–1
  size 69–71, 124 (fig.)
Gerstmann–Straussler syndrome 340

glial-derived nexin 337
globin genes
  α 169
    deletions 170 (fig.)
    mutations 166 (table)
  β 109–10
    mutations 166 (table)
    mutations of promoter regions 63–4
  γ 306
  single point RFLPs 111
glucagon 54
glucose-6-phosphate dehydrogenase
  deficiency 16, 18, 21, 217
  subunits 48
  variants 217
GM-CSF 323, 330 (table)
graft-versus-host disease 289
growth factors 53, 225
growth hormone 322
  deficiency 172
  gene 100

haemoglobin
  A 174
  A$_2$ 174
  Bart's 166 (fig.)
  Constant Spring 143, 144, 145
  E 19, 180
  F 56, 306
  genetic control 56–8
  genetic disorders, prenatal diagnosis 275–7
  Grady 145–6
  Koln 143
  Lepore 146–7, 174
  Long Island 158
  N-terminal end 158
  San Diego 143
  shortened gene products 146
  variants
    fusion 146–8
    structural 142–3, 144–6, 150–1
  Wayne 145
haemoglobin H 168 (fig.)
haemoglobin (Hb)-H mental retardation 315
      (table)
haemophilia 16 (table), 166 (table), 172
  A 34 (table), 166 (table), 167 (table)
  B 166 (table), 167 (table)
  framedrift mutation 182–3
  nonsense mutation 182
  prenatal diagnosis 278
  splice junction mutation associated 180
haemopoietic growth factors 329–33
halothane 216
helix-turn-helix 52
heparin co-factor 153
hepatitis B virus 318
hereditary elliptocytosis 163–4, 167 (table)
hereditary spherocytosis 164
heterozygosity loss 238–9

heterozygotes 7
hexanucleotides 77 (table)
hexosaminidase A 162
high density lipoprotein 201, 203
histones 49
HLA complex, *see* major histocompatibility
    complex
homocystinuria 15 (table)
homozygotes 7
hormones
  lipid soluble 53
  peptide 53
human evolution 342–4
human genome, *see* genome, human
Huntington's disease 34 (table), 188, 279
  clinical features 12 (table)
  frequency 12 (table) 14
  gene 129
  genetic marker 117
  locus assigned by RFLP linkage 119 (table)
  prenatal diagnosis 271 (fig.), 279–80
  racial differences 18 (table)
hybrid arrest 88
hybrid selected translation 88
3-hydroxy-3-methylglutaryl co-enzyme A
    reductase 203
21-hydroxylase deficiency 167, 182
hydroxyurea 307
hypercholesterolaemia 13 (table), 14, 166
    (table), 167 (table)
  familial 34 (table)
  monogenic 155
  nonsense mutation 182
hyperlipidaemias 203–5
hypertension 209–11
hypervariable regions 78–9
hypophosphataemia, locus assigned by RFLP
    linkage 119 (table)

iatrogenic disease 215–17
I cell disease 162
ichthyosis 16 (table), 35 (table)
immunoglobulins 59, 60, 70 (table)
immune system 58–9, 70 (table)
immunity
  cell-mediated 70 (table)
  humoral 70 (table)
immunoglobulin gene superfamily 61–3, 66–9
inborn errors of metabolism 1
infectious disease 217–18
insertional mutagenesis 221
insertions 175–6
in situ hybridization 121–2
insulin 157, 322
  gene 196
  receptor 155–6, 196
insulin-like growth factors (somatomedins)
    329
interferons 324 (table), 330 (table), 334–5
interleukin(s) 330 (table), 333–4

interleukin-2 receptor 324
intermediate density lipoprotein 201, 203
interval mapping 195
inversions 175
islet amyloid polypeptide (amylin; diabetes-
    associated peptide) 198
isoniazid 216

jumping libraries 126–7

Kaposi's sarcoma 246
Klinefelter syndrome (XXY) 23, 24 (fig.), 35
    (table)
kringle 208
kuru 340

Lancer–Gideon syndrome 315 (table)
Laron dwarfism 156
Leber's optic neuropathy 189
lecithin cholesteryl acyl transferase 202 (table)
leprechaunism 156
Lesch–Nyhan syndrome 166 (table), 167
    (table), 172
  carriers 17
  gene therapy 304
  inserts in HGPRT gene 176
  nonsense mutation 182
leucine zippers 52
leukaemia
  acute myeloblastic 231–2, 234–5
  chronic myeloid 231–4
  T cell 244
lipid metabolism 201–3
  'candidate' genes 207 (table)
  exogenous pathway 201
  genetic disorders 203–5
lipoprotein 201
lipoprotein lipase 202 (table)
  deficiency 166 (table), 176
lod score 105
low density lipoprotein 201, 202, (table)
  Lp(a) variant 208
low density lipoprotein receptor gene 154–5
lung cancer 238, 239
lymphokines 63, 329, 333–4
lysosomal hydrolases deficiency 160–1
lysosomal storage diseases 290

major histocompatibility complex
    (MHC: HLA complex) 64, 65
malignant hyperthermia 216
manic-depressive disorders 211–12
map unit (centimorgan) 7
Marfan's syndrome 13 (table), 34 (table), 158,
    159, 166 (table)
  insert in COLA2 gene 176
meiosis, crossovers at 105
Mendel's laws 5, 7
meningioma 238
mental retardation 28–30, 35 (table)

messenger RNA (mRNA) 39
  transcription/processing 43–4
  translation 39
metachromic leucodystrophy 15 (table)
metallothionines 100
methaemoglobinaemia 151
methionine 46, 158
mice
  anaemias 100
  transgenic 99 (fig.), 316–17
Miller–Dieker syndrome 315
microglobulin β_2 66
mitochondria 8, 32
mitochondrial aldehyde dehydrogenase 215
mitochondrial myopathy 189
molecular pathology 312–19
  chromosome disorders 313–14
  congenital malformations 314–17
  polygenic diseases 317–19
  single gene disorders 312–13
monogenic disorders 141–64, 189–91
mucopolysaccaridosis 15 (table)
multifactorial inheritance 25–7
multigene family 55
multiple endocrine neoplasia type 2 119
    (table), 320
multiple polyposis 34 (table)
mutations 140 (fig.)
  causing defective transcription 169–73
    fusion genes 174
    gene deletions 169
    promotor box 176–7
    variation in gene number 169–73
  'distant' from structural genes 184–5
  frameshift 182–3
  initiation codon 181–2
  membrane proteins involvement 163–4
  nonsense 182, 302
  termination codon 183
myasthenia gravis 199
myelodysplastic syndrome 235
myotonic dystrophy 12 (table), 34 (table)

nasopharyngeal carcinoma (China) 318
nerve growth factor 337
neural receptors 336–7
neuroblastoma, n-*myc* in 235
neurofibromatosis 12 (table), 34 (table)
  I 188
  II 188
  loci assigned by RFLP mapping 119 (table)
neurogenic muscular atrophies 15 (table), 35
    (table)
neurology/neurosciences 336–41
  degenerative disorders 340
  developmental studies 388–41
neurotransmitters 336–7
nick translation 74
nexin, glial-derived 337
nonsense mutations 182

obesity 209
oestrogen 248
oligonucleotide probes 75, 76 (fig.), 88, 274–5
oncogenes 222–35
  abnormal function in cancer 234–5
  abnormal function mechanisms 226–8
  cellular, *see* cellular oncogenes
  chromosomal location 228
  fos 339
  transforming properties 222–4
ornithine-δ-aminotransferase deficiency 182
osteogenesis imperfecta (brittle bone
      syndrome) 34 (table), 158, 159, 166
      (table)
  clinical features 13 (table)
  frequency 13 (table)
osteosarcoma 239
otosclerosis 121 (table)

papillomaviruses 319–20
paracrine signalling 53
paraoxonase 278
parental imprinting 188
Parkinson's disease 340
Patau syndrome (trisomy 13) 23, 24 (fig.)
Pelizaeus–Merzbacher syndrome 134
pemphigus vulgaris 199
pentanucleotides 77 (table)
peroneal muscular dystrophy 34 (table)
PERT reaction (phenol-enhanced
    reassociation) 127
phenotypes
  cytoplasmic inheritance associated 188–9
  genetic deletions associated, modification of
    185–6
  modification by mutations that involve
    regulation of transcription/messenger
    RNA processing 186
  modification by parental imprinting 188
  modification by genetic variability at other
    loci 187–8
  X chromosome inactivation 188
phenylbutazone 216
phenylketonuria 34 (table), 166 (table), 180,
    289
  clinical features 15 (table)
  frequency 15 (table)
  prenatal diagnosis 280
phosphatidyl-inositol 4,5-biphosphate 54
photoreceptor mutations 156–7
PI-M 153
PI-Pittsburg 154
PI-S 153
PI-Z 153
plaque hybridization 87 (fig.)
plasmids 80–1
  E. coli 79
  pBR322 98
plasmin 323

plasminogen 208
  activator 322
Plasmodium falciparum malaria 217, 231
platelet-derived growth factor 329
point mutations
  abnormal protein products 142
  consequences for protein structure 143–64
  defective receptor activity 154–6
polyA signal site mutations 181
polycystic disease of the kidney, *see* adult
    polycystic disease
polygenic disease 194–6
polymerase chain reaction 91–3, 94 (fig.),
    263–6
  in diagnostic pathology 319–20, 321
polyposis coli 12 (table), 34 (table)
  locus assigned by RFLP 119 (table)
porphyria
  acute 166 (table)
  acute intermittent 13 (table)
  racial differences 18 (table)
  South African 14, 18 (table)
  variegate 13 (table)
Prader–Willi syndrome 315
prenatal diagnosis 256–9
preproinsulin 46, 157
prions 340
proinsulin 46, 157
proline 148
promotor box mutations 176–7
protein(s)
  activator, G_{m2} 162
  C deficiency 167, 182
  CD3 64
  complement system, class III 65
  G 54, 181, 227
  GAP (GTPase activating protein) 227
  reduced output of particular protein 138
  signal recognition (11S) 158
  structural variants 148–50
    cause of disease 148, 149 (table)
    structure–function relationship 148–50
  surface related 89
  synthesis 44–6
  tertiary configuration 148–9
  unstable 183–4
protein suicide 160
protooncogenes, *see* cellular oncogenes
pseudohypoparathyroidism 167, 181
psychoses 211–14
pulsed-field gel electrophoresis 125

quantitative trait loci 195

recombinant(s) 7
recombinant viruses 98
red blood cell 163
regulatory peptides 337
renin 211

restriction endonucleases 77 (table)
  mapping (gene mapping) 79, 80 (fig.),
    261–6
restriction enzymes 78 (fig.)
restriction fragment length polymorphisms
    78, 107–12 *passim*, 113 (fig.), 266–74
  bridging markers 272
  distribution in α globin gene cluster 111
  due to single base changes 108–9
  haplotypes 110, 111
  human globin gene clusters 109
  intragenic 272
  linkage disequilibrium 272–4
  prenatal diagnosis 266–74
    sources of error 281–2
  single linked 268–70
retinal degeneration 167
retinitis pigmentosa 156, 341
retinoblastoma 34 (table), 236–8, 239, 240,
    242
  cytogenetic change 315
  locus assigned by RFLP linkage 119 (table)
retroviruses 221, 244–6, 296, 297 (fig.)
  insertion technique 296–301
reverse genetics 129–33
  chronic granulomatous disease 131–22
  cystic fibrosis 132–3
  Duchenne muscular dystrophy 129–31
reverse transcriptase (RNA-dependent-DNA-
    polymerase) 73
rheumatoid arthritis 199
rhinitis 218
rhodopsin 156
ribonucleic acid (RNA) 39
rickets, vitamin D-resistant 156
RNA, messenger (mRNA) 128, 139–40
  defective processing 177–81
    consensus sequences mutation 179–80
    cryptic splice sites in exons 180
    cryptic splice sites in introns 177–8
    polyA signal sign mutations 181
    split junction mutations 177, 178 (fig.)
  precursors 139
RNA-dependent-DNA-polymerase (reverse
    transcriptase) 73
Rous sarcoma virus 221
rubella virus genome 199

schizophrenia 31, 119 (table), 212–13
screening programmes 350–2
serpins 153–4
severe combined immunodeficiency, locus
    assigned by RFLP linkage 119 (table)
sickle cell anaemia 15 (table), 21
  haemoglobin 138
  polymerase chain reaction 264, 265 (fig.),
    18 (table)
  prenatal diagnosis 258 (fig.), 273 (fig.),
    275–6
  restriction endonuclease mapping 261–3

signal transmission via receptors 54, 55 (table)
single gene disorders 11, 312–13
  frequency variations 17–21
  molecular pathology 138–91
slow viruses 340
sodium–lithium counter transport 210
somatic cell hybridization 120–1
somatomedins (insulin-like growth factors) 329
spastic paraplegia 34 (table)
  locus assigned by RFLP linkage 119 (table)
spectrin 163–4
spherocytosis 13 (table)
spinal muscular atrophy 15 (table), 119
spinocerebellar ataxia 188
splice junctions mutations 177, 178 (fig.)
storage diseases 160
streptokinase 323
succinylcholine 216
supergene family 55
suxamethonium 216
SV (simian virus) 40-derived plasmid vectors 98
synovial sarcoma 239

Tay–Sachs disease 15 (table), 17–18, 162
T cell(s) 58, 59, 70 (table)
  cytotoxic 63, 65
  helper 63, 65
  interaction with macrophages 66
  receptors 64–5
  suppressor 63
T cell leukaemia 244
T cell specific antigens 89
T cell-specific genes (y) 66
thalassaemia 142, 165–9, 170 (table)
  bone marrow transplantation 290
  gene therapy 305
  HbE/ 19–20
  prenatal diagnosis 258 (fig.)
  racial differences 18 (table)
  world distribution 18–20
thalassaemia, α 165, 166 (table), 167 (table)
  α-globin genes 181
  haplotypes 111
  mutations 166 (table)
thalassaemia, α^+ 165, 169
  crossover giving rise to 171 (fig.)
  deletion of α globin genes 170 (fig.), 264, 265 (fig.)
thalassaemia, α° 20, 165, 185
  deletion of α globin genes 170 (fig.), 264, 265 (fig.)
thalassaemia, β 165, 166 (table), 167 (table)
  carriers 184
  clinical features 15 (table)

'dot-blot' screening for mutations of β globin gene 97 (fig.)
  frequency 15 (table)
  genetic mechanisms modifying phenotype 187
  point mutations 'upstream' from β globin gene 176–7
  prenatal diagnosis 270 (fig.), 274, 276
  Sardinian 274, 276
  transfusion dependent 36
thalassaemia, β° 184, 185, 186
thalassaemia, $\delta\beta$ 166
  deletions responsible for 171 (fig.)
  gene deletion detection 264
  phenotype 169
thanotophoric dwarfism 13 (table)
thymidine kinase gene, mouse cells lacking (Tk$^-$) 97–8
thyroxine 53
tissue-type plasminogen activator 323
topoisomerases 248–9
transforming growth factor 335
transgenic gene transfer 99–100
transgenomes 128
transposons 176
transthyretin (pre-albumin) 162–3
tuberous sclerosis 12 (table), 34 (table)
tumour immunology 246–7
tumour-infiltrating leucocytes 307–8
tumour necrosis factor (cachectin) 330 (table), 332, 334
tumour viruses 221–5
  DNA 224
Turner syndrome (XO) 23
twins 26
type A syndrome 156

vaccine production 325–7
variegate porphyria 13 (table)
vascular amyloid 214
vascular disease 200–1, 205–9
very low density lipoprotein 201, 203
viruses
  human cancer associated 244–6
  slow 340
vision 314

Wilms' tumour 236, 237, 239, 240, 241, 315 (table)

X chromosome 8, 188

Y chromosome 10, 16–17
yeast artificial chromosomes 83–4
yeast cloning 126

zinc fingers 52, 156